BRITISH MEDICAL BULLETIN
VOLUME 56   NUMBER 2   2000

Stroke

09
)09

Scientific Editor
Martin M Brown

Series Editors
L K Borysiewicz PhD FRCP
M J Walport PhD FRCP

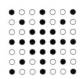

PUBLISHED FOR THE BRITISH COUNCIL BY
THE ROYAL SOCIETY OF MEDICINE PRESS LIMITED

ROYAL SOCIETY OF MEDICINE PRESS LIMITED
1 Wimpole Street, London W1G 0AE, UK
207 E. Westminster Road, Lake Forest, IL 60045, USA

British Library Cataloguing in Publication Data
A catalogue record for this book is available from the British Library
ISBN 1-85315-457-1
ISSN 0007-1420

Subscription information *British Medical Bulletin* is published quarterly in January, April, July and October on behalf of the British Council by the Royal Society of Medicine Press Limited. Subscription rates for Volume 56 (2000), including online access, are £154 Europe (including UK), US$265 USA, £158 elsewhere, £73 developing countries. Prices include postage by surface mail within Europe, by air freight and second class post within the USA*, and by various methods of air-speeded delivery to all other countries. Subscription orders and enquiries should be sent to: Publications Subscription Department, Royal Society of Medicine Press Limited, 1 Wimpole Street, London W1M 8AE, UK (Tel +44 (0)20 7290 2928; Fax +44(0)20 7290 2929; Email rsmjournals@roysocmed.ac.uk).
*Periodicals postage paid at Rahway, NJ. US Postmaster: Send address changes to *British Medical Bulletin*, c/o Mercury Airfreight International Ltd, 365 Blair Road, Avenel, NJ 07001, USA.

Single copies and back numbers of issues published from 1996 are available for purchase directly from the distributors: Hoddle Doyle Meadows Limited, Station Road, Linton, Cambs CB1 6UX, UK (Tel +44 (0)1223 893855; Fax +44 (0)1223 893852). Issues published in 1996 and 1997 cost £24.95/US$41 per copy, and issues published from 1998 cost £34.95/US$57 per copy. Please add £2/US$3.50 for postage.

Pre-1996 back numbers: Orders for any title published prior to 1996 should be sent to Jill Kettley, Subscriptions Manager, Harcourt Brace, Foots Cray, Sidcup, Kent DA14 5HP (Tel +44 (0)181 308 5700; Fax +44 (0)181 309 0807).

This journal is indexed, abstracted and/or published online in the following media: Adonis, Biosis, BRS Colleague (full text), Chemical Abstracts, Colleague (Online), Current Contents/ Clinical Medicine, Current Contents/Life Sciences, Elsevier BIOBASE/Current Awareness in Biological Sciences, EMBASE/Excerpta Medica, Index Medicus/Medline, Medical Documentation Service, Reference Update, Research Alert, Science Citation Index, Scisearch, SIIC-Database Argentina, UMI (Microfilms)

Editorial services and typesetting by BA & GM Haddock, Ford, Midlothian, Scotland
Printed in Great Britain by Bell & Bain Ltd, Glasgow, Scotland.

BRITISH MEDICAL BULLETIN   Volume 56 Number 2 2000

Stroke

Scientific Editor: Martin M Brown

Acknowledgements

The planning committee for this issue of the *British Medical Bulletin* was chaired by Martin Brown and also included John Bamford, Kennedy Lees, Graham Venables and Charles Wolfe.

The British Council and the Royal Society of Medicine Press are most grateful to them for their help and advice and particularly for the valuable work of the Scientific Editor in completing this issue.

Preface

It is an exciting time to be involved in treating patients with stroke. Investment in epidemiology, neuroscience research and clinical trials over the final 20 years of the last century is beginning to show dividends which will improve patient care. The advent of thrombolysis as an acute treatment for stroke and the promise of neuroprotection are transforming the approach to stroke, which is now seen as a 'brain attack' to be treated as an emergency, rather than a 'cerebrovascular accident' for which nothing can be done. There is good evidence that stroke units, where patients can take advantage of optimised medical therapy, surgical treatment and rehabilitation, result in significant benefits in terms of better outcomes compared to routine general medical care. The treatments available to prevent stroke recurrence now include several alternative antiplatelet regimens, anticoagulation, carotid surgery and stenting. Clinical trials provide data to demonstrate the risks and benefit of individual treatments, and to calculate cost. Both surgery and stenting still carry undesirable risks, but recent technical developments are likely to enhance the safety of these procedures. Impressive advancements in imaging, including ultrasound, new CT and MR techniques are making a dramatic difference to our ability to diagnose stroke acutely, image the cerebral blood supply non-invasively and predict prognosis. These advances are reviewed in this millennium volume of the *British Medical Bulletin*, which concentrates on data relevant to clinical management of stroke. We have managed to assemble an impressive collection of neurologists, stroke physicians, radiologists, epidemiologists and surgeons, who all have a special interest in stroke and are experts in their own field. The resulting volume emphasises the British approach to stroke, which involves the practical application of evidence-based medicine, combined with multidisciplinary management and rehabilitation. We hope our readers enjoy reading the volume and find it useful.

Martin M Brown
Professor of Stroke Medicine
Institute of Neurology
University College London
London, UK
E-mail: m.brown@ion.ucl.ac.uk

The impact of stroke

Charles D A Wolfe

Department of Public Health Sciences, Guy's, King's and St Thomas' Hospitals School of Medicine, London, UK

The socio-economic impact of stroke is considerable world-wide. Stroke is assuming an increasing impact in terms of media attention, patient and carer knowledge, service developments and research.

It is estimated that there are 4.5 million deaths a year from stroke in the world and over 9 million stroke survivors. Almost one in four men and nearly one in five women aged 45 years can expect to have a stroke if they live to their 85th year. The overall incidence rate of stroke is around 2–2.5 per thousand population. The risk of recurrence over 5 years is 15–40%. It is estimated that by 2023 there will be an absolute increase in the number of patients experiencing a first ever stroke of about 30% compared with 1983. There is a total prevalence rate of around 5 per thousand population. One year after a stroke, 65% of survivors are functionally independent, stroke comprising the major cause of adult disability.

The socio-economic impact of stroke is considerable world-wide, both in industrialised and non-industrialised countries. Stroke is assuming an increasing impact in terms of media attention, patient and carer knowledge, service developments and research. However, it still remains a 'Cinderella' specialty and is not apportioned relevant resources to allow effective services to be delivered equitably. This is despite considerable advancements in the evidence base to reduce the impact of stroke both in terms of prevention and treatment. Governments around the world have set conservative targets to reduce mortality from stroke, particularly in younger people, and the stroke physicians of Europe have set targets to reduce the impact of stroke over the next 10 years[1,2].

The impact of stroke can be considered from several perspectives which are often overlapping: patients, their families and carers, primary care, acute hospitals and purchasers of healthcare along with policy makers. This chapter will provide an up-date on the impact of stroke focussing on areas that still require considerable attention. A useful description of how to assess the needs of a population for stroke by Wade[3] has been drawn on for this chapter, as have the English inter-collegiate guidelines for stroke[4].

Correspondence to:
Dr Charles D A Wolfe,
Department of Public
Health Sciences,
Guy's Hospital,
42 Weston Street,
London SE1 3QD, UK

The disease

The definition of stroke used in assessing its impact will be that used by the World Health Organization: 'a syndrome of rapidly developing clinical signs of focal (or global) disturbance of cerebral function, with symptoms lasting 24 hours or longer or leading to death, with no apparent cause other than of vascular origin'.

This includes subarachnoid haemorrhage but excludes transient ischaemic attack (TIA), subdural haematoma, and haemorrhage or infarction caused by infection or tumour. It also excludes silent cerebral infarcts. It would appear that studies are likely to underestimate the total burden of cerebrovascular disease, the data discussed being mainly based on symptomatic stroke.

There are a number of classifications of stroke, none of which are ideal. Routine National Health Service data utilise the International Classification of Disease (ICD)[5]. A useful clinically-based classification has been developed by Bamford and colleagues in which prognosis is related to subtype of stroke, although this classification does not adequately describe the risk factors associated with the subtypes, which is important for secondary prevention[6].

Mortality

Mortality data are readily available, reasonably accurate with regard to stroke and used both to assess the overall need for stroke care and, increasingly, by policy makers as outcome measures of health services. When interpreting mortality data, it would be useful to have information on case-severity and incidence of stroke, both of which influence the mortality rate.

The World Health Organization data (1996) indicate that deaths from circulatory diseases are among the world's commonest diseases killing more people than any other disease, and accounting for at least 15 million deaths, or 30% of the annual total, every year[7]. Stroke accounts for 4.5 million of these. In the past, such diseases were thought of as affecting exclusively industrialised nations. However, as non-industrialised countries modernise, cardiovascular diseases are assuming importance, accounting for at least 25% of deaths, *i.e.* 10 million a year. Two-thirds of the stroke deaths occur in non-industrialised countries. There are an estimated 9 million stroke patients world-wide.

In 1997, there were 57,747 deaths in England and Wales from stroke, with 2525 from subarachnoid haemorrhage[5]. Stroke is the third most common cause of death in the UK after myocardial infarction and cancer and is consequently a focus for the UK Government[1]. The target is to reduce deaths from stroke in the under 75-year-olds by two-fifths by 2010 and the White Paper outlines strategies to reduce impact, which include prevention and therapeutic interventions, often without supporting evidence.

There are noticeable differences in the standardised mortality ratios (SMR) for stroke (*i.e.* mortality rates adjusted for age and sex differences in populations) between regions of Europe and in the UK specifically, ranging from 132 in Northumberland to 75 in NW Hertfordshire (national SMR =100)[8]. This implies certain areas would have more difficulty in achieving mortality reduction targets and local knowledge of incidence and case-severity will need to be addressed.

In terms of years of life lost as a result of stroke, in England and Wales in 1993–1994, an average of 28 years of life were lost per 10,000 population and this varied from 21.6 in the South and West region to 34.9 in the North West region[8].

There would appear to be inequities in mortality from stroke between social classes. Kunst *et al* showed that in all countries for men, manual classes had higher stroke mortality rates than non-manual classes, this inequity being relatively large in the UK, Ireland, Finland and small in Sweden, Norway, Denmark, Italy and Spain. These differences probably represent differences in the prevalence of risk factors and access to health services in the different groups[9].

Incidence

The incidence of stroke is defined as the number of first in a life-time strokes occurring per unit time. It is a sensitive measure of the need for stroke services, but is difficult to estimate without considerable resource. The incidence of all acute strokes (first and recurrent) is in the region of 20–30% higher than the first in a life-time. Bonita has estimated that the risk of a person 45 years of age having a stroke within 20 years is very low (about 1 in 30)[10]. However, almost one in four men and nearly one in five women aged 45 years can expect to have a stroke if they live to their 85th year. Although the life-time risk of having an acute stroke is higher in men than women, the converse is true for the life-time risk of dying of a stroke. Thus about 16% of all women are likely to die of a stroke compared with 8% of men; this difference is largely attributable to the higher mean age at stroke onset in women, and to their greater life expectancy.

Sociodemographic influences on incidence

The incidence of stroke doubles with each successive decade over the age of 55 years, with an overall rate 0.2/1000 in those aged 45–54 years and 10/1000 in those aged over 85 years. Men have a 25–30% increased chance of having a stroke. African-Caribbean and African men and women have approximately double the risk of stroke compared to the Caucasian population. People in the lowest social class have a 60% increased chance of having a stroke compared to those in the highest social class[11].

Subarachnoid haemorrhage

The incidence is about 9–14 per 100,000 per year[3]. Other published estimates are as high as 33 per 100,000 per year for men and 25 per 100,000 per year in women.

Cerebral infarction

There have been many population-based studies of stroke, most having had significant methodological flaws[12]. Although the Oxford Community Stroke Project is the gold standard for incidence studies in the UK, it commenced in the mid-1980s when mortality rates were higher and the study area was predominantly in rural Oxfordshire with no ethnic minority groups. The overall crude incidence of first in a life-time stroke was 2.4 per 1000 per year[3]. A south London register reported an overall crude incidence rate of 1.3 per 1000 population (1.28 male. 1.33 female) with a 2.2-fold increased risk in the Black population in 1995[13]. Studies published or presented at conferences covering the years 1995–1997 indicate the incidence rates to be between 119–203 per 100,000 adjusted to the European population, but with significant differences between and within countries.

Incidences of subtypes of cerebral infarction

Intracerebral haemorrhage (excluding SAH) accounts for just over 10% of all stroke, the remainder being cerebral infarction. Using the Bamford classification, the following proportions of first strokes can be expected: cerebral infarction 76% (partial anterior circulation 56%, lacunar 20%, total anterior circulation 15%, posterior circulation 8%, unclassified 1%), primary intracerebral haemorrhage 10%, subarachnoid haemorrhage 4%, not known 10%[6].

Recurrence

The cumulative risk of recurrence over 5 years is high, ranging from 15–42% in community studies and the pathological subtype of recurrence is the same as the index stroke in 88% of cases[14].

Case fatality

Case fatality measures the proportion of people who die within a specified period after the stroke; comparisons are based on the first-ever stroke in a life-time since recurrent strokes have a higher case fatality. One month case fatality rates are dependent on the age structure and health status of the populations studied and vary from 17–49% amongst men in the MONICA studies and 18–57% in women with an average of about 24% from the literature[15]. In the UK, the Oxford 28-day case fatality was 19% overall, that for cerebral infarction being 10%, primary intracerebral haemorrhage 50%, and subarachnoid haemorrhage 46%[3]. Studies reporting rates in the 1990s estimate one month case-fatality of 19–28% and one year case-fatality as 34–41%[11].

Trends in stroke incidence and case fatality

Incidence

There have been few stroke incidence registers that have been maintained over long enough periods of time to document a change in incidence and the results are contradictory. Since stroke rates increase greatly with age and the number of elderly people is increasing world-wide, the burden of stroke on individual families, and the health services is unlikely to fall rapidly. Malmgren *et al* estimated that between 1983 and 2023 there will be an absolute increase in the number of patients experiencing a first ever stroke of about 30%[16]. There will be an increase in the number of deaths from stroke of about 40%, but there will only be an increase of 4–8% in the number of disabled long-term survivors. One can, therefore, anticipate an increase in the need for acute care and early rehabilitation services over this time period, but not an increase in longer term care.

Case fatality

There has been a significant decrease in mortality from stroke over time and in the western world which started in the early 1900s and has accelerated during the past 30 years; this has been attributed by some to better control of hypertension, although this is far from clear[1].

Data on trends in case-fatality rates based on epidemiological studies are scarce and contradictory. Peltonen and colleagues demonstrated marked improvements in short and long-term survival since 1985 in Sweden, equating to a 30% reduction in death rates which they attribute to improved management[17].

Prevalence of stroke

The prevalence is the number of stroke sufferers in the population. There have been very few prevalence surveys of stroke, the prevalence rates being estimated using the incidence and survival data from stroke registers. O'Mahony *et al* validated a simple self-completed questionnaire to screen for cases of stroke in the community and estimated that 10% of respondents reported a history of stroke. The question 'have you ever had a stroke?' had a sensitivity of 95% and a specificity of 96%[18].

Geddes *et al*, in a study in the north of England, estimated the prevalence of stroke to be 46.8 per 10,000 (95% CI 42.5, 51.6). Cognitive impairment (33%), problems with lower limbs (30%) and speech difficulties (27%) were the most common residual impairments[19].

Impairment, disability and handicap

The World Health Organization definitions are used to classify the impact of stroke longer term. The classification is being revised to introduce the concept of 'contextual factors' which impact upon the manifestation of all diseases (social, physical, personal). The revised classification refers to 'activities' and 'participation' rather than 'disability' and 'handicap'[4].

Impairment

Impairment refers to abnormalities arising at the level of the organism. Impairments are usually the external manifestations of the pathology: the symptom and signs. Impairments are 'objective' and cover a wide range of states which carry no personal meaning to the patient: hemianopia, sensory loss, muscle weakness, spasticity, pain, *etc* (Tables 1 & 2).

Disability

Disability refers to changes in the interactions between the patient and the environment. It is the behavioural consequences, which manifest

Table 1 Acute (0–7 days), three week and six month impairment/disability rates

Phenomenon	Acute (%)	3 weeks (%)	6 months (%)
Impairments			
Initial loss/depression of consciousness	5	–	–
Not oriented (or unable to talk)	55	36	27
Marked communication problems (aphasia)	52	29	15
Motor loss (partial or complete)	80	70	53
Disabilities			
Incontinent of faeces	31	13	7
Incontinent of urine	44	24	11
Needs help grooming (teeth, face, hair)	56	27	13
Needs help with toilet/commode	68	39	20
Needs help with feeding	68	38	33
Needs help moving from bed to chair	70	42	19
Unable to walk independently indoors	73	40	15
Needs help dressing	79	51	31
Needs help bathing	86	65	49
Very severely dependent	38	13	4
Severely dependent	20	13	5
Moderately dependent	15	15	12
Mildly dependent	12	28	32
Physically independent	12	31	47

The 'acute' figures are of limited accuracy as many patients were not assessed within the first week; many of these were very ill and probably very dependent. Consequently, the figures relating to acute disability are minimum estimates.
These data relate only to survivors and are summarised from Wade[3].

within the patient's environment, or the personally meaningful functions or activities which are no longer executed, or are altered. Altered behaviours stretch from continence and turning over in bed to dressing and bathing and gardening, interacting with other people and specific work skills. In practical terms, especially in relation to health and social services, disability manifests itself as an increasing dependence upon people and/or environmental adaptations.

Some representative data of disability for the acute phase and 6 months are shown in Tables 1 and 2. The Oxford study estimated that, at 1 year, 65% of survivors were functionally independent.

Handicap

Handicap is the most difficult level to define and measure and is the change in social position which arises from illness; it also refers to the social, societal and personal consequences of the disease. It is the roles and expectations which are performed less readily, if at all.

Table 2 Epidemiology of stroke: the figures are per 100,000 population per year, where relevant

General – SAH, TIAs, stroke – diagnosed	
Cases SAH per year	14
New cases TIA per year	42
– carotid territory TIAs	34
First strokes per year	200
All acute strokes per year	240
Stroke survivors alive in community	600
Presenting for diagnosis	Not known
Impairment/disability presentation (i.e. need acute care), all stroke	
With reduced consciousness	84
Severely dependent	140
Incontinent of urine	106
Disoriented/unable to communicate	132
Unable to get out of bed unaided	168
Impairment/disability at 3 weeks (i.e. need rehabilitation), all stroke	
Needs help dressing	86
Needs help walking	67
Needs help with toilet	66
Communication problems	49
Impairment/disability at 6 months (i.e. needing long-term support)	
Needs help bathing	71
Needs help walking	22
Needs help dressing	45
Difficulty communicating (aphasia)	22
Confused/demented (or severe aphasia)	39
Severely disabled (Barthel < 10/20)	13
Services at 6 months	
Needs long-term institutional care	23
Possibly needs speech therapy	24

This assumes: (i) all stroke, first and recurrent (2.4 per 1000 per year); (ii) 30% die by 3 weeks; (iii) 40% die by 6 months; and (iv) minimal contribution from SAH to care and rehabilitation needs. From Wade[3].

In a population-based survey in south London, the vast majority of stroke survivors, 5 years after their stroke, lived in private accommodation, and the most disabled were only likely to be in private accommodation if they had an identified carer[20]. One-third of survivors were severely or moderately disabled and two-fifths of survivors were more disabled than they had been at 3 months after their stroke. Respite care was only received by a few people. Nearly 75% had an adaptation to the environment and 75% were prescribed treatments aimed at preventing further vascular events. Some 23% were depressed and a further 14% had borderline depression scores. The assessment of quality of life, using the SF36 score and Nottingham Health Profile, suggested that the patients' scores on the various scales were related to their residual disability[20].

Quality of life after stroke is increasingly being measured but published assessments report widely different findings. These differences can be attributed to different methodologies, including the specific quality of life measure and time of investigation.

Needs of families and carers

In recent years, there has been an increasing, but unproven, emphasis on the need for stroke services managed in the community. The strategists and health service planners have not considered the considerable proportion of care undertaken by carers and families. As a result of the pressures, carers suffer from depression and anxiety and family tensions and financial problems are common. Four main areas of concern to carers can be identified through the literature. Carers want information, skills training, emotional support and regular respite. However, these have been highlighted as areas of major deficiency in informal carers' interactions with professionals. Carers frequently mentioned a failure of agencies to supply promised aids or services, a general lack of information and advice and the provision of irrelevant help. These points obviously have great implications for the type of help offered to carers. The nursing literature does suggest the importance of nurses in information giving and counselling: 'the support of informal carers must be seen as a legitimate and important focus for nursing interventions'. Yet the literature also highlights the fact that, on the whole, this has not been happening. The literature also cites the benefits of intervention such as support groups for patients and their carers. However, it has also been shown that these may only benefit certain people and there is a lack of proper evaluation of such groups[21].

Current service provision for stroke

It is estimated that stroke services accounted for at least 4–6% of the NHS budget in the UK, but these figures do not take into account social service and carer costs.

Primary care

The morbidity survey in general practice in the UK estimates that circulatory diseases account for 9% of consultations, 36% of which are 'serious' with the most common reason being essential hypertension[22].

Overall, cerebrovascular disease prevalence was estimated at 5–8 per 1000 individuals. Nearly all patients who consulted for cerebrovascular disease did so for transient cerebral ischaemia or for acute but ill-defined cerebrovascular disease. Comparison of prevalence rates for 1971/2 and 1991/2 shows an overall 64% increase in consultation rates. The number of contacts for follow-up of a stroke would appear from the statistics to be low. These data will vary from country to country depending on the role of primary care in stroke management. Specific stroke surveys in the UK over the last 15 years indicate poor follow-up of patients once discharged. Under half of patients were followed-up by their GPs, less than a third by community nurses and less than 20% had access to other services.

Secondary care

Secondary care services for stroke management span many specialties. The patterns of care vary considerably between and within countries, depending on a variety of local influences such as historic patterns of care, priority of purchasers and providers to modify traditional service provision, and local enthusiasm and expertise in the management of stroke patients[23–25].

Although stroke care usually involves hospitalisation, wide variations have been reported between English districts in the proportion of stroke cases that is admitted to in-patient care (55–90%)[3]. It is estimated that, in terms of acute stroke services, patients consume the following resources: 20% of acute beds, and 25% of all long-term beds, including nursing home places[3]. In a Stroke Association survey in the UK in 1998, consultants responsible for care of stroke patients were questioned. The findings are summarised to illustrate the inequity in impact on health services in the UK of stroke patients[24]: over three-quarters of consultants had access to organised stroke services, yet only half of stroke patients go to them; there was geographical inequity in the provision of organised stroke services; social work support was inadequate; access to neuroradiology remained difficult; stroke consultants are rare; better information and management tools are required.

In a sentinal audit of stroke care in the UK in 1999, Rudd and colleagues re-inforced the survey findings of the Stroke Association but actual practice appeared even more sub-optimal than the consultant survey[25]. Only 18% of patients spent over half their stay in a stroke unit. If care is to be more effective, the changes in stroke service provision will have to be considerable, which will impact on the health services but to the advantage of the patient and their families.

Key points for clinical practice

Table 3 outlines some of the relevant data presented in this chapter that are considered useful information for both patients, families and health care professionals. Stroke has a significant impact on our society and we are only just beginning to be able to quantify it. With increasing opportunities to reduce this impact, it is important that there are reliable baseline figures on the needs of stroke patients and robust tools for monitoring improvements in outcome.

Table 3 Key points for clinical practice

Incidence	
	1 in 4 men and 1 in 5 women will have a stroke if they live to 85 years
	Incidence rate of cerebral infarction 1.2–2 per 1000
	Incidence rate of subarachnoid haemorrhage 9–33 per 100,000
	Recurrence 20–40%
	30% increase in acute strokes between 1983 and 2023
Prevalence	
	9 million stroke patients world-wide
	Prevalence rate 5 per 1000
Survival/mortality	
	4.5 million deaths a year world-wide
	Third most common cause of death
	28 day case fatality 20–28%
	1 year case fatality 34–41%
Health service provision	
	4–6% health service budget
	9% primary care consultations are for 'circulatory' disorders
	55–90% admission rates to hospital
	20% acute beds, 25% long-term beds used for stroke
	Inequity in provision of effective stroke services

References

1   Department of Health. Our Healthier Nation; Saving Lives. London: HMSO, 1999
2   Aboderin I, Venebles G. Stroke management in Europe: Pan European Consensus meeting on stroke management. J Intern Med 1996: **240**: 173–80
3   Wade D. Stroke (acute cerebrovascular disease). In: Stevens A, Raftery J. (eds) Health Care Needs Assessments, vol 1. Oxford: Radcliffe Medical Press, 1994; 111–255
4   Intercollegiate Working Party for Stroke. National Clinical Guidelines for Stroke. London: Royal College of Physicians of England, 2000
5.   Office of National Statistics. Mortality Statistics Causes. England and Wales 1997. Series DH 2 no. 24. London: HMSO, 1998
6   Bamford J, Sandercock P, Dennis M, Warlow C. Classification and natural history of clinically identifiable subtypes of cerebral infarction. Lancet 1991; **337**: 1521–6
7.   Murray CJL, Lopez AD. (eds) The Global Burden of Disease: a comprehensive assessment of mortality and disability from disease, injuries, and risk factors in 1990 and projected to 2020. Boston, MA: Harvard University Press, 1996
8   Department of Health. Public Health Common Data Set 1995. Guildford: Institute of Public Health University of Surrey, 1996

9. Kunst AE, del Rios M, Groenhof F, Mackenbach for the European Union Working Group on Socioeconomic Inequalities in Health. Socioeconomic inequalities in stroke mortality among middle-aged men. An international overview. Stroke 1998; **29**: 2285–91

10 Bonita R. Epidemiology of stroke. Lancet 1992; **339**: 342–4

11 Wolfe CDA. The effectiveness of public health and individual measures in reducing the incidence of stroke. In: Wolfe C, Rudd A, Beech R. (eds) Stroke Services and Research. London: Stroke Association, 1996; 40–87

12 Sudlow CLM, Warlow CP. Comparable studies of the incidence of stroke and its pathological types. Stroke 1997: **28**: 491–9

13 Stewart JA, Dundas R, Howard RS, Rudd AG, Wolfe CDA. Ethnic differences in stroke incidence: prospective study using stroke register. BMJ 1999; **318**: 967–71

14 Hankey G, Jamrozik K, Broadhurst R et al. Long-term risk of first recurrent stroke in the Perth community stroke study. Stroke 1998; **29**: 2491–500

15 Thorvaldsen P, Asplund K, Kuutasmaa K, Rajaknagas AM, Schroll M, for WHO MONICA Project. Stroke incidence, case fatality and mortality in the WHO MONICA project. Stroke 1995; **26**: 361–7

16 Malmgren R, Bamford J, Warlow C, Sandercock P, Slattery J. Projecting the number of patients with first ever strokes and patients newly handicapped by stroke in England and Wales. BMJ 1989; **298**: 656–60

17 Peltonen M, Stegmayr B, Asplund K. Marked improvement since 1985 in short-term and long-term survival after stroke. Cerebrovasc Dis 1999; **9 (Suppl 1)**: 62

18 O'Mahony PG, Dobson R, Rodgers H, James OFW, Thomson RG. Validation of a population screening questionnaire to assess prevalence of stroke. Stroke 1995; **26**: 1334–7

19 Geddes JML, Fear J, Tennant A, Pickering A, Hillman M, Chamberlain MA. Prevalence of self reported stroke in a population in northern England. J Epidemiol Community Health 1996; **50**: 140–3

20 Wilkinson PR, Wolfe CDA, Warburton FG et al. A long-term follow-up of stroke patients. Stroke 1997; **28**: 507–12

21 Bunn F. The needs of families and carers of stroke patients. In: Wolfe C, Rudd A, Beech R. (eds) Stroke Services and Research. London: Stroke Association, 1996; 247–60

22 Office of Population Censuses and Surveys. Morbidity statistics from general practice 1991–1992. London: HMSO, 1995

23 Beech R, Ratcliffe M, Tilling K, Wolfe C. Hospital services for stroke care: a European perspective. Stroke 1996; **27**: 1958–64

24 Ebrahim S, Redfern J. Stroke Care – a matter of chance. A national survey of stroke services. London: Stroke Association, 1999

25 Rudd AG, Irwin P, Rutledge Z et al. The national sentinal audit for stroke: a tool for raising standards of care. J R Coll Physicians 1999; **33**: 460–4

Measuring outcome

Alan Tennant

Rheumatology and Rehabilitation Research Unit, School of Medicine, University of Leeds, Leeds, UK

In the context of health and illness, outcome is usually defined as the extent to which goals are achieved. It is necessary to understand: (i) the conceptual basis of the consequences of stroke; (ii) the context of measurement; and (iii) the calibre of the instruments available. In 1980, the World Health Organization provided an appropriate conceptual framework. The location, for example in-patient or out-patient, must be considered; as should the professional mix of the service; the time since onset and whether or not the setting is routine clinical practice or research. For the calibre of the measuring instruments psychometric studies report on reliability and validity. Other limitations and omissions in current measurement practice are being addressed through Item Response Theory. In clinical practice, current use of outcome measures is limited but it would seem that, by default at least, a core set of outcome measures is emerging.

It is only with the valid transformation of the theoretical domain into an empirical system of relationships and the use of appropriate techniques for assigning numerical values, that measurement can be achieved[1].

In the past, epidemiology has concentrated on establishing the incidence, prevalence and associated mortality of stroke, but during the last decade there has been an increasing focus on the consequence of stroke to the patient and their family. This focus has emerged within Europe and North America as a result of clinical audit, and evidence-based medicine. In the former, routine recording of the process of care, and the outcome and quality of life of the patient, is becoming integral to clinical practice[2]. In the latter, there has been increased emphasis on contracting for healthcare where there is clear evidence of the efficacy of such care[3]. In both cases 'outcome' plays a crucial role and consequently the measurement of outcome has become central to healthcare policy and practice.

The *Shorter Oxford Dictionary*[4] defines outcome as 'that which comes out of something; visible or practical result, effect or product'. Thus there may be many valid 'outcomes' for stroke. It is possible to describe a stroke in terms of the nature and extent of the lesions or, for example, as a range of neurological impairments. Although these are the immediate 'outcome' of the stroke, in the context of health and illness, outcome is usually

Correspondence to:
Dr Alan Tennant,
Rheumatology and
Rehabilitation Research
Unit, School of Medicine,
University of Leeds, 36
Clarendon Road, Leeds
LS2 9NZ, UK

defined as the extent to which goals are achieved[5]. For example, health promotional studies to reduce the risk factors associated with stroke may seek a reduction in the incidence of stroke as a valid outcome. Clinicians and their patients who are undergoing rehabilitation following stroke may expect a recovery in physical function. Younger patients may want to return to work. All are valid goal-orientated outcomes within their chosen context.

Information about the disabling consequences of a stroke to the patient, and the effect upon a patient's life-style is usually derived from health services research studies[6,7]. The principal characteristic of such studies is that they utilise outcome measures, often those which involve a clinician or therapist assigning values to specified tasks undertaken by a patient, or those where the patient, carer or a proxy fill in a questionnaire. The Barthel index[8] is a classic example of the former, the SF-36[9], the latter. This paper sets out to consider the range of valid outcomes, and how to choose relevant outcome measures. This will ensure that any shortfalls, conceptually or methodologically, are understood and that the best choice is made from the measures currently available. In this context the discussion is bounded by three parameters: (i) the conceptual basis for understanding the consequences of stroke; (ii) the context within which measurement is to take place; and (iii) the calibre of the measuring instruments available.

The three parameters for outcome measurement

Conceptual basis for outcome

In 1980, the World Health Organization published its *International Classification of Impairments, Disabilities and Handicaps* (ICIDH)[10]. This provides a conceptual framework for looking at the consequences of disease. The original ICIDH conceptual model shows that disease may give rise to impairment, defined as 'any loss or abnormality of psychological, physiological, or anatomical structure or function'. This may give rise to disability, defined as 'any restriction or lack of ability to perform an activity in the manner or within the range considered normal for a human being'. Impairments directly, or through disability, interact with the physical and social environment to lead to handicap, defined as a 'disadvantage for the given individual...that limits or prevents the fulfilment of a role that is normal'. Badley emphasized that handicap reflects the circumstances that people find themselves in as a result of the interaction between impairment and disability, and the broader physical and cultural environment within which people live[11]. The importance of

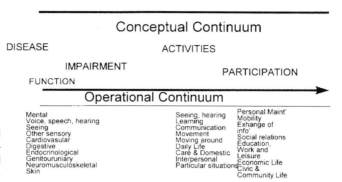

Fig. 1 The international classification of impairments, activities and participation.

Conceptual Continuum

DISEASE   ACTIVITIES

IMPAIRMENT

PARTICIPATION

FUNCTION

Operational Continuum

Mental
Voice, speech, hearing
Seeing
Other sensory
Cardiovasular
Digestive
Endocrinological
Genitouruniary
Neuromusculoskeletal
Skin

Seeing, hearing
Learning
Communication
Movement
Moving around
Daily Life
Care & Domestic
Interpersonal
Particular situations

Personal Maint'
Mobility
Exhange of info'
Social relations
Education,
Work and Leisure
Economic Life
Civic & Community Life

extrinsic factors has been given further emphasis in the most recent revision (ICIDH-2) where the nomenclature has changed to 'impairment, activities and participation'.

Figure 1 shows the generic outcome profile arising from ICIDH-2. The impairments are subdivided into structural and functional domains but just the latter are shown. Activities (disability in ICIDH-1 terms) are, as before, divided into sub-categories. For example, Daily Life Activities is further subdivided into Keeping Self Clean, Washing, Dressing, Activities related to excretion, and so on. Participation (handicap) emphasises the limiting factors placed on the individual by the environment, and society's failure to respond to the needs of the individual. Although ICIDH-2 provides a comprehensive conceptual view of the outcome of disease, it is also important to consider the issue of quality of life (QoL). Measures that address impairment and disability have traditionally been referred to as measures of health status[12,13]. The concept of handicap was also considered as part of health status long before if was set out in the ICIDH[14]. More recently, it has become usual to describe these same dimensions as 'health related quality of life' (HRQoL)[15]. However, there is a tradition of measuring quality of life, grounded in the notions of life satisfaction and well-being, that demonstrates that health status (or HRQoL as it is now called) contributes relatively little to life satisfaction or well-being[16]. In this way, it is quite possible to have a patient who, following stroke, reports a good QoL, despite a range of impairments and disabilities. Thus it is important to note that there may be a fundamental difference between a subjective patient-perceived QoL, and the more 'objective' measurement of health status.

With over a thousand impairments listed in the ICIDH and hundreds of limitations in activities, choosing relevant outcomes is a complex task. What are the most common outcomes? One of a few epidemiological studies which looked at impairment and disability reported that speech and thought processes were the most common impairments, amongst survivors, at the time of the stroke, and approximately 40%

experienced some impairment of movement in arm and leg[17]. While almost a quarter of survivors reported that they had made a full recovery (median time since stroke was 2 years), a wide range of impairments persisted. Arguably the most important of these were impairment of thought processes, reported by a third (33%), and of speech, reported by over a quarter of respondents (27%). Many reported resolution of visual impairments but relatively few of those who experienced impairments in left arm or left leg at the time of their stroke reported that these had returned to normal. Almost half (46%) reported needing help at least daily, including 27% who needed help, or someone to be with them, almost continuously. Consequently, if outcome measures are targeted at these sequelae, it is clear that while temporal trends will affect choice, those measures assessing cognitive impairments, speech and restriction in activities associated with arm and leg movements would dominate, as well as measuring restricted participation in areas of personal maintenance.

The context within which measurement is to take place

Along with the temporal trend of recovery, other factors also play a part in the choice of appropriate outcomes. In all, four aspects need to be considered: (i) the physical location, *e.g.* in-patient or out-patient; (ii) the professional mix of the service; (iii) time since onset; and (iv) routine clinical practice or research.

As time since stroke increases, the measurement of outcome is likely to see a shift in emphasis from survival, through impairment and activities, to participation (including community re-integration) and quality of life. During this time, the balance of professional input is also likely to shift, reflecting the changing focus of intervention as the patient follows the pathway to recovery. Different healthcare settings, for example a general medical ward, an acute stroke ward or a specialist rehabilitation unit, may also have different outcome agendas. Finally, ceteris paribus, more time can be given to measuring outcome within a research programme than in routine clinical practice, usually because there is additional funding for the former. All these aspects may interact to mediate the choice of appropriate outcome and a suitable outcome measure.

The importance of the conceptual basis and the environment, including the time since stroke, within which outcome will be measured, is that they provide a platform from which preliminary choices of outcomes are made. Unless there is a precise understanding of the domain(s) to be measured, where, for example, the intervention is expected to impact, and the context of that intervention, then the choice of measure may be inappropriate, and the measurement may be unreliable or off-target, resulting in all the consequences of imprecise measurement.

The calibre of the measuring instruments

Psychometrics is concerned with the precision of measurement, and expresses this in terms such as reliability and validity[18]. These are the quality parameters of the instruments chosen to measure outcome. Reliability refers to the dispersion of the theoretical (instrument) distribution of measurements while validity refers to its central tendency[19]. There are many books that describe these attributes in detail[20]. At a simple level, it is sufficient to say that outcome measures must give reliable measurement, for example the same result at two time points on stable patients (test–re-test reliability), or the same rating to be given for the same patient by two or more different therapists (inter-rater reliability). Measures must be well-targeted and demonstrate expected associations with other instruments measuring a similar construct (construct validity). More recently, emphasis has also been placed on the ability of an outcome measures to show change when change occurs (responsiveness)[21].

Stroke brings additional problems for self-completion of questionnaires, mostly associated with cognitive and visuospatial impairments. One recent study reported that many patients after a stroke are unable to successfully complete self-report scales, including visual analogue scales[22]. In another study, 214 elderly acute care patients were given the EuroQoL[23] and it was found that the expected probability of needing an interview administration was 0.11 at age 65 years; 0.37 at age 75 years and 0.73 at age 85 years[24]. Under these circumstances, both a validated interview version should be available, and the reliability of the administration should be tested.

In addition to such concerns associated with validity and reliability, there is also an increasing recognition of limitations and omissions in current measurement practice. Rarely is mention made of unidimensionality, the rationale behind the summation procedure in Likert scaling. Here, items are considered to be parallel instruments and through combining item scores targeted at a single dimension, random error that occurs with respect to individual items will be partly averaged away[25]. The responsiveness of a scale may also be compromised by the lack of unidimensionality. For example, where items from different dimensions are summated, overall change scores may be curtailed because items in one dimension are changing at a different rate from another. Thus unidimensionality is a prerequisite both because of the underlying assumptions about summating items, as well as for construct validity, in that the scale is well targeted at the appropriate construct. Internal consistency is a necessary but not sufficient statistic for unidimensionality. Recent work has shown that while coefficient α (Cronbach's alpha) can be used as an indication of the connectedness of items within a scale, it does not confirm unidimensionality[26]. It is quite possible to have two or more dimensions in a large item set which nevertheless give a high α. Despite this, many authors presenting new outcome scales have used this statistic to imply unidimensionality by claiming 'homogeneity' of items. This leads to the prospect that many of the scales in everyday use may have suspect internal construct validity, and thus fail to meet underlying assumptions that underpin their use.

Another major omission is the failure to report on the type of scale produced (ordinal or interval nature). Despite the ways in which these scales are used, *e.g.* by multiplying the raw score to produce a 0–100 scale, it is rare to find empirical proof to sustain this approach in the original, or subsequent papers testing validity and reliability. Yet such proof is crucial to analysis and the choice of appropriate statistical techniques. As additive equal intervals are an explicit requirement of quantitative measurement[27], the absence of testing the assumption of equal intervals for almost all outcome scales must be a cause of concern. Ordinal data 'are seldom in practice, and never in principle, sufficiently interval to justify arithmetical calculations employed by means, variance, regressions and factor analysis'[28].

Another aspect of measurement to consider is differential item functioning (DIF). Originally called 'item bias', an item is biased if equally able individuals, from different groups, do not have equal probabilities of doing the task[29]. In health outcome measurement, DIF may occur in several ways, for example by gender and age, by clinical subgroup or by culture. If DIF is present, then scores cannot be compared across groups.

Some of these shortcomings and omissions can be addressed by the application of item response theory (IRT). IRT offers a supplementary framework for measurement science and is a general statistical theory about item (task) and scale performance and how that performance relates to the abilities that are measured by the items in the scale[30]. By far the greatest application of IRT has been with the one-parameter model Rasch model[31]. A unidimensional model, it assumes that the respondents and items can be uniquely ordered in terms of ability and difficulty. The application of the Rasch model has potentially far reaching consequences for outcome measurement. Fitting data to the Rasch model allows for a re-evaluation of key issues such as internal construct validity through examination of unidimensionality, and a detailed examination of DIF and the scaling properties of the measure. Thus outcome measures are increasingly being subjected to scrutiny by fit of their data to the Rasch model[32].

The principal current outcome measures

In clinical practice, current use of outcome measures is limited. A recent survey of outcome measures in stroke across Europe identified just nine measures in common use in facilities undertaking 63,000 assessments annually on this group of patients[33]. The Barthel index[8] and the functional independence measure (FIM)[34] were the most common, accounting for 46% of all assessments. Thereafter, the mini mental-state exam (MMSE)[35], the modified Ashworth spasticity scale[36] and the Glasgow Coma Score[37] accounted for a further 26% of assessments. Other less frequently used measures included the Rivermead behavioural memory test[38] and the motricity index[39]. It is no coincidence that these common measures target the type of impairments and disabilities that were identified in the epidemiological study as the principal sequelae of stroke. It is also no coincidence that almost all of these scales are completed by professionals observing or interacting with the patient in one way or another. This contrasts sharply with generic instruments that do not address key outcomes, which usually require self-completion and, presumably as a consequence, do not figure in outcome measurement in routine stroke care.

Towards a core set of outcome measures

Some diagnostic groups, *e.g.* the American Spinal Cord Injury Association, have recommended core outcome sets for use in studies and clinical trials[40]. It would seem that, by default at least, a core set of outcome measures is emerging for stroke. These measures focus on those key impairments and disabilities which patients experience following their stroke. The Glasgow Coma Scale determines the extent of impairment of consciousness, while the MMSE and the modified Ashworth spasticity scale determine the extent of cognitive impairment and abnormal tone respectively. The motricity index looks at motor impairment, and the Rivermead behavioural memory test at impairment of memory. The Barthel index and the FIM offer competing scales for physical disability, although the latter has a cognitive component as well. No measures of handicap and quality of life are in routine use at this time. When added to case mix and process indicators that are necessary to allow comparison between different centres[41], an informal 'core set' of outcome measures does appear feasible. However, choice would always be mediated by the focus and context of the intervention. The next task is to subject this potential core set to further methodological examination and to supplement them with adequate measures of handicap and quality of life. When that is complete, the transformation of a theoretical domain into an empirical system of relationships with appropriate scoring systems will, in the terms of Dean *et al*[1], achieve outcome measurement.

References

1   Dean K, Holst E, Kreiner S, Schonborn C, Wilson R. Measurement issues in research on social support and health. *J Epidemiol Community Health* 1994; **48**: 201–6

2   NHS. National Health Service Review. Working Paper No 6 Medical Audit. London: HMSO, 1989

3   Goldstein LB. Evidence-based medicine and stroke. Neuroepidemiology 1999; **18**: 120–4

4   Little W, Fowler HW, Coulson J. The Shorter Oxford Dictionary on Historical Principles. Oxford: Clarenden, 1965

5   Wilkin D, Hallam L, Doggett M-A. Measures of Need and Outcome for Primary Health Care. Oxford: OUP, 1992

6   Osberg JS, DeJong G, Haley S et al. Predicting long-term outcome among post-rehabilitation stroke patients. Am J Phys Med Rehabil 1988; **67**: 94–103

7   Segal ME, Schall RR. Determining functional/health status and its relation to disability in stroke survivors. *Stroke* 1994; **25**: 2391–7

8   Mahoney FI, Barthel DW. Functional evaluation: the Barthel Index. Md State Med J 1965; **14**: 61–5

9   Ware JE, Sherbourne CD. The MOS 36-item short-form health survey (SF-36): I Conceptual framework and item selection. Med Care 1992; **30**: 473–83

10 World Heath Organization. International Classification of Impairments Disabilities, and Handicaps. Geneva: WHO, 1980

11 Badley EM. The genesis of handicap: definition, models of disablement, and role of external factors. Disabil Rehabil 1995; **17**: 53–62

12 Meenan RF, Gertman PM, Mason JH. Measuring health status in arthritis: The Arthritis Impact Measurement Scales. Arthritis Rheum 1980; **23**: 146–52

13 Bergner M. Health status as a measure of health promotion and disease prevention: unresolved issues and the agenda for the 1990's. In: Proceedings of the 1989 Public Health Conference on Records and Statistics. Rockville, MD: National Centre for Health Statistics, 1989

14 Lerner M. Conceptualisation of health and well-being. Health Serv Res 1973; **8**: 6–12

15 Schumaker S, Berzon R. (eds) The International Assessment of Health Related Quality of Life. Oxford: Rapid Communications, 1995

16 Diener E. Subjective well-being. Psychol Bull 1984; **95**: 542–75

17 Geddes JM, Fear J, Pickering A, Tennant A, Hillman M, Chamberlain MA. Prevalence of self-reported stroke in a population in Northern England. J Epidemiol Community Health 1996; **50**: 140–3

18 Nunally JC, Bernstein IH. Psychometric Theory. New York: McGraw Hill, 1994

19 Muir DE. A critique of classical test theory. Psychol Rep 1997; **40**: 383–6

20 Streiner DL, Norman GR. *Health Measurement Scales*, 2nd edn. Oxford: OUP, 1995; 1–231

21 Fitzpatrick R, Ziebland S, Jenkinson C, Mowat A. Importance of sensitivity to change as a criterion for selecting health status measures. Qual Health Care 1992; **1**: 89–93

22 Price CIM, Crless RH, Rodgers H. Can stroke patients use visual analogue scales? Stroke 1999; **30**: 1357–61

23 Kind P. The EuroQoL instrument: an index of health-related quality of life. In: Spiker B. (ed) Quality of Life in Pharmacoeconomics in Clinical Trials, 2nd edn. Philadelphia, PA: Lippincott-Raven, 1996; 191–201

24 Coast J, Peters J, Richards SH, Gunnell DJ. Using the EuroQoL among elderly acute care patients. Qual Life Res 1998; **7**: 1–10

25 van Alphen A, Halfens R, Hasman A, Imtos T. Likert or Rasch? Nothing is more applicable than a good theory. J Adv Nurs 1994; **20**: 196–201

26 Cortina JM. What is coefficient alpha? An examination of theory and applications. J Appl Psychol 1993; **78**: 98–104

27 Fisher WP. Measurement related problems in functional assessment. Am J Occup Ther 1993; **47**: 331–8

28 Wright BD. Comparing Rasch measurement and factor analysis. Struct Equat Model 1996; **3**: 3–24

29 Angoff WH. Perspectives on differential item functioning methodology. In: Holland PW, Wainer H. (eds) Differential Item Functioning. New Jersey: Lawrence Erlbaum, 1993

30 Hambleton RK, Jones RW. Comparison of classical test theory and item response theory their applications to test development. Educ Measure Issues Practice 1993; **12**: 38–47

31 Rasch G. Probabilistic Models for some Intelligence and Attainment Tests. Chicago, IL: University of Chicago Press, 1980

32 Tennant A, Geddes JLM, Chamberlain MA. The Barthel index: an ordinal score or interval level measure? Clin Rehabil 1996; **10**: 301–8

33 Haigh R, Tennant A, Biering-Sørensen F et al. A Survey of Outcome Measures used in Physical Medicine and Rehabilitation across Europe. Contract deliverable to the European Biomedical and Health Research Programme. School of Medicine, The University of Leeds, 1999

34 Granger CV, Hamilton BB, Sherwin FS. Guide for the Use of the uniform Data Set for Medical Rehabilitation. Uniform Data System for Medical Rehabilitation Project Office, Buffalo General Hospital, New York 14203, USA, 1986

35 Folstein ME, Folstein SE, McHugh PR. 'Mini-mental state'. A practical method for grading the cognitive state of patients for the clinician. *J Psychiatr Res* 1975; **12**: 189–98

36 Bohannon RW, Smith MB. Interrater reliability of a modified Ashworth scale of muscle spasticity. *Phys Ther* 1987; **67**: 206–7

37 Teasdale G, Jennet B. Assessment of coma and impaired consciousness: a practical scale. *Lancet* 1974; ii: 81–3

38 Wilson BA, Cockburn J, Baddely AD. The Rivermead Behavioural Memory Test. Titchfield, Hants: Thames Valley Test Company, 1985

39 Demeurisse G, Demol O, Robaye E. Motor evaluation in vascular hemiplegia. *Eur Neurol* 1980; **19**: 382–9

40 American Spinal Injury Association. Standards for Neurological Classification for Spinal Injury Patients. Chicago: ASIA, 1992

41 Irwin P, Rudd A. Casemix and process indicators of outcome in stroke. *J R Coll Physicians Lond* 1998; **32**: 442–4

Pathology of small vessel stroke

G Alistair Lammie

Department of Pathology, University of Wales College of Medicine, Cardiff, UK

Disease of small intracerebral vessels is widely assumed to be responsible for the majority of small, deep-seated (lacunar) infarcts and primary intracerebral haemorrhages. Our present, limited understanding of the pathogenesis of these stroke subtypes, which together constitute up to one-third of all strokes, is based on a limited number of detailed pathology studies, supported by clinical, risk factor and imaging data. Further progress using these traditional approaches has been prevented by a variety of largely technical obstacles. It is suggested that advances in our understanding of the genetic basis of established and new animal stroke models, in turn linked to more focused human genetic stroke surveys, may hold the key to further insights.

An impasse appears to have been reached in our attempts to understand the pathogenesis and, therefore, the prevention, of strokes due to disease of small intracerebral vessels. Current dogma has it that small vessel disease causes a significant proportion of small, deep-seated (lacunar) infarcts and primary (*i.e.* non-traumatic) intracerebral haemorrhage (PICH). This is a problem of clear socio-economic importance, for lacunar strokes constitute approximately 25% of first in-a-lifetime ischaemic stroke[1], and PICH some 10% of all stroke, at least in the West[2]. To this should be added the probable contribution of small vessel disease to global, dementing brain injury, further discussion of which lies outside the scope of this article. I shall describe the central role of pathology in achieving our current, if limited, understanding of small vessel disease related stroke, in particular lacunar stroke, outline the obstacles that have prevented further progress, and suggest how the modern molecular pathologist may offer fresh insights.

Lacunar infarction and the lacunar hypothesis

Correspondence to:
Dr G A Lammie,
Department of
Histopathology,
University Hospital of
Wales, Heath Park,
Cardiff CF4 4XW, UK

The original pathological descriptions of lacunar infarcts were made by the beginning of this century by Durand Fardell and Marie in Paris[3]. Lacunar infarcts vary in maximal dimension from 3–20 mm, and are most commonly found in the putamen, caudate, thalamus, pons, internal capsule and cerebral white matter, in descending order of frequency. By the end of the century, Poirier and Derousne had proposed a neuropathological classification of lacunes. They described old, small infarcts (type I lacunes), old, small haemorrhages (type II) and dilated perivascular spaces (type III)[4]. Type I lacunes are by far the most important clinically. Between times, Fisher had taken the descriptive pathological approach a stage further by his meticulous serial section autopsy reconstructions of the vascular supply of a limited number of lacunar infarcts[5]. His fundamental observation was that lacunar infarcts result from occlusion of small perforating cerebral arteries, in some cases by a destructive process he termed 'segmental arterial disorganisation' or 'lipohyalinosis', and in others by atherosclerosis. In a small minority, he found no occlusive lesion and assumed embolism. Thus arose what became known as the 'lacunar hypothesis', according to which lacunar infarcts are caused by characteristic vascular lesions involving single perforating brain arteries, often in combination with hypertension.

The nature of small vessel lesions causing lacunar infarcts – the legacy of Fisher

There are a large number of potential causes of small vessel occlusion, some autopsy-proven, others inferred (Table 1). These 'causes' may not necessarily be mutually exclusive; for example, small vessel spasm may mediate destructive lesions or exacerbate atheroma[6]. Despite this multiplicity of possible causes, Fisher's work suggested, and there has been no convincing contradictory data since, that there are two small vessel pathologies of major pathogenetic significance to stroke, the first 'lipohyalinosis', the second atherosclerosis.

Lipohyalinosis, as originally described, is a destructive vessel lesion characterised by a loss of normal arterial architecture, mural foam cells and, in acute cases, evidence of fibrinoid vessel wall necrosis. Fisher noted that such vascular lesions involved small arteries of 40–200 µm diameter, and caused correspondingly small (3–7 mm diameter), often asymptomatic, cerebral infarcts, particularly in the striatocapsule[5]. By whatever name, although perhaps less prevalent today in the era of controlled hypertension[5], such vessel lesions are still seen at post mortem in close proximity to lacunar infarcts (Fig. 1b). The important, unresolved questions concerning this lesion are what proportion of lacunar infarcts is it now responsible for and what is the underlying molecular mechanism?

Table 1 Postulated causes of small deep cerebral infarcts

Common (autopsy proven)
    Destructive small vessel disease ('lipohyalinosis')
    Perforating/parent artery atherosclerosis

Uncommon/rare (may be autopsy proven but mechanism often assumed or inferred)
    Embolism
    Vasculitis
        Collagen vascular disease
        Infective
        Recreational drugs (*e.g.* cocaine)
        Isolated CNS angiitis
    Infection
        HIV
        Tuberculosis
        Neurosyphylis
        Cystercicosis
        Lyme disease
    Hypoperfusion
    In situ thrombosis/hypercoaguability
        Antiphospholipid antibodies
        SLE
        Disseminated malignancy
        Thrombocythaemia
        Polycythaemia
    Arterial dissection
    CADASIL
    Cerebral amyloid angiopathy

Speculative (difficult to prove)
    Vasospasm
    Oedema
    Pulsatile trauma
    Destructive ('lytic') agent

The term 'lipohyalinosis' has subsequently been misused to describe almost any cerebral small vessel pathology. It is distinct from, and should not be confused with, the concentric, hyaline wall thickening that is a feature of most aged brains (Fig. 1a), particularly those from the hypertensive and diabetic elderly. Such poorly distensible collagen-rich 'tubes', for which the term 'hyaline arteriosclerosis' is appropriate, are ill-equipped to match cerebral blood supply with demand, particularly if systemic blood pressure is abnormally high or low. They are an almost invariant feature of brains with diffuse, presumed ischaemic, white matter disease or leukoaraiosis. However, although such hyaline arteriosclerosis is often severe in brains harbouring lacunar infarcts, there is no direct evidence that they are a cause of focal brain lesions and lacunar stroke.

The other vascular lesion of pathologically-proven relevance to lacune formation is intracranial atherosclerosis. This is pathologically similar to the disease more familiar in the larger cervicocranial arteries, and affects

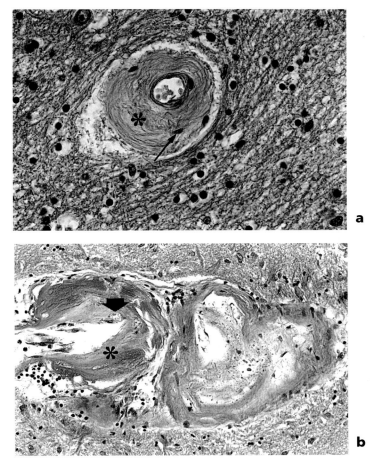

Fig. 1 Photomicrographs illustrating two distinct, but often confused, types of intrinsic cerebral small vessel pathology. (**a**) Hyaline arteriosclerosis ('simple' small vessel disease) in the putamen. Roughly concentric vessel wall thickening by hyaline collagenous material (asterix), with occasional surviving smooth muscle cell nuclei (arrow). (**b**) Healed 'lipohyalinosis' ('complex' small vessel disease) in the putamen of an elderly woman with multiple basal ganglia lacunes. An asymmetrically thickened, disorganised vessel wall with focal fibrosis (asterix) and foam cell infiltration (thick arrow). The vessel is cut in two planes. Haematoxylin and eosin: (a) x430; (b) x200.

somewhat larger perforating arteries than lipohyalinosis (200–800 μm diameter), causing correspondingly larger infarcts, 5 mm or more in diameter, which are more often symptomatic. According to Fisher, the culprit atheromatous plaques were seen in the proximal portion of the perforating artery (microatheroma), at its origin (junctional atheroma) or in the parent artery itself (mural atheroma)[5]. Infarcts were related to stenotic or occlusive plaques, some but not all of which were complicated by overlying thrombus.

Progress in lacune research since Fisher

Since Fisher's landmark pathological observations, most lacune research has been in the clinical arena. Consistent with the lacunar hypothesis, lacunar stroke patients have been found to have a relatively low frequency of cardiac and large vessel atheromatous embolic sources compared to those with cortical infarcts[7]. That lacunar infarcts tend not to have a risk of early recurrence would also seem to mitigate against their being caused by an active embolic source. The risk factor profile for lacunar infarcts continues to be refined, but appears similar to that for ischaemic stroke in general, with the possible exception of hypertension. Hypertension was a more severe disease when Fisher first studied lacunes and he perhaps overestimated its importance in lacune pathogenesis, but it may still be more prevalent in this stroke subtype today[8]. Thus, although not accepted by everyone[9], the lacunar hypothesis has gained general support, not least because the distinct clinical lacunar syndromes have proved useful in patient management[10].

However, it could be argued that this large body of clinical and epidemiological work has not actually advanced our understanding of what actually causes lacunar infarcts. As one eminent stroke physician wrote of lacune research[11], 'attempts to infer the underlying disease by the analysis of clinical risk factors...is at best an approximation of what would be learned by microscopy'. So what of recent pathology research? Perhaps unsurprisingly, there have been no further attempts at serial section analysis, widely held to be the gold standard technique for visualising small vessel anatomy, and there have been few novel technical approaches to visualising the small vessels supplying lacunes[12]. A few large-scale autopsy surveys of lacune brains have been undertaken[13,14], but these have merely confirmed the epidemiological and risk factor trends. A new pathological variant of lacune has been described which is characterised by partially or 'incompletely' infarcted brain tissue, the potential significance of which lies in the fact that it suggests subtotal or temporary stenosis/occlusion as likely causes of lacunar infarcts, for example temporary embolic small vessel occlusion or vessel spasm[15]. Clearly, pathology has contributed little to the debate in recent years, overshadowed perhaps by the promise of the new genetics.

The genetics of lacunar stroke

It is now clear from twin, family and population studies that there is a significant familial or genetic component underlying ischaemic stroke, and there is now increasing effort to identify and characterise the susceptibility genes[16,17]. It is attractive, for example, to speculate that 'cortical' and 'lacunar' stroke patients, who have similar risk factor profiles, suffer different types of stroke because of different genetic predispositions. Of the rare inherited Mendelian disorders with an increased stroke risk, CADASIL and familial variants of cerebral amyloid angiopathy are both associated with specific cerebral small vessel pathologies and cortical/subcortical microinfarcts[18], but neither is likely to contribute significantly to the overall prevalence of lacunar strokes. Gene polymorphism association studies have, however, shown a weak but significant association of the DD genotype of the angiotensin converting enzyme (ACE) gene with ischaemic stroke in general[19]. Two studies have suggested an association between I/D polymorphism status and lacunar stroke in particular[20,21], in one of which there was also suggested to be an association of the GG genotype of the Glu298Asp endothelial nitric oxide synthase gene polymorphism with lacunes[17]. Such genetic studies promise much, but thus far have yielded marginally significant, negative or conflicting results, for reasons which are discussed below.

Obstacles to progress in lacune research

50 years after Fisher began his studies of lacunes, the bulk of clinical, radiological and epidemiological data would appear to support his conclusion that lacunes are caused predominantly by some form of intrinsic small vessel disease. However, we remain largely ignorant as to the underlying cause of the small vessel lesions he described, and so have been powerless to prevent or treat them, apart from managing their associated risk factors. The reasons for this lack of progress are several, and most are intractable.

For the pathologist, the low case fatality[1] means that only rarely does the pathogenetically informative acute small vessel lesion come to autopsy; when it does, it is usually late after the onset of stroke and so is organised and at least partially healed, its appearance perhaps reflecting as much a response to injury as its cause. Even when the fresh lesion does present itself, the technical difficulties inherent in tracing the lesion's vascular supply are formidable. The current climate of research funding would seem to preclude further serial section analysis in a sufficiently large number of informative cases. As discussed, risk factor analysis is unlikely to provide further insight and current methods of imaging small intracerebral vessels during life, lack the necessary resolution. To these problems should be added the limitations inherent in a traditional descriptive pathology approach – the classical descriptions of lipohyalinosis, important though they were, have not of themselves shed light on the underlying cellular or molecular mechanisms. Further, our understanding of the potential contribution of intracranial atheroma is limited, is largely derived from somewhat crude radiological data, and lacks the detailed pathology study which has proved so informative in coronary artery and more recently carotid artery research[22]. A further problem is the clinical and patho-genetic heterogeneity of subcortical, as well as cortical, brain infarction[23]. For example, small infarcts in the centrum ovale may be manifestations of cardiac or large artery disease more commonly than striatocapsular lesions[24]

Faced with these problems, there has not been a satisfactory animal model of lacunar infarction to which the experimental pathologist can turn[25]; most animal stroke models have been used to study the patho-physiology and salvage of ischaemic brain tissue. The stroke-prone spontaneously hypertensive rat (SHRSP) does suffer microinfarcts and haemorrhages, as well as fibrinoid small vessel lesions, and may yet prove to be a useful model of small vessel stroke. However, the SHRSP suffers these lesions only in association with blood pressure levels not commonly encountered in modern clinical practice[25], and in this context may be regarded as a model of malignant hypertension.

Finally, the early genetic studies of human lacunar and other types of stroke have had major limitations which are becoming familiar in other complex or multifactorial diseases[26]. Many studies have had extremely small sample sizes, a lack of adequate numbers of genetically matched controls, an absence of relevant biological data or even of a convincing biological rationale ('fishing'). They too of course have suffered from the difficulties inherent in accurate clinical identification of pathological stroke subtypes.

Primary intracerebral haemorrhage – a related problem

Problems have also beset researchers studying the pathogenesis of PICH. Some of these reflect the same inaccessibility of the culprit intracerebral vessels which has frustrated lacune research, although others are unique.

Apart from those rare cases in which PICH is presumed to follow rupture of structurally normal vessels, usually in association with acute rises in blood pressure or blood flow[27], it is reasonable to assume that rupture of an intracerebral vessel is a consequence of focal vessel wall pathology. As Caplan has pointed out, the so-called Charcot-Bouchard microaneurysm has never been clearly identified as the definitive cause of even a single haematoma[27], and its very existence has now been questioned by elegant histochemical studies suggesting it was an illusion of injection studies produced by complex arteriolar coils and perivascular clots[28]. The consensus view at present is perhaps that the same small vessel lesion observed by Fisher in relation to lacunar infarcts is responsible for the majority of PICH[29,30], a lesion in its acute form characterised by fibrinoid vessel wall necrosis[31]. PICH and lacunar infarction appear to co-localise, often co-exist in the same brain at autopsy, and show broad similarities in risk factor profile[29]. However, why the same or a similar vessel lesion should in some cases lead to a small infarct and in others to an intracerebral haemorrhage is unclear. There is clearly potential for a complex interplay of acute haemodynamic and acquired structural vessel wall changes in the pathogenesis of these stroke subtypes.

Study into the cause of PICH by traditional, observational clinical and autopsy studies have been beset by now familiar difficulties. Intracerebral haemorrhages are a heterogenous stroke type, and it is often difficult to distinguish clinically those cases due, for example, to haemorrhagic transformation of infarcts, haemorrhagic venous infarction, cryptic vascular malformations and cerebral amyloid angiopathy[32]. Clinical series of PICH are, therefore, likely to have included a diversity of patho-genetically unrelated entities. Although a relatively high proportion of severe PICH cases have come to autopsy shortly after the ictus, the problem of causal lesion localisation is the same as for lacunes, and is further complicated by the fact that the vessel lesion is destroyed or at least modified by the rupture itself and the consequent haemorrhage. Yet again, *in vitro* and *in vivo* models of PICH have been sought, but are used mainly to examine the clinical properties of clots and their response to drugs, or the effects of haemorrhage on surrounding brain[33]. There has, to date, been no satisfactory *in vivo* model that sheds light on the mechanism of human PICH.

Future prospects

It is clear from the above that traditional pathological lines of investigation have been pivotal in formulating our current ideas as to how small vessel-strokes occur. There is still much that such an approach can offer, in particular regarding the nature and consequences of cervicocranial atherosclerosis. Stroke researchers have been slow to apply the paradigm of plaque instability to the arteries supplying the brain. Thus, whilst it seems that thrombotic occlusion of the carotid artery usually occurs in a manner directly analogous to coronary artery thrombosis[22], very little is known of the relations between plaque stability, stenosis, plaque pro-gression, thrombosis and embolism. This is particularly true of intracranial vessels, despite the obvious implications for lacunar infarct pathogenesis.

The prospects of such traditional approaches clarifying the role of intracerebral small vessel disease in stroke are by comparison bleak. However, there should be some attempt to standardise pathological terminology in this field, particularly in relation to small vessel lesions. Thereafter, it is perhaps the emerging breed of experimental molecular pathologist who has most to offer[34], ideally in the context of a multidisciplinary stroke research team. Questions which logically pose themselves are 'is there a specific intracerebral vessel lesion associated with lacunar infarction and PICH?' and then, 'is this lesion merely a stochastic event caused by the unfortunate concurrence of multiple risk factors or is it, to an extent at least, (genetically) predictable and hence maybe preventable?' Fisher's work, and the debate it provoked, have provided a provisional answer to the first question – a characteristic destructive cerebral vessel lesion characterised in its acute form by fibrinoid necrosis, does appear to be specifically associated with lacunar infarction, and albeit less convincingly, PICH. The answer to the second question is at one level straightforward – small vessel stroke will, like the vast majority of multi-factorial diseases, prove to be a combination of genetic and environmental risk factors. Advances in our understanding of the genetics of established stroke risk factors, such as hypertension, will complement the search for novel genes predisposing to stroke independent of such factors. Also, small vessel stroke researchers may now begin to take advantage of an improved understanding of the genetic basis of established animal models, such as the SHRSP, in which chromosomal regions have recently been identified containing blood pressure-independent genetic factors predisposing to stroke[16]. In addition, a variety of newer transgenic and gene knock-out animal models[35] have the potential now to model the specific small vessel lesions implicated by human autopsy research. Both approaches will be essential in focusing on biologically plausible candidate genes for association studies in human stroke, an increasingly important concern given the impending availability of the entire human genome sequence and its variability, as well as the development of comprehensive sets of single nucleotide polymorphisms spanning the human genome[36]. These human genetic studies will, of course, continue to require valid stroke subtyping. Finally, more, and more informative, stroke intermediate phenotypes need to be developed. This is partly because such phenotypes are likely to be influenced by a smaller number of genes than stroke itself, thereby improving the power of linkage and association studies, but also as they may provide insights into the mechanisms underlying postulated genetic associations[16]. A well-defined small vessel lesion, modelled in a genetically defined animal, would be an obvious intermediate phenotype which would integrate the fields of Virchowian pathology and molecular genetics in small vessel-related stroke research.

Acknowledgements

The author is grateful to Angela Penman for typing the manuscript, and to Charles Warlow for his consistent support and constructive criticism.

References

1 Bamford J, Sandercock P, Jones L, Warlow CP. The natural history of lacunar infarction: the Oxfordshire Community Stroke Project. *Stroke* 1987; **18**: 545–51
2 Bamford J, Sandercock P, Dennis M, Burn J, Warlow C. A prospective study of acute cerebrovascular disease in the community: The Oxfordshire Community Stroke Project 1981–1986; II: incidence, case fatality rates and overall outcome at one year of cerebral infarction, primary intracerebral and subarachnoid haemorrhage. *J Neurol Neurosurg Psychiatry* 1990; **53**: 16–22
3 Poirier J, Derouesre C. Le concept de lacune cerebrale de 1838 a nos jours. *Rev Neurol (Paris)* 1985; **141**: 3–17
4 Poirier J, Derouesne C. Cerebral lacunae. A proposed new classification. *Clin Neuropathol* 1989; **3**: 266
5 Fisher CM. Lacunar infarcts – a review. *Cerebrovasc Dis* 1991; **1**: 311–20
6 Gutstein WH. Vasospasm, vascular injury and atherogenesis: a perspective. *Hum Pathol* 1999; **30**: 365–71
7 Lodder J, Bamford JM, Sandercock PAG, Jones LN, Warlow CP. Are hypertension or cardiac embolism likely causes of lacunar infarction? *Stroke* 1990; **21**: 375–81
8 Donnan GA. Lacunes and lacunar syndromes. In: Ginsberg MD, Bogousslavsky J. (eds) *Cerebrovascular Disease. Pathophysiology, Diagnosis and Treatment*. Malden, MA: Blackwell Science, 1998; 1090–102
9 Millikan C, Futrell N. The fallacy of the lacune hypothesis. *Stroke* 1990; **21**: 1251–7
10 Bamford JM, Warlow CP. Evolution and testing of the lacunar hypothesis. *Stroke* 1988; **19**: 1074–82
11 Mohr JP. The pathogenesis of single penetrator infarcts. In: Donnan G, Norrving B, Bamford J, Bogousslavsky J. (eds) *Lacunar and other Subcortical Infarctions*. Oxford, OUP, 1995; 29–31
12 Challa VR, Bell MA, Moody DM. A combined haematoxylin-eosin, alkaline phosphatase and high resolution microradiographic study of lacunes. *Clin Neuropathol* 1990; **9**: 196–204
13 Tuszynski MH, Petito CK, Levy DE. Risk factors and clinical manifestations of pathologically verified lacunar infarctions. *Stroke* 1989; **20**: 990–9
14 Dozono K, Ishii N, Nishihara Y, Horie A. An autopsy study of the incidence of lacunes in relation to age, hypertension and arteriosclerosis. *Stroke* 1991; **22**: 993–6
15 Lammie GA, Brannan F, Wardlaw JM. Incomplete lacunar infarction (type 1b lacunes). *Acta Neuropathol* 1998; **96**: 163–71
16 Boerwinkle E, Doris PA, Fornage M. Field of needs. The genetics of stroke. *Circulation* 1999; **99**: 331–3
17 Elbaz A, Amarenco P. Genetic susceptibility and ischaemic stroke. *Curr Opin Neurol* 1999; **12**: 47–55
18 Pullicino P, Greenberg S, Trevisan M. Genetic stroke risk factors. *Curr Opin Neurol* 1997; **10**: 58–63
19 Sharma P. Meta-analysis of the ACE gene in ischaemic stroke. *J Neurol Neurosurg Psychiatry* 1998; **64**: 227–30
20 Elbaz A, Mallet C, Cambien F, Amarenco P. Association between the ACE 4656 (CT) 2/3 polymorphism and plasma ACE level with lacunar stroke in the GENIC study. *Cerebrovasc Dis* 1998; **8** (Suppl 4): 44
21 Markus HS, Barley J, Lunt R *et al*. Angiotensin converting enzyme gene deletion polymorphism: a new risk factor for lacunar stroke but not carotid atheroma. *Stroke* 1995; **26**: 1329–33
22 Lammie GA, Sandercock PAG, Dennis MS. Recently occluded intracranial and extracranial carotid arteries. The relevance of the unstable atherosclerotic plaque. *Stroke* 1999; **30**: 1319–25
23 Bogousslavsky J. The plurality of subcortical infarction. *Stroke* 1992; **23**: 629–31
24 Lammie GA, Wardlaw JM. Small centrum ovale infarcts – a pathological study. *Cerebrovasc Dis* 1999; **9**: 82–90
25 Ginsberg MD, Busto R. Small-animal models of global and focal cerebral ischaemia. In: Ginsberg MD, Bogousslavsky J. (eds) *Cerebrovascular Disease. Pathophysiology, Diagnosis and Management*. Malden, MA: Blackwell Science, 1998; 14–35

26 Todd JA. Interpretation of results from genetic studies of multifactorial diseases. *Lancet* 1999; **354 (suppl 1)**: 15–6

27 Caplan LR. Hypertensive intracerebral haemorrhage. In: Kase CS, Caplan LR. (eds) *Intracerebral Hemorrhage*. Boston, MA: Butterworth-Heinemann, 1994; 99–116

28 Challa VL, Moody DM, Bell MA. The Charcot-Bouchard aneurysm controversy: impact of a new histologic technique. *J Neuropathol Exp Neurol* 1992; **51**: 264–71

29 Norrving B. Cerebral hemorrhage. In: Ginsberg MD, Bogousslavsky J (eds) *Cerebrovascular Disease. Pathophysiology, Diagnosis and Management*. Malden, MA: Blackwell Science, 1998; 1447–73

30 Fisher CM. Pathological observations in hypertensive cerebral hemorrhage. *J Neuropathol Exp Neurol* 1971; **30**: 536–50

31 Rosenblum WI. The importance of fibrinoid necrosis as the cause of cerebral hemorrhage in hypertension. *J Neuropathol Exp Neurol* 1993; **52**: 11–3

32 Garcia JH, Ho K-L, Caccamo DV. Intracerebral hemorrhage: pathology of selected topics. In: Kase CS, Caplan LR. (eds) *Intracerebral Hemorrhage*. Boston, MA: Butterworth-Heinemann, 1994; 45–72

33 Kaufman HH, Schochet SS. Pathology, pathophysiology and modeling. In: Kaufman HH. (ed) *Intracerebral Haematomas*. New York: Raven, 1992; 16–21

34 Quirke P, Mapstone N. The new biology: histopathology. *Lancet* 1999; **354 (suppl 1)**: 26–31

35 Chan PH. The role of transgenic animals in cerebral ischemia. In: Ginsberg MD, Bogousslavsky J. (eds) *Cerebrovascular Disease. Pathophysiology, Diagnosis and Management*. Malden, MA: Blackwell Science, 1998; 481–8

36 Collins FS, Guyer MS, Chakravarti A. Variations on a theme: cataloging human DNA sequence variation. *Science* 1997; **278**: 1580–1

Animal models

Daniel L Small and **Alastair M Buchan**

Institute for Biological Sciences, National Research Council of Canada, Ottawa, Canada

Animal models of cerebral ischaemia mimic at best less than 25% of all strokes. Compounds which prove efficacious in animal models should, therefore, only be expected to improve outcome in a quarter of all strokes. If trials for acute stroke are to succeed, stroke subgroups represented by the animal models should be targeted. For the other subgroups, *e.g.* lacunar stroke, appropriate animal models need to be developed. Moreover, thrombolysis should be included in animal models because it is likely to be used as a first line treatment for ischaemic stroke and any future therapeutics will need to be compatible with it.

The publication of the NINDS tissue plasminogen activator (tPA) Trial in December 1995 demonstrated unequivocally that stroke in humans is treatable. However, the need for an agent which affords neuroprotection and which stabilizes resuscitated brains during reperfusion is paramount, particularly given the very limited window of therapeutic opportunity (<3 h) which thrombolysis offers and the fact that most stroke victims do not seek immediate medical attention. The ability to model cerebral ischaemia and to provide a testing ground for novel compounds has made the utilization of animal models essential prior to launching any clinical trials.

Although many models have been developed, the resulting ischaemia can be broadly classified as either global or focal. Much criticism is levied at the use of the global model, which mimics the human condition of cardiac arrest rather than focal stroke, but the precision with which a global ischaemic insult can induce damage to neurons gives investigators a precise and quantifiable modality in which to assess the efficacy of a neuro-protective agent, before advancing to focal ischaemia where there are many more variables that need to be controlled. There are many compounds which appear to work in focal ischaemia, but a critical review of the last 10 years reveals very few, if any, compounds which consistently achieve neuroprotection in models of severe global ischaemia[1].

Correspondence to:
Dr Daniel L Small,
Institute for Biological
Sciences, National
Research Council of
Canada, Building M-54,
Montreal Road, Ottawa
K1A 0R6, Canada

Global models

The global model of cerebral ischaemia consists of a brief (5–15 min) near complete cessation of cerebral blood flow, followed by reperfusion.

Table 1 Models of global ischaemia

Two-vessel occlusion model in gerbil
Transient bilateral occlusion of common carotids
Two-vessel occlusion model in rat
Transient bilateral occlusion of common carotids plus hypotension (~50 mmHg)
Four-vessel occlusion model in rat
Transient bilateral occlusion of common carotids plus permanent bilateral occlusion of vertebral arteries
Miscellaneous
Cardiac arrest
Decapitation
Neck Tourniquet
Elevated cerebrospinal fluid pressure

Decapitation models do not allow for reperfusion and result in a very different pathology[2]. Cardiac arrest models of global ischaemia most closely mimic cardiac arrest in man, but complicating systemic effects (*e.g.* renal, hepatic and myocardial injury) and the difficulty of resuscitating an animal following brainstem ischaemia, increase the morbidity of these models. These problems have led to the utilization of models where global ischaemia is, in fact, severe forebrain ischaemia. Flow continues to the brainstem allowing animals the ability to spontaneously ventilate and consequently there is an increase in the number of survivors. Although there are many ways of inducing the interruption of flow in severe forebrain ischaemia, most models utilize occlusion of the common carotids (Table 1). There are 3 predominant models.

The simplest, and therefore most popular, global model for screening novel neuroprotectants is the 2 vessel occlusion in gerbils. Bilateral occlusion of the common carotids in this model is sufficient to produce severe forebrain ischaemia, because gerbils lack posterior communicating arteries (PComA) necessary to complete the circle of Willis which, in humans and rats, permits collateral blood flow. The disadvantages of this model are that, although there is delayed and selective neuronal death produced, the results are variable because of variability in the collateral flow and development of the PComA[3]. The small size of gerbils also lends to difficulties in monitoring physiological variables and the behavioural testing following the insult are restricted to simple tests, *e.g.* hyper-locomotor activity[4].

The two-vessel occlusion rat model with hypotension is also surgically simple and, therefore, permits rapid screening. It produces delayed and selective neuronal death and a reliable measure of damage by way of histology and behaviour testing. Monitoring of physiological variables is carried out with relative ease. The only real disadvantages of this model are that, because of the need to induce hypotension, many physiological variables will be altered beyond the control of the experimenter. Modest deviations from the generally accepted 50 mmHg of hypotension required for this model and the variability in the collateral circulation between animals, strains and suppliers can potentially produce profound changes in the severity of the insult[5].

The 4-vessel occlusion rat model is a more difficult surgical procedure. A day before the carotids are occluded, the anterior vertebrals are permanently occluded by electrocauterization. This is often a source of error. Either the vertebrals are insufficiently occluded or the C1 vertebrate is excessively heated, resulting in damage to the medulla and an increase in the mortality resulting from surgery because the animals experience respiratory difficulties. Similarly, problems with gaining access to the vertebrals can result in excess muscle trauma and myoglobinurea post-operatively. There is a marked mortality after the first stage operation but, in laboratories with skilled surgeons, this becomes minimal with experience[5]. The advantage of this model is that there is opportunity to measure physiological variables in the absence of anaesthesia or hypotension. In addition, delayed and selective neuronal death can be combined with reliable measurements of damage which include behavioural testing. This model is associated with less variability than most models, when the surgery is carried out successfully. As with any model there is still some variability which can exist between species of rat and even between batches of animals from the same strain and supplier[6-8]. Differences in vulnerability to ischaemia between strains will be discussed below with reference to transgenic mice.

The delayed and selective death following global ischaemia has been well characterized and is similar among all global models. The histopathology varies with the duration of ischaemia. With a relatively brief insult of 10 min, there is selective damage to the CA1 region of the hippocampus which occurs from about 3–7 days[9]. The rate of death in this region can be accelerated or slowed somewhat by increasing or decreasing the severity of the insult (Fig. 1)[10]. After a critical threshold in duration, death processes, rather than protective preconditioning processes are initiated. The rate of death subsequent to crossing this threshold is accelerated, but there is still a delay of 2–3 days before any death occurs, providing that the threshold in duration is not exceeded beyond a point at which death occurs immediately by necrosis. Within the range sufficient to cause delayed death in the hippocampus, an increase in severity will produce death of small and medium sized striatal neurons as well as pyramidal neurons in layers 3 and 5 of the cortex[9]. The time course of the death in these more resistant regions is, counterintuitively, more rapid (6–12 h in striatum) than that in the more

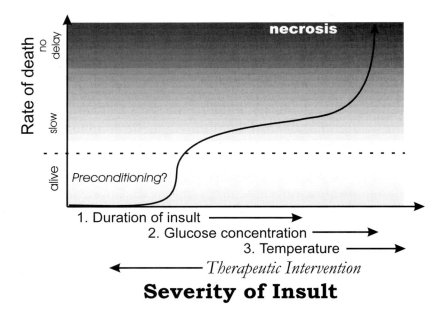

Severity of Insult

Fig. 1 Schematic illustration depicting the relationship between the severity of the ischaemic insult and the temporal profile of cell death. Factors such as the duration of the insult, glucose concentration and temperature all increase the severity of the insult, whereas therapeutic intervention decreases the severity and consequently buys time and prolongs the delay to death or even prevents the death process. With a very extreme insult, death can occur without a delay and is referred to as necrosis.

sensitive hippocampal CA1 region. Interestingly, there is a temporal-spatial vulnerability within the CA1 region. Pyramidal neurons die in an orderly fashion from mesial to lateral and from septal to temporal[9] like a spreading grass fire[10]. The underlying mechanisms of this vulnerability are as yet unknown, but does not seem to correlate with the vasculature of the hippocampus[11].

Focal models

There are several varieties of focal models in rat, many of which are variants of middle cerebral artery occlusion (MCAO) based on various methods of occlusion, including coated or bare thread, clip, photo-thrombosis, clot or endothelin (Table 2). The focal model is a closer approximation to human stroke and produces a heterogeneous pathology which includes a necrotic core and salvageable penumbra, as well as normal, undamaged tissue in both ipsilateral and contralateral hemispheres. In the necrotic core, the area at the centre of the ischaemic territory, there is pan-necrosis in which both neurones and glia die. In

Table 2 Models of focal ischaemia

Permanent or transient

Middle cerebral artery occlusion (MCAO) – methods of occlusion: clip, ligature, intraluminar thread (coated/uncoated), cauterization (not transient)

Use of spontaneously hypertensive rats (SHR) – produces more consistent infarct with MCAO

Permanent – embolism and thrombosis models

Photochemical thrombosis using Rose Bengal (produces a core and no penumbra; not transient)

Carbon microsphere injection into internal carotid artery

Injection of platelet aggregates into common carotid

Injection of small blood clots into common carotid (transient if followed by tPA)

the salvageable penumbra, at the edge of the core, neurones are at risk of dying and can be saved if appropriate interventions are attempted. The penumbra is the area said to be 'at risk' and, although this area represents the smallest volume of tissue, it generates the most attention because it may hold the key to the development of effective stroke therapies. The analogy of a fire can be used, where the core represents the forest already burnt, and the penumbra represents the front of the fire where the fire fighters wage their battle to extinguish the blaze. As with the penumbra, although the front of a fire represents a small fringe of the burnt territory, if the front is left unchecked it will consume more forest leaving a core of burnt territory in its wake.

Focal models are broadly grouped into two categories – permanent and transient occlusion – although even with permanent occlusion there will be some recovery of flow through collaterals, producing, in effect, a transiently ischaemic territory. The transient occlusion models have all the features of the permanent models, as well as the additional complication of reperfusion injury. Reperfused ischaemic tissue is tissue at risk and best represents stroke in man, particularly after spontaneous or therapeutic thrombolysis. The clip models are transcranial and require removal of part of the skull and dura to expose the middle cerebral artery. This affects the intracranial pressure and may reduce the oedema that an intact skull would otherwise cause. There are also extended periods of anaesthesia required in this model. The intraluminal models are less invasive, but experimenters need to visualize the position of the filament either *in situ* postmortem or by staining of endothelium after transient occlusions. Recently, MRI has been used to visualize occlusion during the insult[12], but modifications to the surgery are required because of the restrictions associated with working in a powerful magnet. Clots have been gaining in popularity in focal models because it is thought that they even more closely mimic stroke in man. Photothrombosis,

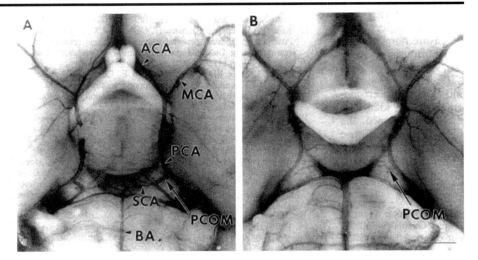

Fig. 2 Photomicrographs of circle of Willis in SV-129 (A) and C57black/6 (B) mice, showing marked difference in posterior communicating arteries after carbon black ink perfusion. Larger posterior communicating arteries were detected in SV-129 mice than in C57black/6 mice (*n* = 10 in each group). There were no significant differences in anterior and middle segments of the circle of Willis between the two strains. ACA indicates anterior cerebral artery; MCA, middle cerebral artery; PCA, posterior cerebral artery; BA, basilar artery; SCA, superior cerebellar artery; PCOM, posterior communicating artery. Scale bar, 1 mm. Reproduced with permission[14].

autoheterologous clots and *in vivo* thrombotic clots are used, but the problem of standardizing clots to minimize the variability of the insult is paramount and needs to be solved before meaningful data can be obtained[13].

Issues for the next millennium

Transgenic mice models

Much attention to models in rats has been recently shifting to mice, despite all of the work which has been carried out in standardizing the rat models and their outcome measures. This is mainly because of the facility with which mouse transgenics can be carried out relative to rats. The standardization and development of ischaemia models has taken a step back and has begun again for mice. Not only are there differences in the patency of the PComA in mice of different strains (Fig. 2)[14] as there are in gerbils[3], but there are very different vascular territories in the different species of mice used to generate the transgenic mice (Fig. 3)[17]. The patency of PComA and cortical microperfusion in three strains of mice commonly used for genetic manipulations were measured and compared to that of gerbils and Wistar rats[18]. The patency of PComA, as

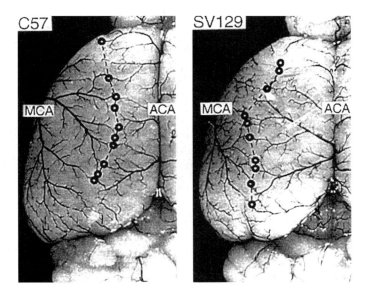

Fig. 3 Dorsal view of the cerebral hemisphere of C57black/6 mice (left) and SV-129 mice (right) after microvascular injection with carbon black stained latex. The points of anastomoses between the middle cerebral artery (MCA) and the anterior cerebral artery (ACA) are marked with circles and connected by the line of anastomoses. Note the marked shift of the line of anastomoses to the midline in C57black/6 mice. Reproduced with permission[17].

measured by diameter relative to the basilar artery, was less than 23% and the baseline cortical microperfusion following bilateral common carotid artery occlusion, was less than 12% in four out of five of the C57BL/6 mice compared to one of five CBA and none of the DBA/2 mice. None of the five gerbils measured had patent PComA in contrast to all five of the Wistar rats used for comparison[18]. In another study, infarct volume measured in three mouse strains, BDF, CFW and BALB/C, varied significantly from 15 mm³ in the BDF mice to 70 mm³ in the BALB/C mice[19]. This has necessitated valiant efforts by experimenters to demonstrate similar vascular territories and vessel patencies in both parental strains used to generate the transgenic mutant. In addition to looking at angioarchitecture and blood flow, another modality of the insult is hypoxia. One way to address this aspect of experimental ischaemia was to use immunohistochemistry to detect macromolecular adducts of a pentafluorinated derivative of 2-nitroimidazole, EF5, which is reduced by hypoxia and, therefore, directly delineates the hypoxic territory[20]. If only one wild-type strain differs from the mutant, then it becomes essential to develop and test wild-type litter-mates. Alternatively, mutant mice can be backcrossed with a single parent strain for at least 12 generations to ensure homogeneity of the genetic background[21]. Other problems have begun to arise as further differences are uncovered between murine species, such as differences in thermoregulation and vascular responsiveness[14] as well as vulnerability to KA excitotoxicity[15] (for review see Steward *et al*[16]).

Should changes be made to models based on trials?

There has been much disappointment resulting from the failure of clinical trials of neuroprotection to replicate the apparent successes of animal models, which has led to questioning of the validity of these models. It should be pointed out, however, that changes in temperature, glucose concentration and blood flow all have striking effects on human stroke (*i.e.* severe stroke, hyperglycaemia, and hyperthermia all predict poor outcome with thrombolysis)[22], and, similarly, all have critical effects on experimental stroke (Fig. 1). Even subtle changes in temperature, and glucose have profound effects on outcome following both human and experimental stroke adding to the validity of the experimental models.

For as long as animal models have been in use, there has been debate as to which model was most representative of stroke in man and/or which model could most accurately forecast the success of a potential therapeutic agent in clinical trials[23–26]. Based on the failure of several recent clinical trials for acute stroke, should animal models be changed to better reflect stroke in man? For example, phase 3 trials for Cerestat were discontinued in December 1997, due to safety and efficacy concerns but a subgroup analysis of patients with a moderate stroke (a score of 17 or less on a modified Rankin stroke scale, 42% of all randomized patients), revealed that 40% achieved a good or better outcome in contrast to 30% of the placebo-treated patients[27]. Similarly, efficacy was not achieved in the phase 3 Clomethiazole Acute Stroke Study (CLASS), but analysis of a subgroup of patients with total anterior infarct circulatory syndrome (TACS; 17% of randomized patients) revealed that clomethiazole-treated patients demonstrated a 37% relative benefit over placebo-treated patients[27]. Although these subgroup analyses may simply reflect the effects of chance, the results argue in favour of designing clinical trials to target a specific subgroup of stroke, *e.g.* TACS, which is well represented by the model in which animal efficacy is observed. The best therapy for TACS may not be equally efficacious in lacunar stroke and a compound which demonstrates efficacy in the MCAO model should not necessarily be expected to work in lacunar stroke.

Changes should also be made to the animal models to better reflect stroke in the clinic. In addition to developing animal models which mimic lacunar stroke or other serious types of stroke, changes should be made to the models to reflect the clinical situation. Consideration should be given to the interaction of potential neuroprotective agents with thrombolytic agents, not to mention the effects of thrombolysis alone on neuronal damage and infarct size in animal models of cerebral ischaemia. The effects of tPA alone have been studied in both global and focal models of ischaemia with varying results[28–30]. There is controversy as to whether tPA is neuroprotective[31] or neurotoxic[26,32,33] and further study is required before the debate can be resolved. With regard to combination therapy with thrombolytics, it is entirely possible that there will come a time when many of the patients being recruited in trials will be given thrombolytics as a primary course of treatment since about 85% of all strokes are ischaemic rather than haemorrhagic. Thrombolytics should, therefore, be used in animal models together with test agents to test for efficacy in the presence of thrombolytic agents as well as testing for potential interactions with the test compound. The future of stroke treatment may well be some form of polytherapy. Given the multiplicity of mechanisms involved in ischaemic neuronal damage, a patient might require multiple pharmacological interventions to affect lasting protection and these agents may be given together or at various times following the event, *e.g.* thrombolytics early to restore blood flow, an excitatory amino acid antagonist together with a sodium channel antagonist, followed by a free radical scavenger and finally a trophic factor to promote regeneration. Animal models have already begun such testing (for review see Buchan *et al*[34]). Although an AMPA receptor antagonist, NBQX, together with an NMDA receptor antagonist, MK-801, proved worse than with NBQX alone[35], both NBQX with tPA[36] and MK-801 with tPA[37] resulted in better protection compared with treating animals with either NBQX, MK-801 or tPA alone. Further studies are required to identify and eliminate combinations which produce adverse effects (*e.g.* MK-801 and NBQX[35] and dextromethorphan and tirilizad[38]) and confirm which combinations demonstrate synergistic neuroprotective effects (*e.g.* tirilizad and magnesium[39], citocholine and MK-801[40], and eliprodil and tPA[41]).

Conclusions

Animal models of cerebral ischaemia mimic at best less than 25% of all strokes. Compounds which prove efficacious in animal models should, therefore, only be expected to improve outcome in a quarter of all strokes. If trials for acute stroke are to succeed, stroke subgroups represented by the animal models should be targeted. For the other subgroups, *e.g.* lacunar stroke, appropriate animal models need to be developed. Moreover, thrombolysis should be included in animal models because it is likely to be used as a first line treatment for ischaemic stroke and any future therapeutics will need to be compatible with it. With the growing interest in developing murine models of cerebral ischaemia, animal models should be refined to better represent clinical stroke. At the same time, those designing clinical trials should focus on targeting stroke of the types best represented by the models currently in use, rather than anticipating a panacea from every compound which has been found to reduce infarct volume by 20% in a rodent.

References

1 Small DL, Buchan AM. NMDA antagonists: Their role in neuroprotection. In: Green AR, Cross AJ. (eds) *Neuroprotective Agents and Cerebral Ischaemia*. San Diego, CA: Academic Press, 1997; 137–71

2 MacManus JP, Hill IE, Preston E, Rasquinha I, Walker T, Buchan AM. Differences in DNA fragmentation following transient cerebral or decapitation ischemia in rats. *J Cereb Blood Flow Metab* 1995; 15: 728–37

3 Berry K, Wisniewski HM, Svarzbein L, Baez S. On the relationship of brain vasculature to production of neurological deficit and morphological changes following acute unilateral common carotid artery ligation in gerbils. *J Neurol Sci* 1975; 25: 75–92

4 Nurse S, Corbett D. Direct measurement of brain temperature during and after intraischemic hypothermia: correlation with behavioral, physiological, and histological endpoints. *J Neurosci* 1994; 14: 7726–34

5 Ginsberg MD, Busto R. Rodent models of cerebral ischemia. *Stroke* 1989; 20: 1627–42

6 Iwasaki H, Ohmachi Y, Kume E, Krieglstein J. Strain differences in vulnerability of hippocampal neurons to transient cerebral ischaemia in the rat. *Int J Exp Pathol* 1995; 76: 171–8

7 Sauter A, Rudin M. Strain-dependent drug effects in rat middle cerebral artery occlusion model of stroke. *J Pharm Exp Ther* 1995; 274: 1008–13

8 Oliff HS, Coyle P, Weber E. Rat strain and vendor differences in collateral anastomoses. *J Cereb Blood Flow Metab* 1997; 17: 571–6

9 Pulsinelli WA, Brierley JB, Plum F. Temporal profile of neuronal damage in a model of transient forebrain ischemia. *Ann Neurol* 1982; 11: 491–8

10 Colbourne F, Li H, Buchan AM, Clemens JA. Continuing postischemic neuronal death in CA1: influence of ischemia duration and cytoprotective doses of NBQX and SNX-111 in rats. *Stroke* 1999; 30: 662–8

11 Marinkovic S, Milisavljevic M, Puskas L. Microvascular anatomy of the hippocampal formation. *Surg Neurol* 1992; 37: 339–49

12 Kohno K, Back T, Hoehn-Berlage M, Hossmann KA. A modified rat model of middle cerebral artery thread occlusion under electrophysiological control for magnetic resonance investigations. *Magn Reson Imaging* 1995; 13: 65–71

13 Kilic E, Hermann DM, Hossmann KA. A reproducible model of thromboembolic stroke in mice. *Neuroreport* 1998; 9: 2967–70

14 Fujii M, Hara H, Meng W, Vonsattel JP, Huang Z, Moskowitz MA. Strain-related differences in susceptibility to transient forebrain ischemia in SV-129 and C57black/6 mice. *Stroke* 1997; 28: 1805–10

15 Schauwecker PE, Steward O. Genetic determinants of susceptibility to excitotoxic cell death: implications for gene targeting approaches. *Proc Natl Acad Sci USA* 1997; 94: 4103–8

16 Steward O, Schauwecker PE, Guth L *et al.* Genetic approaches to neurotrauma research: Opportunities and potential pitfalls of murine models. *Exp Neurol* 1999; 157: 19–42

17 Maeda K, Hata R, Hossmann KA. Differences in the cerebrovascular anatomy of C57black/6 and SV129 mice. *Neuroreport* 1998; 9: 1317–9

18 Kitagawa K, Matsumoto M, Yang G *et al.* Cerebral ischemia after bilateral carotid artery occlusion and intraluminal suture occlusion in mice: evaluation of the patency of the posterior communicating artery. *J Cereb Blood Flow Metab* 1998; 18: 570–9

19 Barone FC, Knudsen DJ, Nelson AH, Feuerstein GZ, Willette RN. Mouse strain differences in susceptibility to cerebral ischemia are related to cerebral vascular anatomy. *J Cereb Blood Flow Metab* 1993; **13**: 683–92

20 MacManus JP, Koch CJ, Jian M, Walker T, Zurakowski B. Decreased brain infarct following focal ischemia in mice lacking the transcription factor E2F1. *Neuroreport* 1999; **10**: 1–4

21 Gerlai R. Gene-targeting studies of mammalian behavior: is it the mutation or the background genotype? *Trends Neurosci* 1996; **19**: 177–81

22 Demchuk AM, Morgenstern LB, Krieger DW *et al.* Serum glucose level and diabetes predict tissue plasminogen activator-related intracerebral hemorrhage in acute ischemic stroke. *Stroke* 1999; **30**: 34–9

23 Hunter AJ, Mackay KB, Rogers DC. To what extent have functional studies of ischaemia in animals been useful in the assessment of potential neuroprotective agents? *Trends Pharmacol Sci* 1998; **19**: 59–66

24 Hunter AJ, Green AR, Cross AJ. Animal models of acute ischaemic stroke: can they predict clinically successful neuroprotective drugs? *Trends Pharmacol Sci* 1995; **16**: 123–8

25 Grotta J. Why do all drugs work in animals but none in stroke patients? 2 Neuroprotective therapy. *J Int Med* 1996; **237**; 89–94

26 del Zoppo GJ. Clinical trials in acute stroke: why have they not been successful? *Neurology* 1998; **51**: S59–61

27 Goldin SM. Recent failures in stroke drug development: Redefining industry strategies. *Drug Market Dev* 1999; **10**: 96–102

28 Wang YF, Tsirka SE, Strickland S, Stieg PE, Soriano SG, Lipton SA. Tissue plasminogen activator (tPA) increases neuronal damage after focal cerebral ischemia in wild-type and tPA-deficient mice. *Nat Med* 1998; **4**: 228–31

29 Kilic E, Hermann DM, Hossmann KA. Recombinant tissue plasminogen activator reduces infarct size after reversible thread occlusion of middle cerebral artery in mice. *Neuroreport* 1999; **10**: 107–11

30 Klein GM, Li H, Sun P, Buchan AM. Tissue plasminogen activator does not increase neuronal damage in rat models of global and focal ischemia. *Neurology* 1999; **52**: 1381–4

31 Kim YH, Park JH, Hong SH, Koh JY. Nonproteolytic neuroprotection by human recombinant tissue plasminogen activator. *Science* 1999; **284**: 647–50

32 Tsirka SE. Clinical implications of the involvement of tPA in neuronal cell death. *J Mol Med* 1997; **75**: 341–7

33 Tsirka SE, Gualandris A, Amaral DG, Strickland S. Excitotoxin-induced neuronal degeneration and seizure are mediated by tissue plasminogen activator. *Nature* 1995; **377**: 340–4

34 Steiner T, Hacke W. Combination therapy with neuroprotectants and thrombolytics in acute ischaemic stroke. *Eur Neurol* 1998; **40**: 1–8

35 Buchan AM, Lesiuk H, Barnes KA *et al.* AMPA antagonists: do they hold more promise for clinical stroke trials than NMDA antagonists? *Stroke* 1993; **24**: I148–52

36 Overgaard K, Sereghy T, Pedersen H, Boysen G. Neuroprotection with NBQX and thrombolysis with rt-PA in rat embolic stroke. *Neurol Res* 1993; **15**: 344–9

37 Sereghy T, Overgaard K, Boysen G. Neuroprotection by excitatory amino acid antagonist augments the benefit of thrombolysis in embolic stroke in rats. *Stroke* 1993; **24**: 1702–8

38 Schmid-Elsaesser R, Zausinger S, Hungerhuber E, Baethmann A, Reulen HJ. Monotherapy with dextromethorphan or tirilizad – but not a combination of both – improves outcome after transient focal cerebral ischemia in rats. *Exp Brain Res* 1998; **122**: 121–7

39 Schmid-Elsaesser R, Zausinger S, Hungerhuber E, Baethmann A, Reulen HJ. Neuroprotective effects of combination therapy with tirilizad and magnesium in rats subjected to reversible focal cerebral ischemia. *Neurosurgery* 1999; **44**:163–71

40 Onal MZ, Li F, Tatlisumak T, Locke KW, Sandage BW, Fisher M. Synergistic effects of citicholine and MK-801 in temporary experimental focal ischemia in rats. *Stroke* 1997; **28**: 1060–5

41 Lekieffre D, Benavides J, Scatton B, Nowicki JP. Neuroprotection afforded by a combination of eliprodil and a thrombolytic agent, rt-PA, in a rat thrombolytic stroke model. *Brain Res* 1997; **776**: 88–95

Diagnosis of stroke with advanced CT and MR imaging

H R Jäger

Institute of Neurology and The National Hospital of Neurology and Neurosurgery, London, UK

There have been important advances in stroke imaging, including CT perfusion imaging, xenon-CT, CT angiography, MR diffusion imaging, MR perfusion imaging, MR angiography and haemorrhage-sensitive gradient echo MR sequences.

The technical principles and clinical applications of these methods are explained. An emphasis is made on the diagnosis of hyperacute cerebral ischaemia and issues surrounding the differentiation of reversible from irreversible ischaemic damage with modern imaging modalities, which has implications for thrombolytic therapy. This is followed by an overview of the role of imaging in patients with chronic stroke and transient ischaemic attack. In these patients, the diagnostic contribution of MRI in detecting the underlying pathology and the assessment of cerebrovascular reserve with perfusion imaging form an important part in the secondary prevention of stroke.

Technical advances in cross-sectional imaging

Computed tomography (CT) of the brain has been the mainstay of imaging patients with an acute neurological deficit. In recent years, magnetic resonance imaging (MRI) has been increasingly used in addition to CT. There have been important technological advances in both modalities. This development has been driven to a large extent by the need for early stroke detection prompted by the fact that active treatment with thrombolytic agents was beneficial and is beginning to be more widely used. An overview of technical advances will precede a discussion of the imaging in acute ischaemia, which is the main focus of this chapter, followed by considerations pertaining to the imaging of subacute and chronic cerebral ischaemia.

Correspondence to:
Dr H R Jäger, Lysholm
Radiological Department,
The National Hospital
for Neurology and
Neurosurgery,
Queen Square, London
WC1N 3BG, UK

Advances in CT scanning

Spiral CT scanning

All modern CT scanners provide now a facility for spiral CT scanning. In conventional incremental CT scanning, slices are acquired individually with a time delay between them for table repositioning and tube cooling. Spiral (or helical) scanning is performed with a continuous rotation of the X-ray tube during simultaneous movement of the CT table at a pre-selected speed. This allows the acquisition of a volumetric 3D data set, which can subsequently be divided into individual slices of variable thickness[1]. Spiral scanning provides a considerable increase in scanning speed and allows coverage of the entire head in approximately 15 s. This can be of advantage in restless patients with acute stroke and represents a prerequisite for CT angiography where imaging is performed during the relatively short intravascular phase of a contrast medium (see below). The most recent developments in this field are multi-slice spiral CT scanners, which use multiple detectors for simultaneous data collection at different locations and can acquire images at 3 times the speed of single detector spiral CT scanners[2].

CT perfusion imaging

There are two fundamentally different methods by which CT scanning can be used to assess cerebral perfusion. One uses the inhalation of xenon, the other a bolus injection of an iodinated contrast medium[3,4].

Xenon is a stable gas, which has an atomic number close to iodine and, therefore, attenuates the X-ray beam in a similar fashion. Unlike iodine, xenon is freely diffusable and penetrates the blood–brain barrier. Current set-ups for xenon CT scanning consist of the inhalation of a gas containing 28% xenon during sequential acquisition of CT images over a period of approximately 6 min. The distribution of xenon in the brain depends on the regional blood flow and is slightly quicker in grey matter than in white matter. The change of the Hounsfield numbers (CT numbers) over time during inhalation of xenon forms the basis of blood flow calculations, which are usually displayed as colour maps. The wash-out of xenon occurs relatively rapidly, allowing a repeat examination after 15–20 min. A disadvantage of this method is that any patient movement during the 6 min period causes misregistration of data. Xenon uptake may also be impaired in patients with severe pulmonary disease.

The second technique of CT perfusion imaging, tracks transients changes in the blood vessels and brain parenchyma during the first pass passage of an intravenously injected contrast medium, similar to MR perfusion imaging (see below). A series of images is acquired at a predetermined level with a temporal resolution of one image every 1 or 2 s. The passage of the contrast-medium bolus causes a transient increase in Hounsfield units, which is proportional to the iodine concentration in the perfused tissue. Maps of cerebral blood volume (CBV), mean transit time (MTT) and cerebral blood flow (CBF) can be obtained from a pixel-by-pixel analysis of the density changes over time.

Absolute quantification of cerebral blood flow is theoretically possible with this method because of the linear relationship between iodine concentration and Hounsfield numbers, but there remains some doubt about its accuracy in practice. Blood flow measurements of cortical grey matter using the bolus perfusion technique were systematically lower compared to data from xenon CT studies[4].

CT angiography

Selective imaging of blood vessels with CT has become possible with the introduction of spiral CT scanners. The image quality of CT angiography is likely to improve dramatically with the advent of the new multi-slice spiral CT scanners[5]. Data are acquired during the vascular phase of an iodinated contrast, which is injected intravenously, typically at a rate of 3 ml/s. The enhanced blood vessels are extracted from 3D data sets by applying specific density thresholds during the post-processing. The vessels can then be displayed as 2D projectional images, which resemble convent-ional angiograms, or as 3D surface rendered structures[6]. CT angiography can be performed rapidly and can be easily 'tagged onto' a routine diagnostic CT. It has the disadvantage of using iodinated contrast medium, which carries a small risk of adverse reactions. It may also be difficult to isolate blood vessels running close to bone during post processing.

Advances in MR imaging

MR perfusion imaging

MR perfusion imaging exploits magnetic susceptibility effects within the brain tissue during the first pass of an intravenously injected gadolinium-based contrast agent. During its first pass through the brain, the contrast medium causes a transient signal drop on T_2^*-weighted (susceptibility-weighted) MR images (Fig. 1)[7]. Images are typically acquired with a temporal resolution of one image every 1–2 s, similar to CT perfusion. The use of single-shot echoplanar imaging (EPI), however, allows multi-slice imaging with full brain coverage, which represents a distinct advantage compared to the single slice technique in CT perfusion imaging. MR perfusion imaging is, however, at present only semiquantitative and cannot provide absolute values[8]. The sequential changes in signal intensity can by plotted as a time-signal intensity curve of a chosen region of interest or reproduced as pixel based colour maps (Fig. 1). The relative cerebral blood volume (rCBV) is proportional to the area under the curve on the time-signal intensity graph. Other measurements that can be derived are arrival time (T_0) and mean transit time (MTT) of the gadolinium bolus. Using tracer kinetics, the relative cerebral blood flow (rCBF) can be estimated by dividing the relative blood volume by the

Fig. 1 MR perfusion study in a patient with bilateral carotid artery occlusion. An MRA of the intracranial circulation (**a**) does not demonstrate any internal carotid arteries. Both middle meningeal arteries (arrows) are prominent and provide collateral supply to the brain. The right posterior cerebral artery (curved arrow) is normal but only the proximal part of the left posterior cerebral artery is seen. T_2* weighted EPI images before (**b**) and 20 s after injection of a gadolinium bolus (**c**) demonstrate the magnetic susceptibility effects of the passing gadolinium bolus, which leads to a decrease in signal intensity of the blood vessels and brain parenchyma in (c) compared to (b). The time course of this signal change is shown in a time-signal intensity graph (**d**) for two separate regions of interest: the right occipital lobe (region 1) and left frontal lobe (region 2). The signal drop in the right occipital occurs much earlier and is more marked than in the left frontal region, where perfusion is impaired. A colour map (**e**) of the mean transit time (MTT) shows areas with a prolonged transit time in green and red. Prolongation of the MTT, which corresponds to a delayed passage of the bolus, is found in watershed areas at the boundaries between the anterior and middle and between the middle and posterior cerebral arteries.

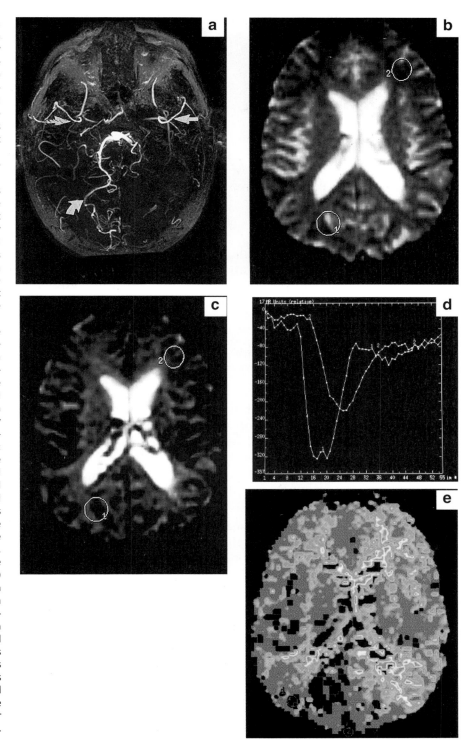

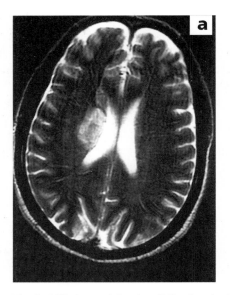 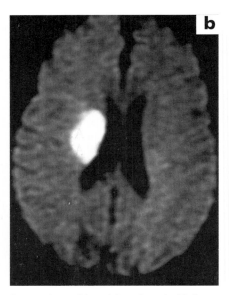

Fig. 2 Diffusion-weighted and T2 spin-echo images in a patient with a right subcortical infarct. Although the lesion is seen on the T_2-weighted image (**a**), it is much more conspicuous on the diffusion-weighted image (**b**), which confirms that the lesion is acute. The diffusion of water molecules is restricted in an area of acute ischaemia, which appears therefore a bright on diffusion-weighted images ('light bulb sign'). Note that the CSF, which has a high degree of molecular motion, appears dark.

mean transit time $(rCBF = rCBV/MTT)$[8]. In the absence of absolute quantification of the cerebral blood flow, comparison with the contralateral hemisphere provides the easiest way to analyse MR perfusion images. However, this becomes problematic if the perfusion of the contralateral hemisphere is not normal, as in the presence of bilateral carotid artery disease.

MR diffusion imaging

Diffusion-weighted MR imaging exploits the presence of random motion (Brownian motion) of water molecules to produce image contrast, thereby providing information not available on standard T_1- or T_2-weighted images[9]. This is achieved by applying a pair of 'diffusion' gradients symmetrically around a 180° refocusing radio frequency (RF) pulse of a T_2-weighted MR sequence. Mobile molecules acquire phase shifts, which prevent their complete rephasing and result in signal loss. The loss of signal is proportional to the degree of microscopic motion that occurs during the pulse sequence. On diffusion-weighted images, regions of relatively stationary water molecules appear much brighter than areas with a higher molecular diffusion (Fig. 2). The degree of phase shift and signal loss depends also on the strength and duration of the 'diffusion' gradient, which is expressed by the 'b value'. B-values used for imaging of acute stroke lie typically around 1000 s/mm^2. Quantitative analysis of the apparent diffusion coefficient (ADC) requires scanning with at least two different b-values and additional postprocessing. ADC maps are solely based on differences of tissue diffusion, independent of any T$_2$ effects[9]. The ADC in the normal brain ranges from 2.94 x 10^{-3} mm^2/s for CSF to 0.22 x 10^{-3} mm^2/s for white matter; grey matter lying in between with a ADC of 0.76 x 10^{-3} mm^2/s[10]. Areas with a decreased ADC appear dark on ADC maps, which is the converse to diffusion-weighted images where areas of decreased diffusion appear bright[9].

MR angiography

MR angiography can be performed at the same time as MR imaging of the brain parenchyma and forms an important part in the work-up of acute and chronic stroke. Its technical principles and applications are discussed by Clifton elsewhere in this issue.

Imaging of acute stroke

Pathophysiological considerations

The pathophysiology of acute stroke represents a chain of rather complex events, which can be simplified into three consecutive stages for the purpose of explaining the evolution of imaging findings: (i) flow abnormalities; (ii) cellular dysfunction; and (iii) structural breakdown[11,12]. Flow abnormalities represent a kinetic phenomenon, which can be detected immediately after the onset of stroke, both at the macrovascular and at microvascular level; the former by MRA and CTA, the latter by CT perfusion and MR perfusion imaging.

The second stage, cellular dysfunction, occurs if the cerebral blood flow falls below a critical level. At 20 ml/100 g/min, the electrical activity in the brain ceases and the water homeostasis begins to be disrupted. At 10–15 ml/100 mg, failure of the energy-dependent sodium pump leads to an accumulation of intracellular sodium and water moves into intracellular compartments causing swelling of neurons (cytotoxic oedema). Cytotoxic oedema predominates during the first 6 h following the onset of ischaemia. It is most conspicuous on diffusion-weighted MR images, but is also responsible for the early CT signs. Energy failure leads to an accumulation of lactate, which can be detected with spectroscopy (see Saunders elsewhere in this issue). As time proceeds, structural breakdown of the blood–brain barrier occurs with leakage of intravascular fluid and protein into the extracellular space (vasogenic oedema). The breakdown of the blood–brain barrier is a result of ischaemic damage to the endothelial lining of the capillaries, which is less oxygen dependent than neurons. Vasogenic oedema therefore develops after 6 h, reaching its peak between 24–48 h after the onset of ischaemia. Vasogenic oedema causes brain swelling, produces low-attenuation on CT and high signal on T_2-weighted and fluid-attenuated inversion recovery (FLAIR) images.

CT imaging of acute stroke

Exclusion of haemorrhage

CT scanning has been the modality of choice for imaging patients with acute stroke. Its major advantage, apart from wide-spread accessibility, is its reliability in detecting intracerebral and subarachnoid haemorrhage. It is, therefore, highly sensitive in distinguishing haemorrhagic from non-haemorrhagic stroke. Rare exceptions are very anaemic patients with a haematocrit of 20% or less, in whom haematomas can be isointense[13]. All major thrombolysis trial to date have used CT as primary imaging modality to exclude haemorrhage or extended infarction[14].

Large vessel occlusion

A 'dense middle cerebral artery sign' is the earliest detectable change on CT and can be seen at the onset of the ictus[15]. It is the result of increased attenuation of the horizontal first segment of the middle cerebral artery, which contains thrombus. The presence of a 'dense middle cerebral artery sign' correlates with large infarcts and worse patient outcome. One pitfall in diagnosing a dense middle cerebral artery sign is the presence of heavily calcified intracranial arteries, but these are usually bilateral.

CT angiography appears promising in the detection of acute middle cerebral artery occlusion and can be combined with delayed phase imaging, which shows enhancement of the collateral circulation[16,17].

CT perfusion imaging

The effects of a proximal artery occlusion on the microvascular circulation can be assessed with CT perfusion. Xenon CT studies have been used to produce quantitative perfusion data in patients with angiographically proven acute MCA occlusions, 55% of whom had a normal CT[18]: patients with a M1 segment occlusion had a mean CBF of 12 ml/100 g/min compared to 30 ml/100 g/min in patients without a M1 occlusion. Xenon CT also proved to be a useful predictor for the development of severe oedema with life-threatening brain herniation[19]. This was observed in patients with a mean CBF of 8.6 ml/100 g/min compared to a mean CBF of 18 ml/100 g/min in patients with only mild oedema. Koenig[4] used CT perfusion imaging following an intervenous bolus injection in patients presenting within 6 h after onset of an acute stroke. He demonstrated a reduction of CBF in 25 of 28 patients who subsequently progressed to develop an infarct. The 3 patients missed with this technique developed the infarct outside the scanned level, which demonstrates the limitation of a single slice technique.

Early signs on conventional CT

Early signs of parenchymal change in acute ischaemia are obscuration of the lentiform nucleus, loss of the insular ribbon and loss of the differentiation between cortical grey and subcortical white matter. These changes reflect neurotoxic oedema with accumulation of water in grey matter structures, which decreases their Hounsfield number and makes them no longer distinguishable from the adjacent white matter. A change of 4 Hounsfield units or more is visually detectable and corresponds to a change in water content of approximately 1.5%. In cases of severe ischaemia with poor collateral circulation, cytotoxic oedema produces a 3% increase in water content within 1 h and a 6% increase within 4 h. Severe ischaemia can, therefore, be detectable on a CT performed at 1 h but areas with marginal cerebral blood flow between 15–20 ml/100 g/min may remain undetected on early CT[20]. Later, vasogenic oedema causes effacement of the cerebral sulci and diffuse parenchymal hypodensity. Extensive diffuse hypodensity on early CT scans involving over 50% of the MCA territory is associated with a high mortality from malignant brain oedema[21].

It must be emphasised that early ischaemic changes on CT scans are subtle and may easily be overlooked by less experienced observers. The CT scans of patients entered into the European Cooperative Acute Stroke Study (ECASS) underwent a *post hoc* review by experts, which showed that the initial 'on site' interpretation overlooked an early infarct in 11% of the patients[22].

MR imaging of acute stroke

Exclusion of haemorrhage

Detection of hyperacute haemorrhage on conventional spin echo MR sequences is more difficult than on CT. The MR appearances of haemorrhage depend on the presence of paramagnetic haemoglobin breakdown products such as deoxyhaemoglobin, methaemoglobin and haemosiderin. Conventional spin echo sequences are sensitive to subacute and chronic haemorrhage, but the detection of hyperacute and acute haemorrhage can be greatly improved by using a T_2*-weighted gradient echo sequence[23]. It is much more susceptible to paramagnetic breakdown products, which cause signal loss and appear as areas of low intensity. Whether T_2*-weighted GRE is as sensitive as CT in excluding haemorrhage remains to be proven.

Occlusion of large vessels

Occlusion of a major intracerebral blood vessel may evident by a lack of flow void on conventional spin echo images or can be diagnosed with MRA (see Fig. 1). MRA is discussed in detail in a separate chapter. It is worth mentioning that, in the context of acute stroke, MRA has been shown to correlate well with conventional angiography in demonstrating vascular occlusion prior to and recanalisation following thrombolytic treatment[24].

MR perfusion imaging

MR perfusion imaging provides immediate and direct evidence of the repercussions of proximal vessel occlusion on the microcirculation[12]. A prolongation of the mean transit time (MTT) is the earliest and most consistent sign of an impairment in perfusion[14,25]. The relative cerebral blood volume (rCBV) may be normal or increased in the presence of adequate collateral supply, but is decreased if the collateral circulation is insufficient[26]. The response of rCBV to a prolongation of MTT provides information about the autoregulatory capacity, which aims to maintain the cerebral blood flow (rCBF) by increasing rCBV (rCBF = MTT/rCBV) by vasodilatation and recruitment of collaterals[27].

Sorenson[25] initially studied patients in the first 10 h and showed abnormalities on MTT maps to be more extensive than on rCBV maps. In a subsequent study[26], he performed rCBF measurements from MR perfusion studies and showed that, in the hyperacute state, blood flow maps revealed abnormalities not visible on blood volume maps, but that the final infarct in these untreated patients corresponded more closely to the blood volume maps. Ueda[28] showed that the size of the final infarct was grossly over-estimated on MTT maps, but correlated well with the extent of abnormality shown on rCBV maps.

MR diffusion imaging

MR diffusion imaging is by far the most sensitive MR technique for the detection of early parenchymal change following an ischaemic insult. Water diffusion is restricted in areas of ischaemic damage which appear therefore bright on diffusion weighted images ('light bulb sign') or dark on ADC maps. The precise mechanisms leading to a reduction in diffusion are actively debated, but redistribution of extracellular water into the intra-cellular compartment (cytotoxic oedema), resulting in shrinkage of the extracellular space appears the most likely explanation[9,29]. Diffusion-weighted imaging is highly sensitive and specific for the detection of early ischaemia and infarcts within the first 6 h of onset[30]. MR diffusion imaging has, therefore, a pre-eminent role in the assessments of patients presenting within the therapeutic window for thrombolysis, as routine T_2-weighted images will be normal at this stage (Fig. 3). Diffusion-weighted

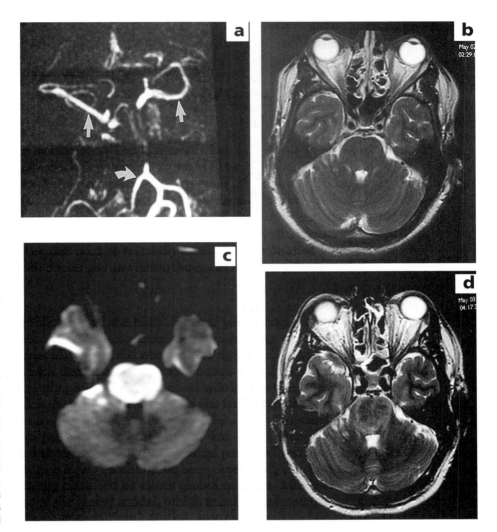

Fig. 3 34-year-old patient with a locked-in syndrome. The frontal projection of an MRA of the posterior circulation (**a**) shows occlusion of the basilar artery distal to the right anterior inferior cerebellar artery (curved arrow) with filling of the posterior cerebral arteries through collaterals (arrows). The T$_2$-weighted image in the hyperacute phase (**b**) is normal but the diffusion-weighted image shows high signal in the pons (**c**), which is becomes visible on T$_2$-weighted image after 48 h (**d**).

images may also be useful in differentiating between a transient ischaemic attack (TIA) and an infarct, since they appear to be normal in the former[9].

MRI diffusion imaging was also shown to be useful in subacute infarcts. In the presence of several abnormalities on T$_2$-weighted images, diffusion-weighted images can pinpoint the acute lesion and determine its vascular territory, which was felt to be clinically relevant in 48% of the cases in a recent clinical study[31].

Combined MR perfusion and diffusion imaging

Cerebral ischaemia is a complex disease process. Current therapeutic efforts are directed towards preventing tissue in with reversible ischaemia (the ischaemic penumbra) progressing to full infarction. Without rapid treatment or spontaneous recanalisation, the penumbra will eventually infarct. There is currently debate regarding the imaging equivalent of the ischaemic penumbra and it has been suggested that combining diffusion-weighted and perfusion-weighted MR imaging might be helpful. The initial concept was based on the observation that abnormalities are often more extensive on perfusion imaging than on diffusion-weighted images. It was assumed that the abnormalities on diffusion-weighted images (DWI) were irreversible and represented the core of infarct. The ischaemic penumbra was thought to be the area of perfusion/diffusion mismatch surrounding the core[8,25,26]. This concept has been challenged[11,32] and recent reports showed that abnormalities on diffusion weighted images could be reversible[9,14]. It appears likely that diffusion can already be impaired if the blood flow lies between 10–20 ml/100 g/min and not only below 10 ml/100 g/min, which is associated with irreversible ischaemic damage. This theory has been supported by animal experiments[9]. There is a feeling that abnormalities on diffusion-weighted imaging should be interpreted with caution and may prove to be more frequently reversible with the more wide-spread use of thrombolysis[11]. Others emphasise the need for better quantification of perfusion and diffusion parameters in order to differentiate reversible from irreversible ischaemia[32].

Imaging of subacute and chronic stroke

Subacute stroke

In the subacute phase, brain swelling may improve gradually but low attenuation change on CT and T_2 hyperintensities on MR persist. Gyriform contrast enhancement can be seen on CT and MR indicating disruption of the blood–brain barrier. Haemorrhagic transformation, defined as secondary bleeding into the ischaemic zone, is much more frequently detected on MRI than on CT. The occurrence and severity of haemorrhagic transformation correlates with the size of the infarct and degree of contrast-enhancement in the early stage and has been shown in up to 80% of infarcts on MRI[33].

A study using serial MR perfusion scans[34] showed an increase of rCBV in the infarcted region in the subacute stage, often associated with recanalisation of the occluded vessel on MRA, which was followed by a decrease in rCBV in the chronic stage.

Abnormalities on diffusion-weighted imaging begin to normalise between 7–14 days; after this period, there is increased water mobility in gliotic tissue, which appears dark on diffusion-weighted images and bright on ADC maps[29,35].

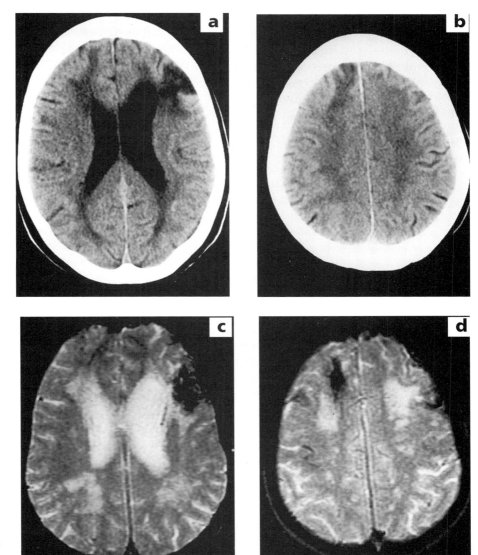

Fig. 4 CT scans of a 75-year-old patient at the level of the lateral ventricles (**a**) and the vertex (**b**) showing evidence of small vessel ischaemic disease and two mature cortical infarcts, in the left and right frontal lobes. The T_2*-weighted gradient-echo images at corresponding levels (**c,d**) show areas of low signal, consistent with haemosiderin staining, which indicates previous haemorrhage. The presence of multiple lobar haemorrhages is typical of amyloid angiopathy. Additional periventricular high signal areas are consistent with small vessel ischaemic disease.

Chronic stroke and transient ischaemic attack

The purpose of imaging in patients presenting with chronic stroke is not guidance of an acute therapeutic intervention, but secondary prevention of recurrent stroke.

In this context, it is important to establish the aetiology of the stroke. A distinction has to be made between previous haemorrhage, small vessel disease, large vessel disease and cardiac emboli. Establishing the diagnosis of an old haemorrhage is not possible with CT, since blood clots become hypodense within a few weeks and may resemble infarcts. MRI is much more sensitive in showing evidence of previous haemorrhage because haemosiderin is taken up by macrophages and can persist for years, appearing as a characteristic low signal area on T_2-weighted images. The sensitivity for detection of haemosiderin can be increased by using T_2*-weighted gradient-echo or echo planar imaging (EPI) sequences. Evidence of multiple peripheral haemorrhages in elderly patients is suggestive of amyloid angiopathy (Fig. 4)[36].

Small vessel ischaemic disease may be evident as hypodense white matter lesions on CT, but MRI is more sensitive to small vessel ischaemic changes, particularly if a FLAIR sequence is used[39]. White matter lesions are more frequently seen in patients with hypertension, but may also be a feature of vasculitic diseases[37,38].

To determine the vascular territory of an infarct, one has to take into account variations of the circle of Willis, which can be readily assessed with MRA. One of the more frequently encountered variants is a fetal origin of the posterior cerebral artery from the internal carotid artery, which has been described in up to 31% of subjects[40]. It is worth remembering that, in patients with this variant, occipital infarcts can be caused by carotid stenosis rather than vertebrobasilar disease.

Watershed infarcts at the boundaries between the anterior, middle and posterior cerebral artery territories (and between the deep and superficial cerebral circulation) may be the result of global ischaemia following an episode of hypotension or represent haemodymanic failure distal to a critically stenosed carotid artery.

Multiple infarcts in different vascular territories suggest cardiogenic emboli. Infarcts, which do not correspond to an arterial territory, have to raise the suspicion of venous infarcts, particularly if there is evidence of extensive haemorrhagic transformation. Patency of the major dural sinuses can be easily assessed with phase-contrast MR venography in these cases[41].

Assessment of the carotid bifurcation is crucial in the diagnostic work-up of chronic stroke and secondary prevention of a recurrent stroke. This can be performed non-invasively with Doppler ultrasound and MR angiography, which are discussed elsewhere in this issue.

Dissection of the carotid arteries is an important cause of stroke in young and middle aged adults. The characteristic MRI findings are a rim of high signal expanding the outer diameter of the artery and narrowing its lumen. The high signal represents subacute intramural haematoma, which becomes apparent after a few days. In the acute stage, the intramural haematoma is isointense to muscle and may be more difficult to detect[42].

MR perfusion imaging can also be useful in patients with chronic cerebrovascular disease and severe carotid artery stenosis[43]. In cases with established infarcts on T_2-weighted images, perfusion imaging can show more extensive abnormalities in regions that appear normal on T_2-weighted images, such as a prolongation of the MTT which may indicate tissue at risk. In the presence of bilateral carotid artery stenosis/occlusion, MR perfusion imaging may show impaired perfusion in a watershed distribution (see Fig. 1). In these cases, perfusion imaging can be used to monitor the results of an intra-extracranial bypass operation.

With significant carotid artery stenosis, cerebral perfusion imaging may be normal at rest, but show impairment following a challenge of the vascular reserve with acetazolamide. Normally, the cerebral flow increases following acetazolamide administration. Some patients with severe steno-occlusive disease have a decreased response to the acetazolamide challenge[44]. Demonstration of this unilateral vascular steal on xenon CT perfusion studies has been shown to be associated with a 30% stroke rate during follow-up[45].

Finally, one can assess recovery from stroke with functional MRI using cortical activation studies. This can provide evidence of the plasticity of the brain, *e.g.* when the function of areas damaged by ischaemia is taken over by adjacent or contralateral cortical regions[46].

References

1 Napel S. Basic principles of spiral CT. In: Fishman E, Jeffrey B. (eds) *Spiral CT: Principles, Techniques, Clinical Applications*. New York: Raven, 1995; 1–9

2 Hu H. Multi-slice helical CT: scan and reconstruction. *Med Phys* 1999; **26**: 5–18

3 Jungreis CA, Yonas H, Firlik AD, Wechsler LR. Advanced CT imaging (functional CT). *Neuroimaging Clin North Am* 1999; **9**: 455–64

4 Koenig M, Klotz E, Luka B, Vanderink D, Spittler J, Heuser L. Perfusion CT of the brain: diagnostic approach for early detection of ischaemic stroke. *Radiology* 1998; **209**: 85–93

5 Rubin GD, Shiau MC, Schmidt AJ *et al*. Computed tomographic angiography: historical perspective and new state-of-the-art using multi-detector-row helical computed tomography. *J Comput Assist Tomogr* 1999; **23 (Suppl 1)**: S83–90

6 Napel S. Principles and techniques of 3D spiral CT angiography. In: Fishman E, Jeffrey B. (eds) *Spiral CT: Principles, Techniques, Clinical Applications*. New York: Raven, 1995; 167–82

7 Sorensen AG, Rosen BR. Functional MRI of the brain. Magnetic Resonance Imaging of The Brain and Spine. In: Atlas SW, ed. *Magnetic Resonance Imaging of the Brain and Spine*, 2 edn, Lippincott-Raven, Philadelphia, USA. 1996; 1501–45

8 Yoshiura T, Wu O, Sorensen A. Advanced MR techniques. Diffusion MR imaging, perfusion MR imaging, and spectroscopy. *Neuroimaging Clin North Am* 1999; **9**: 439–53

9 Provenzale J, Sorensen G. Diffusion-weighted MR imaging in acute stroke: theoretic considerations and clinical applications. *AJR Am J Roentgenol* 1999; **173**: 1459–67

10 LeBihan D. *Diffusion and Perfusion Magnetic Resonance Imaging: Applications to Functional MRI*. New York: Raven, 1995

11 Yuh W, Ueda T, White M, Schuster M, Taoka T. The need for objective assessment of the new imaging techniques and understanding the expanding roles of stroke imaging. *AJNR Am J Neuroradiol* 1999; **20**: 1779–884

12 Ueda T, Yuh W, Taoka T. Clinical application of perfusion and diffusion MR imaging in acute ischemic stroke. *J Magn Reson Imaging* 1999; **10**: 305–9

13 Culebras A, Kase CS, Masdeu JC. Practice guidelines for the use of imaging in transient ischaemic attacks and acute stroke: a report of the Stroke Council, American Heart Association. *Stroke* 1997; **28**: 1480–97

14 Beauchamp N, Barker P, Wang P, van Zijl P. Imaging of acute cerebral ischaemia. *Radiology* 1999; **212**: 307–24

15 Leys D, Pruvo JP, Godefroy O, Rondepierre P, Leclerc X. Prevalence and significance of hyperdense middle cerebral artery in acute stroke. *Stroke* 1992; **23**: 317–24

16 Shrier D, Tanaka H, Numaguchi Y, Konno S, Patel U, Shibata D. CT angiography in the evaluation of acute stroke. *AJNR Am J Neuroradiol* 1997; **18**: 1011–20

17 Na DG, Byun HS, Lee KH *et al.* Acute occlusion of the middle cerebral artery: early evaluation with triphasic helical CT – preliminary results. *Radiology* 1998; **207**: 113–22

18 Firlik A, Kaufmann A, Wechsler L, Firlik K, Fului M, Yonas H. Quantitive cerebral blood flow determinations in acute ischemic stroke. Relationship to computed tomography and angiography. *Stroke* 1997; **28**: 2208–13

19 Firlik A, Yonas H, Kaufmann A *et al.* Relationship between cerebral blood flow and the development of swelling and life-threatening herniation in acute ischemic stroke. *J Neurosurg* 1998; **89**: 243–9

20 Gaskill-Shipley M. Routine CT evaluation of acute stroke. *Neuroimaging Clin North Am* 1999; **9**: 411–64

21 Kummer R, Meyding-Lamade U, Forsting M *et al.* Sensitivity and prognostic value of early CT in occlusion of the middle cerebral artery trunk. *AJNR Am J Neuroradiol* 1994; **15**: 9–15

22 Hacke W, Kaste M, Fieschi C *et al.* Intravenous thrombolysis with recombinant tissue plasminogen activator for acute hemispheric stroke. The European Cooperative Acute Stroke Study (ECASS). *JAMA* 1995; **274**: 1017–25

23 Atlas SW, Mark AS, Grossman RI, Gomori JM. Intracranial hemorrhage: gradient-echo MR imaging at 1.5 T. Comparison with spin-echo imaging and clinical applications. *Radiology* 1988; **168**: 803–7

24 Ohue S, Kohno K, Kusunoki K *et al.* Magnetic resonance angiography in patients with acute stroke treated by local thrombolysis. *Neuroradiology* 1998; **40**: 536–40

25 Sorensen A, Buonanno F, Gonzalez R *et al.* Hyperacute stroke: evaluation with combined multisection diffusion-weighted and hemodynamically weighted echo-planar MR imaging. *Radiology* 1996; **199**: 391–401

26 Sorensen AG, Copen WA, Ostergaard L *et al.* Hyperacute stroke: simultaneous measurement of relative cerebral blood volume, relative cerebral blood flow, and mean tissue transit time. *Radiology* 1999; **210**: 519–27

27 Powers W. Cerebral hemodynamics in ischemic cerebrovascular disease. *Ann Neurol* 1991; **29**: 1–9

28 Ueda T, Yuh W, Maley J, Quets J, Hahn P, Magnotta V. Outcome of acute ischemic lesions evaluated by diffusion and perfusion MR imaging. *AJNR Am J Neuroradiol* 1999; **20**: 983–9

29 Beauchamp N, Ulug A, Passe T, van Zijl P. MR diffusion imaging in stroke: review and controversies. *Radiographics* 1998; **18**: 1269–83

30 Gonzalez RG, Schaefer PW, Buonanno FS *et al.* Diffusion-weighted MR imaging: diagnostic accuracy in patients imaged within 6 hours of stroke symptom onset. *Radiology* 1999; **210**: 155–62

31 Albers GW, Lansberg MG, Norbash AM *et al.* Yield of diffusion-weighted MRI for detection of potentially relevant findings in stroke patients. *Neurology* 2000; **54**: 1562–7

32 Latchaw R. The roles of diffusion and perfusion imaging in acute stroke management. *AJNR Am J Neuroradiol* 1999; **20**: 957–9

33 Mayer TE, Schuffe-Altedorneburg G, Droste DW, Bruckmann H. Serial CT and MRI of ischaemic cerebral infarcts: frequency and clinical impact of haemorrhagic transformation. *Neuroradiology* 2000; **42**: 233–9

34 Kim JH, Shin T, Chung JD *et al.* Temporal pattern of blood volume change in cerebral infarction: evaluation with dynamic contrast-enhanced T2-weighted MR imaging. *AJR Am J Roentgenol* 1998; **170**: 765–70

35 Schlaug G, Siewert B, Benfield A, Edelman RR, Warach S. Time course of the apparent diffusion coefficient (ADC) abnormality in human stroke. *Neurology* 1997; **49**: 113–9

36 Greenberg SM. Cerebral amyloid angiopathy: prospects for clinical diagnosis and treatment. *Neurology* 1998; **51**: 690–4

37 Pomper M, Miller T, Stone H, Tidmore W, Hellman D. CNS vasculitis in autoimmune disease : MR imaging findings and correlation with angiography. *AJNR Am J Neuroradiol* 1999; **20**: 75–85

38 Jäger H, Albrecht T, Curati-Alasonatti W, Williams E, Haskard D. MRI in neuro-Behçet's syndrome: comparison of conventional spin echo and FLAIR sequences. *Neuroradiology* 1999; **41**: 750–8

39 Alexander JA, Sheppard S, Davies PC, Salverda P. Adult cerebrovascular disease: role of modified rapid fluid-attenuated inversion-recovery sequences. *AJNR Am J Neuroradiol* 1996; **17**: 1507–13

40 Bisaria KK. Anomalies of the posterior communicating artery and their potential clinical significance. *J Neurosurg* 1984; **60**: 572–6

41 Provenzale JM, Joseph GJ, Barboriak DP. Dural sinus thrombosis: findings on CT and MR imaging and diagnostic pitfalls. *AJR Am J Roentgenol* 1998; **170**: 777–83

42 Provenzale JM. Dissection of the internal carotid and vertebral arteries: imaging features. *AJR Am J Roentgenol* 1995; **165**: 1099–104

43 Maeda M, Yuh W, Ueda T *et al*. Severe occlusive carotid artery disease: hemodynamic assessment by MR imaging in symptomatic patients. *AJNR Am J Neuroradiol* 1999; **20**: 43–51

44 Gückel FJ, Brix G, Schmiedek P *et al*. Cerebrovascular reserve capacity in patients with occlusive cerebrovascular disease: assessment with dynamic susceptibility contrast-enhanced MR imaging and the acetazolamide stimulation test. *Radiology* 1996; **201**: 405–12

45 Webster M, Makaroon M, Steed D, Smith H, Johnson D, Yonas H. Compromised cerebral blood flow reactivity is a predictor of stroke in patients with symptomatic carotid artery occlusive disease. *J Vasc Surg* 1995; **21**: 338–45

46 Frackowiak R. Functional imaging of recovery from stroke: A review of personal experience. *Cerebrovasc Dis* 1999; **9** (**Suppl 5**): 23–8

MR spectroscopy in stroke

Dawn E Saunders

Department of Radiology, King's College Hospital, London, UK

Magnetic resonance spectroscopy (MRS) is a non-invasive *in vivo* method that allows the investigation of biochemical changes in both animals and humans. The application of MRS to the study of stroke has made possible dynamic studies of intracellular metabolism of cerebral ischaemia. The majority of the stroke studies have been carried out using proton [¹H]-MRS which allows the detection of N-acetyl aspartate (NAA), a neuronal marker. [¹H]-MRS changes in humans demonstrate that after an infarct, lactate appears, while NAA and total creatine are reduced compared to the contralateral hemisphere. Longitudinal studies demonstrate a further reduction of NAA suggesting that ischaemic injury continues for more than a week following infarction.

Major advances in the treatment of acute stroke require the accurate prediction of the mortality of stroke patients. Patients with large infarcts are known to do badly. In patients with small infarcts, less than 80 cm³, the addition of core NAA concentrations and cerebral blood flow have enabled the identification of some of the patients likely to benefit from new drug treatment.

Conventional magnetic resonance imaging (MRI) is a well-developed and much utilised method for visualising the radiological extent of disorders involving cerebral ischaemia. Magnetic resonance spectroscopy (MRS) is a non-invasive *in vivo* method that allows the investigation of biochemical changes in both animals and humans. The application of MRS to the study of stroke has made possible dynamic studies of intracellular metabolism of cerebral ischaemia. The concentrations of metabolites detected by MRS are relatively low (2–20 mM) compared to the concentration of water (83.4 M) detected by MRI, and the sensitivity to local magnetic field inhomogeneities and difficulties in quantitation of peak areas has until recently limited the technique to use as a research tool. Despite the relatively low signal-to-noise ratio of spectroscopy, improvements in magnet and gradient design, and the wider availability of magnets at high field strength (1.5 T) now enable good quality brain [¹H]-MRS spectra to be recorded on most modern clinical instruments.

[¹H]-MRS and phosphorus [³¹P]-MRS are most commonly carried out in humans. In the brain, [¹H]-MRS has two great advantages: the proton is 15 more times sensitive than ³¹P, and almost every compound in living

*Correspondence to:
Dr Dawn E Saunders,
Department of
Neuroradiology, Atkinson
Morley's Hospital, Copse
Hill, Wimbledon,
London SW20 0NE, UK*

tissue contains hydrogen. The study of cerebral ischaemia in humans is predominantly confined to [^{1}H]-MRS, the subject of this chapter.

Until recently, data acquisition required the skills of experienced spectroscopists and physicists for manual adjustment of parameters for each and every scan resulting in long examination times. The development of automated software programs, like the single voxel proton brain exam (PROBE, General Electric, Milwaukee, USA)[1], and their implementation on clinical systems has gone a long way to overcoming some of the problems of data collection. The small concentrations of visible metabolites requires the collection of data from a single voxel many times larger than that required for MR imaging.

Chemical shift imaging (CSI) or multivoxel MR spectroscopic imaging is a more advanced form of spectroscopy that uses phase encoding to subdivide a large volume of interest into smaller acquisition voxels, thereby allowing the study of large and heterogeneous areas of brain. The major disadvantages of CSI include complicated acquisition techniques, longer scan times, and a large volume of generated data. CSI is ideally suited to the study of stroke, particularly in the detection of the ischaemic penumbra. However, the complexity of image acquisition and data processing often necessitates the availability of a dedicated spectroscopist and has limited the number of stroke studies carried out using CSI.

The normal [^{1}H]-MRS spectrum

Histochemical and cell culture studies have shown that specific cell types or structures have metabolites that give rise to [^{1}H]-MRS peaks. A change in the resonance intensity of these marker compounds may reflect loss or damage to a specific cell type or compound.

The acquisition of long echo data (TE = 270 ms, TR = 3 s) only allows the detection of NAA, Cr/PCr and Cho in normal brain, and lactate in regions of abnormality. T_2 losses results in lower signal-to-noise and increases the complexity of quantitation methods. The acquisition of short echo time data (TE = 30 ms, TR = 2s) reduces the effects of signal loss due to T_2 relaxation and, therefore, provides spectra with increased signal-to-noise. In addition, short echo time spectroscopy detects additional resonances from metabolites with complex MR spectra such as *myo*-inositol, glutamate and glutamine. Signals from these metabolites cancel at long echo times due to phase modulation ('J-coupling'). Whilst providing us with more information, short echo time data include a broad background signal consisting of low concentration metabolites, and macromolecules and lipids with short T_2 relaxation times, which increases the difficulty of accurate peak area estimation.

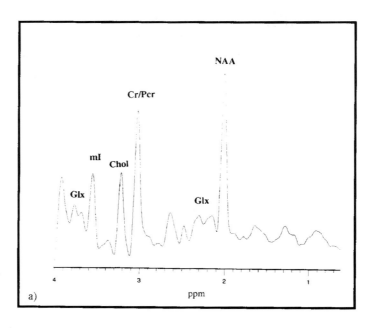

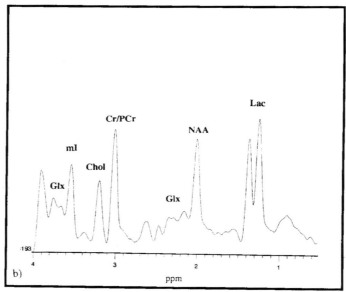

Fig. 1 Proton spectra (TE = 30 ms, TR = 2020 ms) obtained in the acute phase from the (a) contralateral and (b) infarct centre. Resonance peaks are: glutamate and glutamine (Glx) at 3.8 and 2.1–2.45 parts per million (ppm), *myo*-inositol (mI) at 3.56 ppm, choline containing compounds (Cho) at 3.22 ppm, creatine and phosphocreatine (Cr/PCr) methyl singlet at 3.03 ppm, N-acetyl aspartate (NAA) methyl singlet at 2.01 ppm, and lactate doublet (Lac) at 1.33 ppm. The concentration of NAA and Cr/PCr are reduced and lactate is elevated in the infarct centre compared with the contralateral hemisphere.

Short echo [¹H]-MRS spectra acquired from an infarct and the contralateral hemisphere are shown in Figure 1. The chemical shift of the peaks are assigned with respect to water which has been removed from the spectra.

N-acetyl aspartate (2.01 ppm)

The methyl resonance of N-acetyl aspartate (NAA) produces a large sharp peak at 2.01 ppm and acts as a neuronal marker as it is almost exclusively confined to neurones in the human brain, where it is found predominantly in the axons and nerve processes[2]. It has also been found in the oligodendrocyte type II astrocyte progenitor cells in rats[3], but these cells represent only 2–3% of the glial population in man[4]. Since the discovery of NAA in 1956[2], there has been a large body of literature on the synthesis, distribution and function, which has been reviewed by Birken and Oldendorf[5] and Williams[6]. However, despite a large body of work, the function of NAA remains unknown.

The interpretation of NAA signal in the brain of children is complicated by increases in the concentration during development[7] when it is thought to have a role in supplying acetyl groups for myelin synthesis[6]. In adults, the concentration of NAA is known to vary in different areas of the brain[8]. This can be overcome in the study of stroke patients by using the contralateral hemisphere for comparison[9].

Creatine (3.94 & 3.03 ppm)

Both creatine and phosphocreatine have signals at 3.94 ppm (methylene singlet) and 3.03 ppm (methyl singlet) which makes it impossible to distinguish between the two compounds and therefore total creatine (Cr/PCr) signal changes are considered by [¹H]-MRS. Other resonances seen at 3.03 ppm arise from γ-amino butyric acid (GABA)[10] and cytosolic macromolecules become incorporated into the Cr/PCr peak[11,12].

Cr/PCr is found in both neurones and glial cells[4] and acts as a phosphate transport system and energy buffer within the cell. As the signal comes from the sum of creatine and phosphocreatine, little information can be gleaned about phosphocreatine metabolism. The complete absence of creatine signal probably reflects necrotic tissue, but the interpretation of reduced total creatine levels requires more work.

Choline (3.22 ppm)

The trimethylamine resonance of choline-containing compounds is present at 3.2 ppm and has been proposed as a marker of membrane damage.

In normal brain, the choline (Cho) peak is thought to consist predominantly of glycerolphosphocholine and phosphocholine; both compounds are involved in membrane synthesis and degradation[13].

Lipid/macromolecule resonances

Lipid peaks are detectable by short echo proton spectroscopy but not seen at long echo due to T_2 losses. Peaks assigned to lipids/macromolecules have been detected at 0.9, 1.3 and 1.45 ppm in normal appearing brains[14,15]. Increases in these peaks have been reported in stroke[15], and demyelination[14,16].

The 0.9 and 1.3 ppm resonances are assigned to the methylene and methyl groups of lipid, respectively[17]. Recent work in animal models has shown that contributions to these resonances also arise from mobile proteins[12], and correlate with peaks found in humans[18]. The significance of the appearances of these peaks is as yet unknown and may only represent increased MRS visibility of cell membrane lipids following cell breakdown. The assignment of these signals will, however, influence the interpretation of proton spectra obtained from the cerebral cortex.

[¹H]-MRS changes in cerebral ischaemia

[¹H]-MRS studies in humans demonstrate that after acute cerebral infarction, lactate appears, while NAA and total Cr/PCr are reduced within the infarct compared to the contralateral hemisphere[9]. Large variations in the initial concentrations of Cho have been observed in the region of infarction[9,19].

Lactate (doublet at 1.33 ppm)

Lactate is not normally detected within the brain and, as the end product of glycolysis, is a particularly useful measure of metabolism. The concentration of lactate rises when the glycolytic rate exceeds the tissue's capacity to catabolise it or remove it from the blood stream. The rise in brain lactate that results from the mismatch between glycolysis and oxygen supply has been demonstrated by numerous [¹H]-MRS experiments[9,19,20] making it a hallmark for the detection of cerebral ischaemia.

The persistence of lactate weeks or months following stroke onset has been observed[9,20]. Removal of lactate depends on tissue perfusion, the permeability of the blood brain barrier (BBB) and diffusion of the metabolite through the damaged tissue. The fall of lactate concentration has been shown to occur during a period of hyperaemia[20]. Using [1-^{13}C]-labelled glucose, the metabolic activity of the lactate pool associated with a 32-day-old stroke has demonstrated that all the cerebral lactate arises from glycolysis of serum glucose. This supports the hypothesis that elevated lactate, present weeks after a stroke, is the product of ongoing lactate synthesis in the brain[21]. It is not possible to establish whether the lactate is being produced by on-going ischaemic tissue or metabolically active macrophages. The presence of lactate beyond the time in which active phagocytosis occurs supports the theory of persistently ischaemic tissue[22].

Spectroscopic imaging studies have demonstrated that lactate levels in regions adjacent to the T_2 hyperintensities were not significantly different from those found in the infarcted brain and that lactate is not confined to areas of infarction determined by T_2-weighted imaging and were even found in the contralateral hemisphere in patients with large infarcts[23].

NAA (2.01 ppm)

Longitudinal studies in humans demonstrated a decline in NAA following initial reductions in NAA detected in the first spectra after the onset of cerebral infarction[9,19,20]. The continuing fall in NAA concentration over the course of the first week after stroke onset cannot be explained simply by an increase in oedema because changes in the concentration of water within the infarct have been corrected for by using the contralateral water signal as the internal standard[9]. It has been suggested that NAA is actively degraded by enzymes within the injured neurones in the first few days or hours following infarction[16]. This remains a possibility, but it would appear unlikely that enzymes would remain active for up to 7–10 days within an ischaemic neurone. The gradual decline in NAA concentration and the persistence of lactate within the region of infarction over a period of a number of days is suggestive of ongoing ischaemia[9] (Fig. 2) and has important implications in the timing of therapeutic intervention.

Cr/PCr (3.94 & 3.03 ppm)

Initial reductions in Cr/PCr are identified following infarction and further reductions have been demonstrated up to 10 days following the time of onset[9]. The reduction in NAA in the infarct region is more marked than the reduction in Cr/PCR and this is thought to reflect the increased sensitivity of neurones to ischaemia.

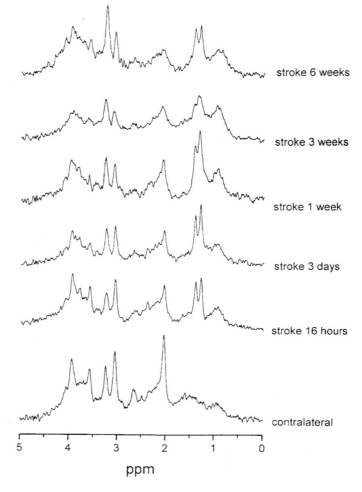

Fig. 2 A longitudinal study of the infarct core in a 32-year-old lady. NAA and Cr/PCr continue to fall over 6 weeks following infarction. Lactate is visible within 16 h and persists for 6 weeks. The lactate peaks can be seen to increase further with some contribution from underlying lipids. Choline increases up to 6 weeks which reflects increased visibility of choline containing compounds within the membrane due to cell necrosis. (see Fig. 1 for peak assignments).

stroke 6 weeks

stroke 3 weeks

stroke 1 week

stroke 3 days

stroke 16 hours

contralateral

ppm

Choline (3.22 ppm)

Changes in the choline peak have been shown to be increase, decrease and stay the same following infarction[9,19,20]. The changes in the choline peak are thought to reflect changes in the MR visibility of the choline containing compounds that make up the cell membrane.

Glutamate and other amino acids

Measurements of amino acids, such as glutamate and glutamine, are difficult due to their complex peak structures. Other amino acids, such as GABA, aspartate and alanine are difficult to detect because of their low concentration and/or overlap with more intense resonances from other

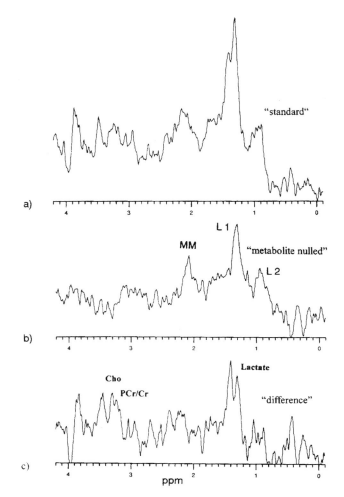

Fig. 3 Spectra acquired from a 62-year-old stroke patient 4 weeks following stroke onset. The top spectrum is the 'standard' spectrum showing a large lipid peak underlying the asymmetrical peaks of the lactate doublet. The centre spectrum is the metabolite 'nulled' spectrum acquired from underlying lipid/macromolecules and showing a large lipid peak at the position of the lactate peak (1.3 ppm). The bottom spectrum is the 'pure' metabolite or 'difference' spectrum and shows the lactate signal as a doublet without the underlying baseline. NAA = N-acetyl aspartate, Cr/PCr = total creatine, Cho = choline, Lac = lactate, L1 and L2 = lipids, MM = macromolecule peak.

compounds[24]. To date, there is very little work in cerebral ischaemia on the detection of glutamate and glutamine, reflecting the difficulty of spectral analysis.

Lipid/macromolecules

Signals from lipids pose particular problems in [¹H]-MRS by obscuring the resonance from the methyl group of lactate. It has been postulated that membrane lipids in the brain under normal conditions are not mobile enough to generate sharp peaks in *in vivo* spectra. During ischaemia, degradation of the membrane leads to the release of free fatty acids that produce well defined but broad resonances in the region of the lactate peak resulting in difficulties in the accurate quantitation of lactate. The metabolite nulling technique has been used to separate the lipid from the lactate signal (Fig. 3)[15,18].

Reversible changes detected by [¹H]-MRS

The identification of the ischaemic penumbra by [¹H]-MRS depends on the observation of the reversibility of metabolic changes within the region of infarction. Spectroscopy studies have reported a reversible reduction of NAA in acute multiple sclerosis lesions[14,16,25], and mitochondrial encephalopathy with lactic acidosis and stroke-like episodes (MELAS)[25]. No convincing reports of reversible NAA in cerebral infarction have been published. In MELAS, the primary defect is mitochondrial and, as NAA is synthesised in mitochondria, it has been suggested that in demyelinating lesions, the function of the mito-chondria is reversibly impaired during inflammation resulting in the reversible reduction of the production of NAA within the damaged neurone[14]. CSI studies have observed high levels of lactate return to undetectable levels, in normal appearing regions of the brain separate from the area of infarction. Although, slight reductions in NAA were later observed, the presence of high lactate concentrations did not result in complete infarction[23].

Quantitation methods in [¹H]-MRS

To move MRS further into the clinical domain and allow the compari-son of metabolite concentrations within and between institutions, automated methods of quantitation need to be implemented to provide data analysis protocols for clinical studies. Previously, peak area metabolite ratios calculated from long echo time spectra were used to study metabolic changes in both animal and man. Ratios can be misleading when metabolite concentrations in the numerator and denominator change in disease states. Although the majority of stroke studies have been carried out using metabolite ratios, some studies have used absolute quantitation of brain metabolites[9,15].

The accuracy of the metabolite estimation depends on the fitting of the accuracy of the fitting method. Various fitting routines have been incorporated in the frequency domain[26] (the conventional domain of MRS data analysis) and the time domain to overcome the problem of contributions to peak area estimates from the underlying baseline and adjacent peaks to improve the accuracy of metabolite quantitation[27,28].

'Metabolite nulling' has been employed to simplify the spectrum and overcome the problems of the incorporation of the broad background signal into the peak area estimates of short echo proton spectroscopy[18].

[^{1}H]-MRS as a predictor of outcome

Major advances in the treatment of acute stroke require the accurate prediction of the mortality of stroke patients and, therefore, the identification of patients likely to benefit from drug treatment. Single voxel and CSI studies of stroke have attempted to provide information about the possible outcome of stroke.

Infarct volume determined by T_2-weighted MR imaging has been shown to be a good predictor of outcome. All patients with small infarcts (<80 cm^3) survived 3 months[29]. The addition of the NAA concentration to infarct volume allows a better prediction of patients' morbidity, than either the NAA concentration or infarct volume alone[30]. In a small number of serially studied patients, the best recovery was seen in those patients with relatively preserved NAA, total creatine and choline peaks[31]. Large cerebral infarcts have been shown to be associated with reduced NAA concentration and raised lactate as well as reduced blood velocity. The best predictor of outcome was infarct volume and not metabolite concentration alone[32].

The importance of lactate in the pathogenesis of cerebral infarction has been studied extensively in animals. The degree and extent of tissue damage has been correlated with the content of lactic acid in animals[33], and an increase in morbidity and mortality in hyperglycaemic animals has been linked to excessive lactate production and the resulting acidosis[34]. The correlation of lactate with outcome in humans, has been variable. Although a single study has shown lactate to correlate with acute stroke severity and outcome[19], other studies have failed to demonstrate a relationship between outcome and infarct lactate concentration alone[30,32].

Application of [^{1}H]-MRS to the clinical study of cerebral ischaemia

MR spectroscopy and multivoxel MR spectroscopic imaging have proven to be valuable tools in the study of cerebral vascular disease. Their role in the detection of potentially salvageable ischaemic tissue suitable for treatment with thrombolytic and neuroprotective agents has not yet been fully realised. The combined use of diffusion-weighted and perfusion imaging with [^{1}H]-MRS may prove more valuable, especially in light of the growing observation of the negative diffusion-weighted images in acute stroke[35]. The ability of multivoxel chemical shift imaging to detect changes throughout the brain makes it the most suited spectroscopy technique for the study of cerebral ischaemia. Further development of the CSI and data processing techniques are required to move the use of spectroscopy further into the clinical domain.

Acknowledgement

I thank Prof. S R Williams, Department of Imaging Science and Engineering, University of Manchester, UK for reading the manuscript.

References

1   Webb PG, Sailasuta N, Kohler SJ et al. Automated single-voxel proton MRS: technical development and multisite verification. Magn Reson Med 1994; 31: 365–73

2   Tallan HH, Moore S, Stein WH. N-acetyl-L-aspartic acid in brain. J Biochem 1956; 219: 257–64

3   Urenjak J, Williams SR, Gadian DG, Noble M. Proton nuclear magnetic resonance spectroscopy unambiguously identifies different neural cell types. J Neurosci 1993; 13: 981–9

4   Wolswijk G, Munro PMG, Riddle PN, Noble M. Origin, growth factor responses, and ultra structure characteristics of an adult-specific glial progenitor-cell. Ann N Y Acad Sci 1991; 633; 502–4

5   Birken DL, Oldendorf WH. N-acetyl-L-aspartic acid: a literature review of a compound prominent in ¹H-NMR spectroscopic studies of brain. Neurosci Biobehav Rev 1989; 13: 23–31

6   Williams SR. In vivo proton spectroscopy. Experimental aspects and potentials. In: Rudin M, Seelig J. (eds) NMR – Basic Principles and Progress: In vivo magnetic resonance spectroscopy. Heidelberg: Springer, 1992; 55–72

7   Kreis R, Ernst T, Ross BD. Development of the human brain: in vivo quantification of metabolite and water content with proton magnetic resonance spectroscopy. Magn Reson Med 1993; 30: 424–37

8   Kreis R, Ernst T, Ross BD. Absolute quantitation of water and metabolites in the human brain. II Metabolite concentrations. J Magn Reson 1993; 102: 9–19

9   Saunders DE, Howe FA, van den Boogaart A, McLean MA, Griffiths JG, Brown MM. Continuing ischaemic damage after acute middle cerebral artery infarction in humans demonstrated by short-echo proton spectroscopy. Stroke 1995; 26: 1007–13

10 Rothman DL, Petroff OAC, Behar KL, Mattson RH. Localised ¹H-NMR measurements of γ-amino butyric acid in human brain in vivo. Proc Natl Acad Sci USA 1993; 90; 5662–6

11 Behar KL, Ogino T. Characterisation of macromolecule resonances in the ¹H-NMR spectrum of rat brain. Magn Reson Med 1993; 30: 38–44

12 Kauppinen RA, Kokko H, Williams SR. Detection of mobile proteins by proton magnetic resonance spectroscopy in the guinea pig brain ex vivo and their partial purification. J Neurochem 1992; 58: 967–74

13 Miller BL. A review of chemical issues in ¹H-NMR spectroscopy; N-acetyl-L-aspartate, creatine and choline. NMR Biomed 1991; 4: 47–52

14 Davie CA, Hawkins CP, Barker GJ, Tofts PS, Miller DH, McDonald WI. Serial proton magnetic resonance spectroscopy in acute multiple sclerosis lesions. Brain 1994; 117: 49–58

15 Saunders DE, Howe FA, van den Boogaart A, Griffiths JG, Brown MM. Discrimination of metabolites from lipid and macromolecule resonances in cerebral infarction in humans using short echo proton spectroscopy. J Magn Reson Imaging 1997; 7: 1116–21

16 Arnold DL, Matthews PM, Francis GS, O'Connor J, Antel JP. Proton magnetic resonance spectroscopic imaging for metabolic characterization of demyelinating plaques. *Ann Neurol* 1992; **31**: 235–41

17 May GL, Wright LC, Holmes KT *et al*. Assignment of methylene proton magnetic resonances in NMR spectra of embryonic and transformed cells to plasma triglyceride. *J Biol Chem* 1986; **261**: 3048–53

18 Behar KL, Rothman DL, Spencer DD, Petroff OAC. Analysis of macromolecule resonances in ^{1}H-NMR spectra in human brain. *Magn Reson Med* 1994; **32**: 294–302

19 Graham GD, Blamire AM, Rothman DL *et al*. Early temporal variation of cerebral metabolites after human stroke: a proton magnetic resonance spectroscopy study. *Stroke* 1993; **24**: 1891–6

20 Gideon P, Henriksen O, Sperling B *et al*. Early time course of N-acetyl aspartate, creatine and phosphocreatine, and compounds containing choline in the brain after acute stroke. *Stroke* 1992; **11**: 1566–72

21 Rothman DL, Howseman A, Graham GD *et al*. Localised proton NMR observation of [3-^{13}C]-lactate in stroke after [1-^{13}C]-glucose infusion. *Magn Reson Med* 1991; **21**: 302–7

22 Houkin K, Kwee IL, Nakada T. Persistent high lactate level as a sensitive MR spectroscopy indicator of complete infarction. *Brain Pathol* 1994; **4**: 23–36

23 Gillard JH, Barker PB, van Zijl PCM, Bryan RN, Oppenheimer SM. Proton MR spectroscopy in acute middle cerebral artery stroke. *AJNR Am J Neuroradiol* 1996; **17**: 873–86

24 Williams SR. Cerebral amino acids studied by nuclear magnetic resonance spectroscopy *in vivo*. *Prog Nuclear Magn Reson Spect* 1999; **34**: 301–26

25 De Stafano N, Matthews PM, Arnold DL. Reversible decreases in N-acetyl-aspartate after acute brain injury. *Magn Reson Med* 1995; **34**: 721–7

26 Provencher SW. Estimation of metabolite concentrations from localised *in vivo* proton NMR spectra. *Magn Reson Med* 1993; **30**: 672–9

27 de Beer R, van Ormondt D, Pijnappel WWF, van der Veen JWC. Quantitative analysis of magnetic resonance signals in the time domain. *Isr J Chem* 1988; **28**: 249–61

28 van der Veen JWC, de Beer R, Luyten PR, van Ormondt D. Accurate quantification of *in vivo* ^{31}P NMR signals using the variable projection method and prior knowledge. *Magn Reson Med* 1988; **6**: 92–8

29 Saunders DE, Clifton AG, Brown MB. Measurement of infarct size using MRI predicts prognosis in middle cerebral artery infarction. *Stroke* 1995; **26**: 2272–6

30 Pereira AC, Saunders DE, Doyle VL *et al*. Measurement of initial N-acetyl aspartate using magnetic resonance spectroscopy and initial infarct volume using MRI predicts outcome in patients with middle cerebral artery territory infarction. *Stroke* 1999; **30**: 1577–82

31 Ford CC, Griffey RH, Matwiywoff NA, Rosenberg GA. Multi-voxel ^{1}H-MRS of stroke. *Neurology* 1992; **42**: 1408–12

32 Wardlaw JM, Marshall I, Wild J, Dennis MS, Cannon J, Lewis SC. Studies of acute ischaemic stroke with proton magnetic resonance spectroscopy. Relation between time from onset, neurological deficit, metabolite abnormalities in the infarct, blood flow and clinical outcome. *Stroke* 1998; **29**: 1618–24

33 Pulsinelli WA, Waldman S, Rawlinson D, Plum F. Moderate hyperglycaemia augments ischaemic brain damage: a neuropathologic study in the rat. *Neurology* 1982; **32**: 1239–46

34 Siemkowicz E, Gjedde A. Post ishcaemic coma in rats: effect of different pre-ischaemic blood glucose levels on cerebral metabolic recovery after ischaemia. *Acta Physiol Scand* 1980; **110**: 225–32

35 Wang PY, Beauchamp NJ, Ulag AM, Barker PB, van Zijl PCM. Diffusion negative MR in acute stroke [abstract]. In: *Proceedings of the Annual Meeting of the American Society of Neuroradiology*. Philadelphia PA: American Society of Neuroradiology, 1997

Ultrasound of the carotid and vertebral arteries

Paul S Sidhu

University Department of Neurosurgery, National Hospital for Neurology and Neurosurgery, London and Department of Diagnostic Radiology, King's College Hospital, London, UK

Ultrasound plays an important role in the assessment of carotid arterial disease, complimentary to other imaging modalities. However, ultrasound does have limitations, not least the requirement of a high degree of operator skill. Recent advances in ultrasound technology will strengthen its role by improving accuracy. This review discusses the role of ultrasound in assessing the carotid arterial system with emphasis on evaluating stenosis

Historically, non-invasive ultrasound (US) of the extra-cranial carotid circulation became possible with oculopneumoplethysmography, in which alterations in peri-orbital vascular beds distal to the carotid bifurcation were detected. Although highly specific, the technique gave no indication as to the site of the abnormality[1]. Increased sophistication of ultrasound, in particular Doppler probes, has allowed direct interrogation of the neck vessels to detect stenotic lesions. Doppler and B-mode US were first linked as 'duplex machines' in 1974[2]. Colour Doppler is now an integral part of the US examination and enables the assessment of flow in vessels and spectral waveform analysis at the point of maximum stenosis[3]. Doppler-derived velocity parameters may be used to detect and quantify stenoses of the internal carotid artery. Indeed, colour Doppler ultrasound (CDUS) is the most cost-effective method of evaluating patients with symptoms of carotid transient ischaemic attacks[4]. This review discusses the role of ultrasound in assessing the carotid arterial system with emphasis on evaluating stenosis.

Correspondence to:
Dr Paul S Sidhu,
Department of
Diagnostic Radiology,
King's College Hospital,
Denmark Hill, London
SE5 9RS, UK

Ultrasound assessment of stenosis: technique

The common carotid artery divides into its internal and the external branches at the level of the fourth cervical vertebrae, although the level of this division may vary from T2 to C1[5]. Several centimetres of the internal carotid artery and external carotid artery may be examined

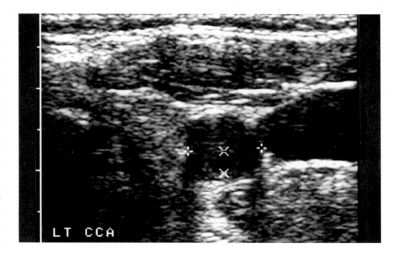

Fig. 1 Transverse section through the distal left common carotid artery (LT CCA) demonstrating a measured diameter reduction of the artery (x–x; residual lumen, +–+; vessel walls with internal circumferential atheroma). This method of calculation of a stenosis is rarely possible.

when the bifurcation is at the normal level. In the majority of patients, the internal carotid artery lies posterior and lateral to the external carotid artery. Both vessels have a number of distinguishing US features which aid differentiation. Ideally, the area reduction of an internal carotid artery stenosis should be estimated in the transverse plane with the probe perpendicular to the vessel walls (Fig. 1). However, for a variety of reasons not all internal carotid artery luminal stenoses are amenable to assessment in this manner. A measurement of the velocity of flow in the longitudinal direction is invariably required and constitutes an indirect estimate of the degree of luminal narrowing.

Grey-scale imaging in the longitudinal direction should precede colour Doppler imaging to avoid obscuring subtle areas of plaque. The common carotid artery is generally imaged as far proximal as possible and followed distally to the level of the bifurcation. In most patients, it is not possible to examine the external carotid artery, internal carotid artery and carotid bulb at the same time and each vessel should be examined sequentially. It may be possible to identify the region of maximal internal carotid artery narrowing on grey-scale images thereby allowing accurate placement of the pulsed-Doppler sample volume. However, an area of colour turbulence on CDUS allows accurate placement of the pulsed-Doppler sample volume at the point of maximum narrowing (Fig. 2) and improves the sensitivity and speed of the examination[6,7]. A spectral waveform is obtained from which a velocity measurement is generated using the Doppler equation (Appendix 1).

The angle of insonation must remain constant (*i.e.* less than 60°) for velocity measurement, since small changes in angle may affect absolute velocity readings. The extent of atherosclerotic narrowing is calculated from measurements of the peak systolic and end diastolic velocities in

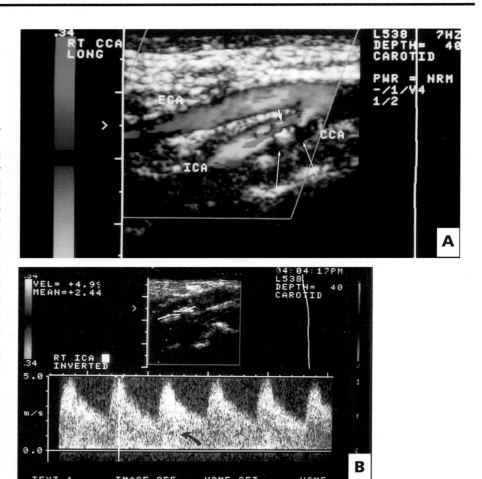

Fig. 2 (**A**) Colour disturbance (blue, arrow) in the proximal internal carotid artery (ICA). This indicates an area of stenosis caused by heterogeneous plaque disease in the carotid bulb (long arrow, ECA; external carotid artery, CCA; common carotid artery). (**B**) With the spectral gate placed at the region of greatest colour disturbance, a spectral Doppler waveform shows an elevated velocity of 4.99 m/s (normal < 1.0 m/s). The 'in-filling' beneath the outline of the spectral trace (curved arrow) is called spectral broadening and represents a multitude of different velocities.

the common carotid artery and internal carotid artery. It is important to identify and record the spectral waveform in the external carotid artery, so that it is clear that the velocities have been measured in the correct vessels. Flow reversal, manifest as colour change from red to blue separated by a thin black line in the carotid bulb opposite to the origin of the external carotid artery, is commonly seen and should not be mistaken for turbulence.

The vertebral arteries may also be interrogated during the examination. By moving the probe laterally beyond the common carotid artery, the arteries are identified between the transverse processes of the cervical spine. The vertebral artery can normally be examined in three segments: the proximal (pre-transverse) portion, the inter-transverse portion and the atlas loop[8]. The more anteriorly located vertebral vein should be readily identified on spectral and colour Doppler. Failure to show the vertebral arteries may be due to absence or occlusion which will not be

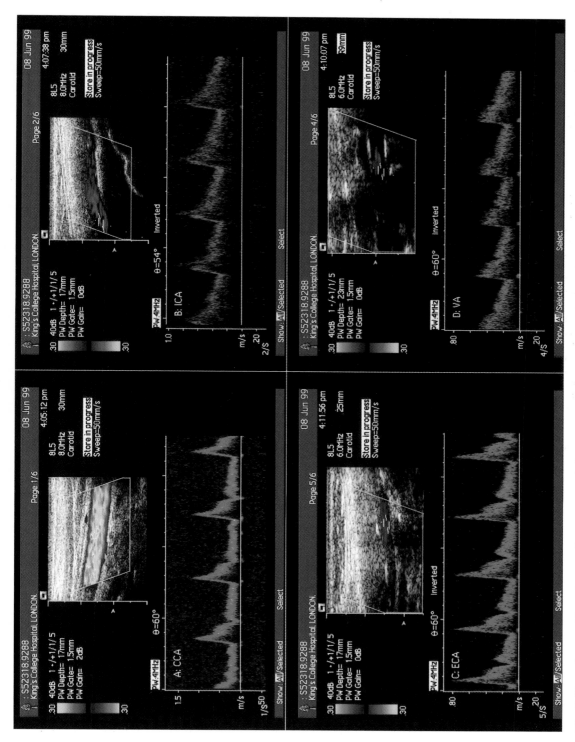

Fig. 3 Normal spectral Doppler waveform patterns. (A) Common carotid artery (CCA). (B) Internal carotid artery (ICA). (C) External carotid artery (ECA). (D) Vertebral artery (VA).

clear from the ultrasound examination. The calibre of the vertebral arteries may be asymmetrical in up to 25% of normal individuals, with the left usually the larger[9].

The normal spectral waveform patterns of the common carotid artery, internal carotid artery, external carotid artery and the vertebral artery are shown in Figure 3. In general, both the internal carotid artery and the vertebral artery, which directly supply brain parenchyma, have a 'low resistance' pattern on spectral analysis which contrasts with the 'high resistance' external carotid artery, which supplies the facial muscles and the scalp. There is a wide systolic peak and high diastolic flow in the internal carotid artery and vertebral artery, whereas the external carotid artery has a narrow systolic peak and absence of diastolic flow. The common carotid artery is a hybrid of the two patterns with a narrow systolic peak and some forward diastolic flow. Velocity measurements are calculated using the Doppler equation from the frequency shift (Appendix 1)[10]. However, it should be remembered that the accuracy and reproducibility of velocity measurements between ultrasound machines has been questioned; differences of up to 15% have been documented[11].

Numerous velocity measurements to grade stenoses have been suggested[12-15]. The most commonly used criteria are the internal carotid peak systolic velocity (ICPSV) and the ICPSV to common carotid peak systolic (CCPSV) ratio, with the end diastolic velocity used to discriminate in borderline measurements.

Velocity parameters, in the crucial 60–70% diameter reduction range, have been re-assessed in line with the conclusions of the North American Symptomatic Carotid Endarterectomy Trial (NASCET)[16] and European Carotid Surgery Trial[17]. In one retrospective study, a variety of ultrasound parameters were compared with those at angiography[18]. The authors concluded that the single most useful measurement was the ICPSV, which when greater than a measurement of 230 cm/s, indicated a diameter reduction of greater than 70%. Moneta et al have prospectively studied 100 angiograms, measuring the degree of diameter reduction based on NASCET criteria and correlating this with findings on CDUS[19]. An ICPSV/CCPSV ratio of greater than 4.0 provided the best combination of sensitivity, specificity, positive predictive value, negative predictive value and overall accuracy for detection of a 70–99% stenosis. An ICPSV of greater than 130 cm/s and an ICPSV/CCPSV ratio of greater than 3.2 suggests a reduction in diameter of greater than 60%. A guide to these measurement indices is shown in Table 1.

In practice, these figures should only be the basis from which to develop criteria specific for individual vascular departments and the type of equipment used. Ideally each centre should be constantly auditing CDUS findings, comparing these to angiography and findings at surgery. The particular criteria chosen to assess a stenosis should be carefully

Table 1 Suggested duplex Doppler ultrasound criteria for grading internal carotid artery (ICA) diameter reduction, based on derived figures[19,105]

Diameter reduction (%)	PSV	EDV	PSV$_{ICA}$/PSV$_{CCA}$
0–29	< 100	< 40	< 3.2
30–49	110–130	< 40	< 3.2
50–59	> 130	< 40	< 3.2
60–69	> 130	40–110	3.2–4.0
70–79	> 230	110–140	> 4.0
80–95	> 230	> 140	> 4.0
96–99	'String flow'		
100	'No flow'		

CCA, common carotid artery; PSV, peak systolic velocity; EDV, end diastolic velocity; PSV$_{ICA}$/PSV$_{CCA}$, ratio of the velocities. Velocity measurements are in cm/s.

considered. For example, employing a single ICPSV measurement instead of a ratio measurement does not eliminate the problems of variable cardiac output, cardiac arrhythmia, the presence of a proximal common carotid artery narrowing (the so-called 'tandem' lesion[20]) and interval changes of myocardial function. Often a combination of measurements will increase the accuracy of estimation of the stenosis.

Comparison of imaging modalities

Conventional arteriography, magnetic resonance arteriography and contrast enhanced dynamic computed tomography provide an assessment of the luminal size but are unable to characterize the vessel wall or associated plaques. Early plaque formation is accompanied by compensatory arterial enlargement, a phenomenon seen both in the coronary[21] and the carotid arteries[22], and significant plaque formation may occur before detectable luminal narrowing on arteriography. A comparison between ultrasound and arteriography in 900 patients demonstrated that half of the 345 arteries considered normal at arteriography were shown to have a lesion at ultrasound[23]. It would seem, therefore, that ultrasound may be of value in evaluating atherosclerosis in the carotid arteries. The accuracy of colour Doppler ultrasound in comparison with conventional angiography is not disputed[7,24].

Limitations of carotid Doppler ultrasound

A number of technical factors may limit the value of ultrasound examination. With extensive plaque disease, particularly if calcified, acoustic shadowing may hamper insonation of the area distal to the

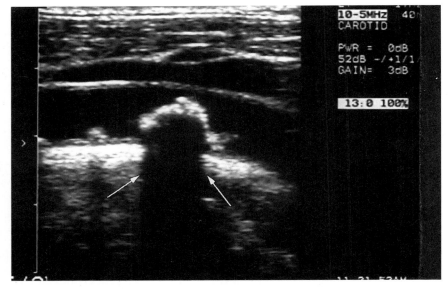

Fig. 4 An area of plaque in the common carotid artery containing a substantial amount of calcification causes marked distal acoustic shadowing (arrows). The acoustic shadowing precludes interrogation of the area beneath the plaque.

calcification (Fig. 4). Significant narrowing of the underlying vessel may be present in the absence of a high velocity jet. Varying the angle of insonation (*e.g.* posteriorly) may be helpful, but often the examination is inconclusive and another imaging modality is necessary. Similarly, a bifurcation at the level of the mandible may be obscured. Finally, a tortuous vessel may result in a spurious increase in velocity. In practice, this is less of a problem with colour Doppler imaging since the vessel is completely filled with colour and no narrowing is demonstrated.

Detection of carotid occlusion

The distinction between a total occlusion and a 99% diameter reduction is crucial, since the former is a contra-indication to surgery[25]. In high-grade internal carotid artery lesions, a reduction in volume flow causes the velocity measured at the stenosis to decrease and normal velocity criteria no longer apply. Internal carotid artery occlusion on US can be inferred on the basis of the lack of pulsation or expansion of vessel walls but this is unreliable[26]. The diagnosis of occlusion based on the detection of a thrombus-filled lumen, the absence of wall motion characteristics and the lack of Doppler flow signal has a high reported accuracy[27]. Characteristic flow reversal, with dampening of flow in the common carotid artery, may also be present in the patent vessel just proximal to the occlusion. With long-standing occlusion, the external carotid artery may become 'internalized' with the development of collaterals, particularly around the orbit, producing a hypertrophied external carotid artery with a high forward

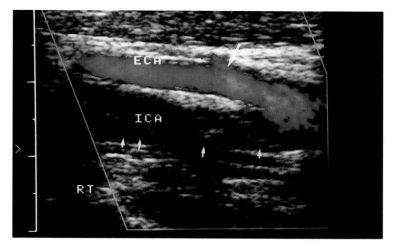

Fig. 5 No colour signal is obtained from the lumen of the internal carotid artery (ICA) which is filled with echo poor thrombus (arrows). The external carotid artery (ECA) is hypertrophied with a prominent branch (long arrow). These appearances are those of a long-standing ICA occlusion.

diastolic component in the spectral waveform (Fig. 5). The ipsilateral vertebral artery may then become dominant.

Colour Doppler has improved the ability of US to distinguish between an occlusion and severe stenosis by allowing a narrow channel to be identified. However, technical difficulties remain (Fig. 6). The accuracy in detection of a very narrow patent channel of severe stenosis and the distinction from a total occlusion is likely to improve in the future with the use of 'power' Doppler and intravenous ultrasound contrast media[28].

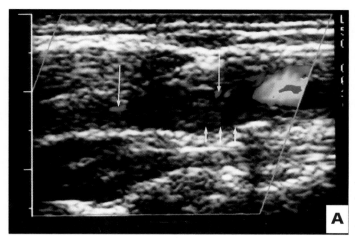

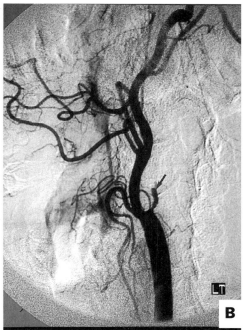

Fig. 6 (**A**) The lumen of the internal carotid artery (short arrows) is filled with echo-poor thrombus but some flow is demonstrated on colour Doppler ultrasound (long arrows) with optimized flow settings, indicating a near occlusion. (**B**) Angiography confirms a short patent segment of internal carotid artery (arrow).

Plaque morphology

The extent of plaque disease has been positively correlated with an increasing likelihood of cerebrovascular events[29–31]. Plaque disease associated with haemorrhage and ulceration may be associated with cerebrovascular symptoms[32]. Many patients with symptoms of carotid disease do not have a significant stenosis of the ipsilateral internal carotid artery and those with a significant stenosis do not necessarily have symptoms. In one study, the number of patients with a significant stenosis and symptoms of stroke attributable to the stenosis was estimated at 20% of the total number of stroke patients[33]. The potential for atherosclerotic plaques to produce cerebral ischaemic events is dependent not only on flow-reduction through the stenosis but also the embologenic property of atherosclerotic plaque[34].

The importance of plaque morphology in assessing risk has received less attention than quantifying stenosis. The morphological characteristics of plaque, as seen on US, may provide important information on the type of plaque and the risk for neurological events. As discussed above, arteriography, magnetic resonance arteriography and contrast enhanced dynamic computed tomography provide an assessment of the luminal size but are unable to characterize the vessel wall or associated plaque[35].

Classification of plaque

A classification of plaque morphology has been suggested[36]. Four categories are recognized: predominantly echolucent (type 1), uniformly echogenic (type 4), with the intermediate forms being more echolucent (type 2) and more echogenic (type 3). Calcification may occur in all plaque types[37]. More recently, a classification of plaque has been proposed by the Committee on Standards in Non–invasive Vascular Testing of the Joint Council of the Society for Vascular Surgery and the International Society for Cardiovascular Surgery[26]. Put simply, plaques may be characterized as homogeneous or heterogeneous (Fig. 7). The division is subjective with heterogeneous plaques being those in which major differences in echogenicity are identified.

In an attempt to classify carotid bifurcation disease to take account of both the grade of diameter stenosis and plaque characteristics, the same committee has suggested a classification system modelled on the TNM classification of tumours. The plaque is characterized by 'P' where P1 = homogeneous and P2 = heterogeneous, the surface character by 'S' where S1 = smooth, S2 = irregular and S3 = ulcerated and the luminal narrowing by 'H' (H1–H5: degree of stenosis), taking into account all clinically important features.

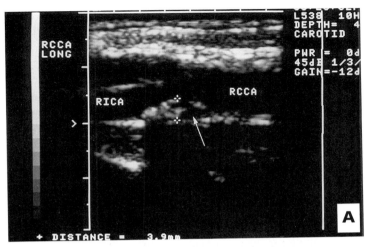

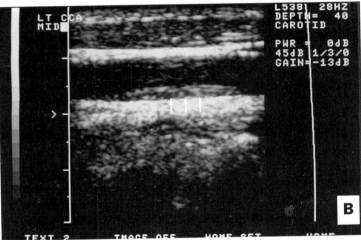

Fig. 7 (**A**) Heterogeneous plaque (cursors) in the right carotid bulb. Echolucent areas (arrow) correspond to lipid deposits or areas of intraplaque haemorrhage. (RCCA; right common carotid artery, RICA; right internal carotid artery. (**B**) Homogenous plaque with a uniform echogenic appearance (arrows).

Complications of plaque disease

Clinicopathological studies of carotid atheroma have implicated plaque structure, more specifically intraplaque haemorrhage, as an aetiological factor in symptomatic carotid artery disease[38-40]. However, disagreement exists about the relationship between the histological nature of plaque and US features. A study which correlated histology with US suggested that fibrous plaques are highly echogenic. As the lipid content increased, plaque became more echolucent[41]. It is suggested that the increased lipid and cholesterol content of echolucent plaque renders these plaques unstable[42]; echogenic plaques contain significantly more fibrin and collagen, rendering them more stable[43,44]. Other studies have suggested that low echogenic areas in plaque demonstrate a high correlation with areas of intraplaque haemorrhage on histological examination[37,45]. These low echogenic areas, thought to represent intraplaque haemorrhage, have been associated with an increased risk of cerebrovascular events[34]. A recent study found a specificity of only 78% and a sensitivity of only 44% for detecting intra-plaque haemorrhage as echolucent areas on US[46]. However, the concept of a haemorrhage-containing plaque, has been questioned[47]. Indeed, the value of US in the detection of plaque haemorrhage remains controversial.

Whatever the histological correlate of the echolucent areas within atherosclerotic plaques, this ultrasound feature seems to identify patients with a greater risk of symptomatic cerebrovascular disease. Hetero-geneous plaques have been shown to be the dominant plaque type in symptomatic patients with a greater than 70% stenosis[48]; these patients have an increase in neurological deficits over a 3 year follow–up period[49]. Heterogeneous plaques are also the dominant plaque in asymptomatic patients who are subsequently symptomatic[50]. Fibrous plaques may predict a tendency to remain clinically stable[51].

The surface morphology of plaque may be categorized as smooth, irregular or ulcerated (Fig. 8)[52]. Ulcerated plaques have been associated with an increase in the number of infarcts detected on computed tomo-graphy and, therefore, represent a more sinister finding than a smooth fibrotic plaque[53]; plaque ulceration predisposes to the development of thrombus and subsequent emboli. Lipid emboli may also arise from the ulcerated surface[54]. A comparison of US and arteriography with surgical specimens, in the assessment of plaque surface ulceration and irregularity, has shown that US detection is superior to that of arteriography[55,56]. However, even US does not consistently evaluate ulceration[57]. It is, therefore, better to classify lesions seen on US as either smooth or irregular and only if a crater depth of greater than 2 mm is seen can ulceration be considered present and more likely to initiate an embolus[26].

Intima-medial thickness

The development of plaque disease and the consequent arterial narrowing are late manifestations of atherosclerotic disease; minor alterations in the inner arterial wall predate these changes. Ultrasound can be used to image the boundaries of the inner arterial wall with clarity[58]. The inner echogenic line represents the luminal–intimal inter-face and the outer echogenic line represents the media-adventitia inter-face; the distance between the two lines is a measure of the thickness of the combined intima and media[59]. These interfaces can be seen on both the near and far walls of larger arteries when the US beam is perpendicular to the wall, but more clearly on the far wall in vessels

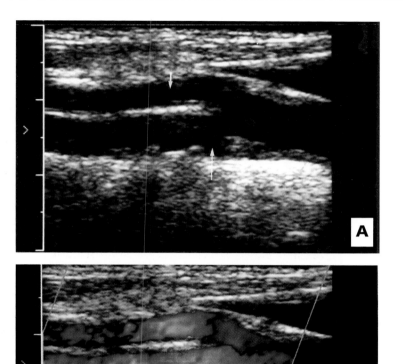

Fig. 8 **(A)** An ulcerated plaque (arrow) is demonstrated in the carotid bulb (short arrow; external carotid artery). **(B)** The ulcer crater fills with turbulent flow on colour Doppler ultrasound (arrow).

running parallel to the skin surface (Fig. 9). An increase in the distance between these two lines, the intima-media thickness (IMT) predicts atherosclerosis in other vessels, especially the coronary arteries[60].

A number of risk factors have been associated with an increased IMT in the carotid artery. Patients with hypercholesterolaemia are at higher risk of developing cardiovascular disease and elevated levels of cholesterol, independent of other risk factors, have been related to an increased IMT[61,62]. Other factors have been linked to increased IMT measurements and are detailed in Table 2[61-69]. It has been demonstrated that HDL-cholesterol levels have a negative correlation with IMT measurements suggesting a protective effect at the arterial wall level[70]. Increased IMT is associated with the presence of severe angiographically-detected coronary heart disease[63] and has been related to the presence of coronary artery calcification, itself a marker of early coronary artery disease, on ultra-fast computed tomography[71].

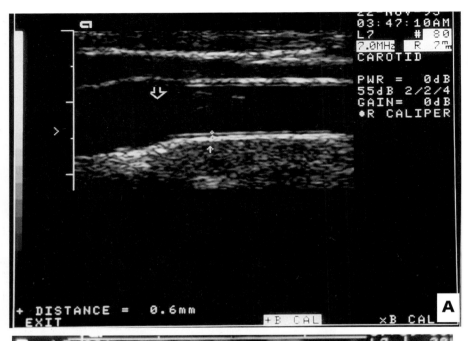

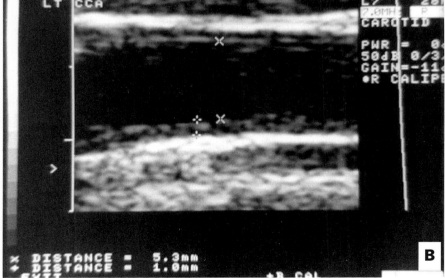

Fig. 9 (**A**) Longitudinal image of the distal common carotid artery and bulb (open arrow) demonstrating the inner arterial wall complex (arrow, between cursors) in a normal young person. (**B**) Same position in the distal common carotid artery in a patient with hypercholesterolaemia. The intima-media layer is thickened (+−+, 1.0 mm). The lumen of the common carotid is between the cursors (x–x).

More recently[72], the measurement of IMT has been used to document the regression of atherosclerotic disease in patients treated with the 3-hydroxy-3-methylglutaryl-coenzyme-A reductase inhibitors, such as lovastatin™. A lowering of serum cholesterol has a direct effect on the arterial wall, suggesting that increased IMT may be used as a marker of regression or progression of atherosclerosis.

Table 2 Risk factors for an increase in intimal-medial thickness (IMT) of the inner arterial wall as seen on ultrasound

Age
Familial hypercholesterolaemia
LDL-cholesterol
Lipoprotein (a)
Active and passive smoking
Homocysteine
Chronic exposure to elevated levels of serum angiotensin converting enzyme
Hypertension
Diabetes mellitus

Currently, there is no consensus on the ideal location for the measurement of IMT. In practice, it is appropriate to measure at a site that is readily visualized so that reproducible measurements may be made. Typically, IMT is measured along the far wall of the common carotid artery bilaterally, within 1 cm proximal to the carotid bulb[73]. The median wall thickness in adults ranges between 0.5–1.0 mm, with an increase with advancing age[74]. In general, IMT is thicker in men[75]. Values of greater than 1.0 mm are considered abnormal by most observers[76].

Vertebral artery

Reversal of flow in the vertebral artery ipsilateral to a proximal subclavian artery stenosis was demonstrated separately by Contorni[77] and Reivich[78] in 1960, and termed the subclavian steal syndrome by Fisher[79]. Initially, a large spectrum of symptoms were thought to be a result of this disorder, arising from brainstem ischaemia and stroke; these were considered to occur spontaneously or secondary to arm exercise[80]. More recent observations have raised doubts as to the significance of retrograde vertebral artery flow in producing cerebrovascular events. Like internal carotid artery stenosis, the subclavian steal phenomenon represents generalized atherosclerosis and may be a harmless haemodynamic phenomenon[81,82].

Demonstration of reversed flow in the vertebral artery by CDUS is accepted practice and is a valid substitute to arteriography as the first line investigation. However, arteriography is still sometimes necessary to delineate the proximal subclavian artery abnormality[83]. Routine examination of the vertebral arteries during a CDUS examination is rapid and ascertains the presence of vertebral artery flow reversal. The detection of reversal or biphasic flow at rest in the vertebral artery allows the diagnosis of subclavian steal to be made without any further investigation. In some cases, steal from the basilar artery does not occur at rest and blood flow to the arm must be increased to demonstrate vertebral flow reversal[84].

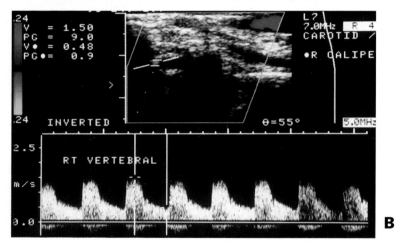

Fig. 10 (**A**) Colour Doppler ultrasound of the vertebral right vertebral artery demonstrating an area of colour disturbance corresponding to a stenosis (arrow). The open arrows indicate the transverse processes of the cervical vertebral bodies through which the vertebral courses (short arrow; vertebral vein). (**B**) Spectral Doppler waveform indicates a velocity of 1.50 m/s, confirming a stenosis.

Stenosis on vertebral artery US may be seen as turbulent flow or waveform dampening[85]. The relationship between the severity of a vertebral artery stenosis and the peak systolic velocity has not been fully assessed. The average peak systolic velocity in the normal vertebral artery is estimated at 56 cm/s (range 19–98 cm/s)[9]; a focal velocity greater than 100 cm/s, accompanied by disturbed flow is suggestive of a stenosis (Fig. 10). Transcranial US is able to image the distal vertebral arteries to the level of the basilar artery and this may extend the value of US in the assessment of the posterior fossa circulation[86].

Dissection of the carotid and vertebral artery

Angiography has been the method of choice for imaging an internal carotid artery dissection[87]. The most common angiographic feature is a tapered stenosis, less often an occlusion or an aneurysm is seen[88]. Ultrasound is capable of imaging the flow dynamics of a dissection, establishing the patency of a false lumen as well as defining the extent of thrombus in the vessel wall. Imaging with dynamic contrast enhanced spiral computed tomography and magnetic resonance, do not allow the interrogation of flow dynamics; demonstrating a peri-arterial rim of intramural haematoma surrounding either a normal or narrowed flow void[89].

In two series of internal carotid artery dissections imaged with US, the commonest spectral Doppler finding was either a bi-directional high resistance pattern or absence of a signal in a total occlusion[90,91]. Further-more, resolution occurred in a high proportion of patients – 68% over a mean time of 51 days. Flow reversal[92], bi-directional flow[93] and forward flow[94] may occur in the false lumen during the cardiac cycle. Vertebral artery dissections are less common, occurring secondary to neck trauma and spontaneously[95]. Vertebral artery dissections have been analyzed using both transcranial and extracranial US, but patterns are non-characteristic[96,97].

Other vascular diseases

A non-specific response to terminal internal carotid artery occlusion of any cause is the development of a fine system of collateral vessels around the base of the brain, the angiographic features described as a 'puff of smoke'[98]. Classically, these appearances are associated with moya-moya disease[99]. In an assessment of the ultrasound appearances associated with moya-moya disease, abnormal spectral waveforms were obtained from the ipsilateral internal carotid artery showing either no flow or a high-resistance flow pattern[100]. The US appearances in the extracranial internal carotid artery can mimic a dissection[101].

In Takayasu's disease, US demonstrates a characteristic circumferential arterial wall thickening, described as a 'macaroni-like' diffusely thickened intima-medial complex[102]. Ultrasound was found to be superior to arteriography in delineating this abnormality and, therefore, able to detect disease at an earlier stage[103]. Furthermore, US was found to be more sensitive than magnetic resonance in resolving wall thickening. Spectral Doppler usually shows a high resistance pattern[103]. Follow-up with US allows the monitoring of the regression of the wall abnormalities while on treatment, greatly reducing the need for repeated angiography.

Conclusion

Ultrasound plays an important role in the assessment of carotid arterial disease, complimentary to other imaging modalities. However, ultrasound does have limitations, not least the requirement of a high degree of operator skill. Recent advances in ultrasound technology will strengthen its role by improving accuracy[104]. Carotid Doppler ultrasound is an essential tool in the armamentarium of the stroke physician.

References

1 O'Leary DH, Person AV, Clouse ME. Noninvasive testing for carotid artery stenosis: 1. Prospective analysis of three methods. *Am J Neuroradiol* 1981; **2**: 437–42

2 Barber FE, Baker DW, Nation AWC, Strandness DE, Reid JM. Ultrasonic duplex echo-Doppler scanner. *IEEE Trans Biomed Engineer* 1974; **21**: 109–13

3 Polak JF, Dobkin GR, O'Leary DH, Wang AM, Cutler SS. Internal carotid artery stenosis: Accuracy and reproducibility of color-Doppler assisted duplex imaging. *Radiology* 1989; **173**: 793–8

4 Hankey GJ, Warlow CP. Symptomatic carotid ischaemic events: safest and most cost effective way of selecting patients for angiography, before carotid endarterectomy. *BMJ* 1990; **300**: 1485–91

5 Zwiebel WJ, Knighton R. Duplex examination of the carotid arteries. *Semin Ultrasound CT MR* 1990; **11**: 97–135

6 Hallam MJ, Reid JM, Cooperberg PL. Color-flow Doppler and conventional duplex scanning of the carotid bifurcation: Prospective, double-blind, correlative study. *Am J Roentgenol* 1989; **152**: 1101–5

7 Steinke W, Kloetzsch C, Hennerici M. Carotid artery disease assessed by color Doppler flow imaging: correlation with standard Doppler sonography and angiography. *Am J Roentgenol* 1990; **154**: 1061–8

8 Trattnig S, Schwaighofer B, Hubsch P, Schwarz M, Kainberger F. Color-coded Doppler sonography of vertebral arteries. *J Ultrasound Med* 1991; **10**: 221–6

9 Trattnig S, Hubsch P, Schuster H, Polzleitner D. Color-coded Doppler imaging of normal vertebral arteries. *Stroke* 1990; **21**: 1222–5

10 Jacobs NM, Grant EG, Schellinger D, Byrd MC, Richardson JD, Cohan SL. Duplex carotid sonography: Criteria for stenosis, accuracy, and pitfalls. *Radiology* 1985; **154**: 385–91

11 Hoskins PR. Accuracy of maximum velocity estimates made using Doppler ultrasound systems. *Br J Radiol* 1996; **69**: 172–7

12 Spencer MP, Reid JM. Quantification of carotid stenosis with continuous-wave (CW) Doppler ultrasound. *Stroke* 1979; **10**: 326–30

13 Roederer GO, Langlois YE, Jaeger KA. A simple parameter for accurate classification of severe carotid disease. *Bruit* 1984; **8**: 174–8

14 Moneta GL, Taylor DC, Zierler RE, Kazmers A, Beach K, Strandness DE. Asymptomatic high-grade internal carotid stenosis: is stratification to risk factors or duplex spectral analysis possible? *J Vasc Surg* 1989; **10**: 475–83

15 Keagy BA, Pharr WF, Thomas D, Bowles DE. Evaluation of peak frequency ratio (PFR) measurement in the detection of internal carotid artery stenosis. *J Clin Ultrasound* 1982; **10**: 109–12

16 North American Symptomatic Carotid Endarterectomy Trial Collaborators. Beneficial effect of carotid endarterectomy in symptomatic patients with high-grade carotid stenosis. *N Engl J Med* 1991; **325**: 445–53

17 European Carotid Surgery Trialists Collaboration Group. MRC European Carotid Surgery Trial: interim results for symptomatic patients with severe (70–99%) or with mild (0–29%) carotid stenosis. *Lancet* 1991; **337**: 1235–43

18 Hunink MGM, Polak JF, Barlan MM, O'Leary DH. Detection and quantification of carotid artery stenosis: Efficacy of various Doppler velocity parameters. *Am J Roentgenol* 1993; **160**: 619–25

19 Moneta GL, Edwards JM, Chitwood RW *et al*. Correlation of North American Symptomatic carotid Endarterectomy Trial (NASCET) angiographic definition of 70% to 99% internal carotid artery stenosis with duplex scanning. *J Vasc Surg* 1993; **17**: 152–9

20 Khaw KT. Does carotid duplex imaging render angiography redundant before carotid endarterectomy? *Br J Radiol* 1997; **70**: 235–8

21 Glagov S, Weisenberg E, Zarins CK, Stankunavicius R, Kolettis GJ. Compensatory enlargement of human atherosclerotic coronary arteries. *N Engl J Med* 1987; **316**: 1371–5

22 Crouse JR, Goldbourt U, Evans G *et al*. Arterial enlargement in the atherosclerosis risk in communities (ARIC) cohort. *In vivo* quantification of carotid arterial enlargement. *Stroke* 1994; **25**: 1354–9

23 Ricotta JJ, Bryan FA, Bond MG *et al*. Multicenter validation study of real-time (B-mode) ultrasound, arteriography, and pathologic examination. *J Vasc Surg* 1987; **6**: 512–20

24 Erickson SJ, Mewissen MW, Foley WD *et al*. Stenosis of the internal carotid artery: assessment using color Doppler imaging compared with angiography. *Am J Roentgenol* 1989; **152**: 1299–305

25 Berman S, Devine J, Erodes L. Distinguishing carotid artery pseudo-occlusion with color flow Doppler. *Stroke* 1997; **26**: 434–8

26 Theile BL, Jones AM, Hobson RW *et al*. Standards in noninvasive cerebrovascular testing. Report from the Committee on Standards for Noninvasive Testing of the Joint Council of the Society for Vascular Surgery and the North American Chapter of the International Society for Cardiovascular Surgery. *J Vasc Surg* 1992; **15**: 495–503

27 Lee TH, Ryu JE, Chen ST, Tseng KJ. Comparison between carotid duplex sonography and angiography in the diagnosis of extracranial internal carotid artery occlusion. *J Formosa Med Assoc* 1992; **91**: 575–9

28 Sitzer M, Furst G, Siebler M, Steinmetz H. Usefulness of an intravenous contrast medium in the characterization of high-grade internal carotid stenosis with color Doppler-assisted duplex imaging. *Stroke* 1994; **25**: 385–9

29 May AG, Vandeberg L, DeWeese JA, Rob CG. Critical arterial stenosis. *Surgery* 1963; **54**: 250–7

30 Norris JW, Zhu CZ, Bornstein NM, Chambers BR. Vascular risks of asymptomatic carotid stenosis. *Stroke* 1991; **22**: 1485–90

31 Roederer GO, Langlois YE, Jaeger KA *et al*. The natural history of carotid arterial diseases in asymptomatic patients with cervical bruits. *Stroke* 1984; **15**: 605–13

32 de Bray JM, Baud JM, Dauzat M. Consensus concerning the morphology and the risk of carotid plaques. *Cerebrovasc Dis* 1997; **7**: 289–96

33 Brown PB, Zwiebel WJ, Call GK. Degree of cervical carotid artery stenosis and hemispheric stroke: duplex US findings. *Radiology* 1989; **170**: 541–3

34 Gomez CR. Carotid plaque morphology and the risk of stroke. *Stroke* 1990; **21**: 148–51

35 Wasserman BA, Haacke EM, Li D. Carotid plaque formation and its evaluation with angiography, ultrasound, and MR angiography. *J Magn Reson Imaging* 1994; **4**: 515–27

36 Steffen CM, Gray-Weale AC, Byrne KE, Lusby RJ. Carotid artery atheroma: ultrasound appearance in symptomatic and asymptomatic vessels. *Aust N Z J Surg* 1989; **59**: 529–34

37 Reilly LM, Lusby RJ, Hughes L, Ferrell LD, Stoney RJ, Ehrenfeld WK. Carotid plaque histology using real-time ultrasonography. Clinical and therapeutic implications. *Am J Surg* 1983; **146**: 188–93

38 Imparato A, Riles T, Gorstein F. The carotid bifurcation plaque: pathologic findings associated with cerebral ischemia. *Stroke* 1979; **10**: 238–44

39 Imparato A, Riles T, Mintzer R, Baumann F. The importance of hemorrhage in the relationship between gross morphologic characteristics and cerebral symptoms in 376 carotid artery plaques. *Ann Surg* 1983; **197**: 195–203

40 Lusby R, Ferell L, Ehrenfeld WK, Stoney R, Wylie EJ. Carotid plaque hemorrhage. Its role in production of cerebral ischemia. *Arch Surg* 1982; **117**: 1479–88

41 O'Donnell TF, Erodes L, Mackey WC *et al*. Correlation of B-mode ultrasound imaging and arteriography with pathologic findings at carotid endarterectomy. *Arch Surg* 1985; **120**: 443–9

42 Hatsukami TS, Ferguson MS, Beach KW *et al*. Carotid plaque morphology and clinical events. *Stroke* 1997; **28**: 95–100

43 Seeger J, Klingman N. The relationship between carotid plaque composition and neurological symptoms. *J Surg Res* 1987; **43**: 78–85

44 Wolverson MK, Bashiti HM, Peterson GJ. Ultrasonic tissue characterisation of atheromatous plaques using a high resolution real time scanner. *Ultrasound Med Biol* 1983; **9**: 599–609

45 Bluth EI, Kay D, Merritt CR *et al*. Sonographic characterization of carotid plaque: detection of hemorrhage. *Am J Roentgenol* 1986; **146**: 1061–5

46 Barry R, Pienaar C, Nel CJ. Accuracy of B-mode ultrasonography in detecting carotid plaque hemorrhage and ulceration. *Ann Vasc Surg* 1990; **4**: 466–70

47 Leen EJ, Feeley TM, Colgan MP *et al*. 'Haemorrhagic' carotid plaque does not contain haemorrhage. *Eur J Vasc Surg* 1990; **4**: 123–8

48 Geroulakos G, Ramaswami G, Nicolaides A *et al*. Characterization of symptomatic and asymptomatic carotid plaques using high-resolution real-time ultrasonography. *Br J Surg* 1993; **80**: 1274–7

49 Sterpetti AV, Schultz RD, Feldhaus RJ *et al*. Ultrasonographic features of carotid plaque and the risk of subsequent neurologic deficits. *Surgery* 1988; **104**: 652–60

50 Johnson JM, Kennelly MM, Decesare D, Morgan S, Sparrow A. Natural history of asymptomatic carotid plaque. *Arch Surg* 1985; **120**: 1110–2

51 Hennerici M, Rautenberg W, Trockel U, Kladetzky RG. Spontaneous progression and regression of small carotid atheroma. *Lancet* 1985; i: 1415–9

52 Ricotta JJ. Plaque characterisation by B-mode scan. *Surg Clin North Am* 1990; **70**: 191–9

53 Zukowski AJ, Nicolaides AN, Lewis RT *et al*. The correlation between carotid plaque ulceration and cerebral infarction seen on CT scan. *J Vasc Surg* 1984; **1**: 782–6

54 Constantinides P. Cause of thrombosis in human atherosclerotic arteries. *Am J Cardiol* 1990; **66**: 37G–40G

55 Comerota AJ, Katz ML, White JV, Grosh JD. The preoperative diagnosis of ulcerated carotid atheroma. *J Vasc Surg* 1990; **11**: 505–10

56 Rubin JR, Bondi JA, Rhodes RS. Duplex scanning versus conventional arteriography for the evaluation of carotid artery plaque morphology. *Surgery* 1987; **102**: 749–55

57 Davenport KL, Sterpetti AV, Hunter WJ. Real-time B-mode carotid imaging and plaque morphology. *J Vasc Technol* 1987; **11**: 176–82

58 James EM, Earnest F, Forbes GS, Reese DF, Houser ON, Folger WN. High resolution dynamic ultrasound of the carotid bifurcation: a prospective evaluation. *Radiology* 1982; **144**: 853–8

59 Pignoli P, Tremoli E, Poli A, Oreste P, Paoletti R. Intimal plus medial thickness of the arterial wall: a direct measurement with ultrasound imaging. *Circulation* 1986; **74**: 1399-406

60 Salonen JT, Salonen R. Ultrasound B-mode imaging in observational studies of atherosclerotic progression. *Circulation* 1993; **87**: II-56–65

61 Poli A, Tremoli E, Colombo A, Sirtori M, Pignoli P, Paoletti R. Ultrasonographic measurement of the common carotid artery wall thickness in hypercholesterolemic patients. *Atherosclerosis* 1988; **70**: 253–61

62 Wendelhag I, Wiklund O, Wikstrand J. Arterial wall thickness in familial hypercholesterolaemia. Ultrasound measurement of the intima-media thickness in the common carotid artery. *Arterioscler Thromb Vasc Biol* 1992; **12**: 70–7

63 Geroulakos G, O'Gorman DJ, Kalodiki E, Sheridan DJ, Nicolaides AN. The carotid intima-media thickness as a marker of the presence of severe symptomatic coronary artery disease. *Eur Heart J* 1994; **15**: 781–5

64 Pauciullo P, Iannuzzi A, Sartorio R *et al*. Increased intima-media thickness of the common carotid artery in hypercholesterolaemic children. *Arterioscler Thromb Vasc Biol* 1994; **14**: 1075–9

65 Sinclair AM, Hughes AD, Geroulakos G *et al*. Structural changes in the heart and carotid arteries associated with hypertension in humans. *J Hum Hypertens* 1995; **7**: 1–13

66 Howard G, Burke GL, Szklo M *et al*. Active and passive smoking are associated with increased carotid wall thickness. The Atherosclerosis Risk in Communities Study. *Arch Intern Med* 1994; **154**: 1277–82

67 Malinow MR, Nieto J, Szklo M, Chambless LE, Bond G. Carotid artery intimal-medial wall thickening and plasma homocyst(e)ine in asymptomatic adults. The Atherosclerosis Risk in Communities Study. *Circulation* 1993; **87**: 1107–13

68 Bonithon-Kopp C, Ducimetiere P, Touboul PJ et al. Plasma angiotensin-converting enzyme activity and carotid wall thickening. Circulation 1994; 89: 952–4

69 Veller M, Fisher C, Nicolaides A. Measurement of the ultrasonic intima-media complex thickness in normal subjects. J Vasc Surg 1993; 17: 719–25

70 Sidhu PS, Naoumova RP, Maher VMG et al. The extracranial carotid artery in familial hypercholesterolaemia: relationship of intimal-medial thickness and plaque morphology with plasma lipids and coronary heart disease. J Cardiovasc Risk 1996; 3: 61–7

71 Sidhu PS, Naoumova RP, Forbat SM, Neuwirth CKY, Underwood SR, Thompson GR. The association of intima-media thickening and plaque morphology of the extracranial carotid arteries with coronary artery calcificaton in hypercholesterolaemia [abstract]. Br J Radiol 1995; 68: 803

72 Furberg CD, Adams HP, Applegate WB et al. Effect of lovastatin on early carotid atherosclerosis and cardiovascular events. Asymptomatic Carotid Artery Progression Study (ACAPS) Research Group. Circulation 1994; 90: 1679–87

73 Sidhu PS, Desai SR. A simple and reproducible method of assessing intimal-medial thickness of the common carotid artery. Br J Radiol 1997; 70: 85–9

74 Howard G, Manolio TA, Burke GL, Wolfson SK, O'Leary DH. Does the association of risk factors and atherosclerosis change with age? An analysis of the combined ARIC and CHS cohorts. Stroke 1997; 28: 1693–701

75 Salonen R, Salonen JT. Progression of carotid atherosclerosis and its determinants: a population-based ultrasonography study. Atherosclerosis 1990; 81: 33–40

76 Shah E. Use of B-mode ultrasound of peripheral arteries as an end point in clinical trials. Br Heart J 1994; 72: 501–3

77 Controni L. Il circolo collaterale vertebro-vertebro nell' obliterazione dell'arteria succlavia alla sua origine. Minerva Chir 1960; 15: 268–71

78 Reivich M, Holling HE, Roberts B, Toole JF. Reversal of blood flow through the vertebral artery and its effect on cerebral circulation. N Engl J Med 1961; 265: 878–85

79 Fisher CM. A new vascular syndrome 'the subclavian steal'. N Engl J Med 1961; 265: 912–3

80 Herring M. The subclavian steal syndrome: a review. Am Surg 1977; 43: 220–8

81 Borstein NM, Norris JW. Subclavian steal: a harmless haemodynamic phenomenon? Lancet 1986; ii: 303–5

82 Hennerici M, Klemm C, Rautenberg W. The subclavian steal phenomenon: a common vascular disorder with rare neurologic deficits. Neurology 1988; 38: 669–73

83 Walker DW, Acker JD, Cole CA. Subclavian steal syndrome detected with duplex pulsed Doppler sonography. Am J Neuroradiol 1982; 3: 615–8

84 Bendick PJ, Glover JL. Hemodynamic evaluation of vertebral arteries by duplex ultrasound. Surg Clin North Am 1990; 70: 235–44

85 Zwiebel WJ. Duplex vertebral examination. In: Zwiebel WJ. (ed) Introduction to Vascular Ultrasound. New York: Saunders, 1992; 133–43

86 Schoning M, Walter J. Evaluation of the vertebrobasilar-posterior system by transcranial color Duplex sonography in adults. Stroke 1992; 23: 1280–6

87 Fisher CM, Ojemann RG, Roberson GH. Spontaneous dissection of cervico-cerebral arteries. Can J Neurol Sci 1978; 5: 9–19

88 Biller J, Hingtgen WL, Adams HP, Smoker WRK, Godersky JC, Toffol GJ. Cervicocephalic arterial dissections. A ten-year experience. Arch Neurol 1986; 43: 1234–8

89 Zuber M, Meary E, Meder JF, Mas JL. Magnetic resonance imaging and dynamic CT scan in cervical dissections. Stroke 1994; 25: 576–81

90 Sturzenegger M, Mattle HP, Rivoir A, Baumgartner RW. Ultrasound findings in carotid artery dissection: analysis of 43 patients. Neurology 1995; 45: 691–8

91 Steinke W, Rautenberg W, Schwartz A, Hennerici M. Noninvasive monitoring of internal carotid artery dissection. Stroke 1994; 25: 998–1005

92 Bluth EI, Shyn PB, Sullivan M, Merritt CR. Doppler color flow imaging of carotid artery dissection. J Ultrasound Med 1989; 8: 149–53

93 Kotval PS, Babu SC, Fakhry J, Cozzi A, Barakat K. Role of the intimal flap in arterial dissection: Sonographic demonstration. Am J Roentgenol 1988; 150 : 1181–2

94 Sidhu PS, Jonker ND, Khaw KT et al. Spontaneous dissections of the internal carotid artery: Appearances on color Doppler ultrasound. Br J Radiol 1997; 70: 50–7

95 Hinse P, Thie A, Lachenmayer L. Dissection of the extracranial vertebral artery: a report of four cases and a review of the literature. *J Neurol Neurosurg Psychiatry* 1991; **54**: 863–9

96 Sturzenegger M, Mattle HP, Rivoir A, Rihs F, Schmid C. Ultrasound findings in spontaneous extracranial vertebral artery dissection. *Stroke* 1993; **24**: 1910–21

97 Hoffmann M, Sacco RL, Chan S, Mohr JP. Noninvasive detection of vertebral artery dissection. *Stroke* 1993; **24**: 815–9

98 Poor G, Gias G. The so-called 'Moyamoya disease'. *J Neurol* 1974; **37**: 370–7

99 Suzuki J, Kodama N. Moyamoya disease: a review. *Stroke* 1983; **14**: 104–9

100 Muppala M, Castaldo JE. Unilateral supraclinoid internal carotid artery stenosis with moyamoya like vasculopathy. Noninvasive assessments. *J Neuroimaging* 1994; **4**: 11–6

101 Sidhu PS, Ray-Chaudhuri K, Khaw KT. Case report: moyamoya disease mimicking a spontaneous internal carotid artery dissection on Doppler ultrasound. *Eur Radiol* 2000; **10**: 149–53

102 Maeda H, Handa N, Matsumoto M *et al*. Carotid lesions detected by B-mode ultrasonography in Takayasu's arteritis: 'macaroni sign' as an indicator of the disease. *Ultrasound Med Biol* 1991; **17**: 695–701

103 Buckley A, Southwood T, Culham G, Nadel H, Malleson P, Petty R. The role of ultrasound in evaluation of Takayasu's arteritis. *J Rheumatol* 1991; **18**: 1073–80

104 Whittingham TA. Broadband transducers. *Eur Radiol* 1999; **9**: 5298–303

105 Moneta GL, Edwards JM, Papanicolaou G *et al*. Screening for asymptomatic internal carotid artery stenosis: Duplex criteria for discriminating 60% to 99% stenosis. *J Vasc Surg* 1995; **21**: 989–94

Appendix 1

Doppler equation

$$f_D = 2v \, (\cos \theta) \, f/c$$

Where, f_D = difference between received and transmitted ultrasound frequency; v = speed of the target; θ = angle between the direction of the ultrasound beam and the target; c = speed of sound in tissue; and f = frequency of the transmitted ultrasound.

MR angiography

Andrew G Clifton

Department of Neuroradiology, Atkinson Morley's Hospital, London, UK

The primary use of angiography in the neck, either conventional catheter angiography or non-invasive techniques (MR angiography, CT angiography and ultrasound), is for the evaluation of the presence and severity of carotid stenosis. Other conditions such as vertebral artery stenosis, carotid and vertebral artery dissection and fibromuscular dysplasia are much less common but easily detectable with conventional angiography and are becoming increasingly reliably evaluated by non-invasive imaging. Intracranially, the value of MR angiography is less clear cut. It is certainly of use presurgery to look for vessel occlusion and encasement of vessels by tumour. It is also useful in excluding venous thrombosis as a cause of stroke. MR angiography for the detection and screening of intracranial aneurysms is less clear cut and, at present, it is the author's belief that MR angiography cannot replace conventional catheter angiography. Straightforward spin echo imaging is the most accurate way of detecting arteriovenous malformations (AVMs) with magnetic resonance.

Extracranial MR angiography

Angiography, either conventional catheter angiography or non-invasive techniques (MR and CT angiography and ultrasound), is used for the investigation of arterial and venous pathology in the neck. Its primary use is for the evaluation of the presence and severity of carotid stenosis. Other conditions such as vertebral artery stenosis and occlusion, carotid and vertebral artery dissection, fibromuscular dysplasia are less common but easily detectable with conventional angiography and are becoming increasingly reliably evaluated by non-invasive imaging.

Conventional angiography

Correspondence to:
Dr A G Clifton,
Consultant Neuro-
radiologist, Atkinson
Morley's Hospital, Copse
Hill, Wimbledon,
London SW20 0NE, UK

The ideal investigation is non-invasive, has no morbidity, has a high sensitivity and specificity, and is low cost. All non-invasive tests strive to achieve this ideal. Conventional angiography, the gold standard, is invasive and has morbidity, including locally at the puncture site, systemic complications and stroke. Conventional angiography is relatively safe in patients without atherosclerotic disease. Berenstein reports in the 4 years (1992–1995) in 1802 angiograms complications occurred in four procedures, three with temporary neurological deficit (0.17%) and one with permanent neurological deficit (0.05%)[1]. However, a study looking at patients with cerebrovascular disease, the Asymptomatic Carotid Atherosclerosis Study (ACAS)[2] reports stroke rates from angiography of 1.2% and 1.6%. This is significant morbidity.

The majority of patients being investigated are those with carotid stenosis. Recent multicentre clinical trials, the European Carotid Surgery Trial (ECST) and the North American Symptomatic Endarterectomy Trial (NASCET), have shown that the risks of stroke are significantly reduced in medically fit patients with recent symptoms with severe carotid stenosis and consequently an increasing number of patients with TIA and stroke are being investigated, up to 10% of these having a source from the carotid artery[3]. Thus a non-invasive technique is ideal. It is our practice to use a combination of screening with ultrasound, followed by magnetic resonance angiography (MRA) if the ultrasound detects a significant stenosis. Doppler ultrasound has been fully discussed elsewhere in this issue, and will not be dealt with further here. In our practice, if a Doppler study is positive, *i.e.* showing stenosis greater than 70%, this then needs to be confirmed with an MRA study. The combination of both results has been shown to give sensitivities of 100% and specificities between 90–98%. This is based on data from 1995 and before[4]. Further technological improvements in ultrasound and MRI will improve these figures. If there is discordance between the two tests, conventional angiography is performed. We perform angiography in less than 5% of patients, although other authors report angiography rates of 16–21%[5–7]. The latter is higher than desirable and should be reduced because advances in technology since 1995 have made MRA more accurate.

Pitfalls and advantages of MRA

Artefacts and over-estimation of a stenosis

Turbulent flow can cause pseudostenosis in a normal bulbous bifurcation and a tight focal stenosis can cause distal turbulence and a large flow gap, mimicking a long 2–3 cm stenosis. Swallowing can cause marked artefact. Any metal, such as a stent or clips, can degrade the image. Review of the source images with the post processing images (maximum intensity projection, MIP) is always essential.

Differentiation of complete occlusion of the ICA from a very severe stenosis or string sign

This is important as a complete occlusion is treated medically, but a very severe, greater than 95% stenosis with a string sign may be treated surgically. MRA is 100% sensitive and specific in differentiating carotid occlusion from a string sign, but it is vital to analyse the cross sectional source images[8].

Tandem and intracranial lesions

Controversy exists in the vascular surgical community as to whether it is worth looking for tandem lesions. Many surgeons are happy to operate on carotid stenosis after ultrasound alone or ultrasound and MRA. Others still require full angiography, looking at the intracranial circulation. With conventional angiography, intracranial stenoses are easily and accurately detected. MRA is relatively sensitive, particularly with severe stenoses but MIPs should be interpreted with care. Stenoses can often be greatly overestimated and tortuous vessels coursing in and out of the scan plane can also suggest stenosis when it is not really there. It is our experience that significant tandem stenosis is rare and we do not routinely image the intracranial circulation with MRA. Similar arguments apply to the origin of the great vessels from the aortic arch with the incidence of stenoses in this region being quoted as high as 5%[9]. Success in imaging the aortic arch with MRA has been poor to date but newer techniques involving Gadolinium-enhanced MRA, as discussed below, show great promise.

Techniques

I will now give a brief overview of techniques of MRA. These equally well apply to intracranial MRA, discussed later.

Until recently, the mainstay of MRA has been time of flight or phased contrast angiography. The objective in both techniques is to maximise the signal from rapidly flowing blood and to minimise signal from background stationary tissues. Keller[10] and Rosovsky et al[11] provide excellent reviews of the physics which will not be discussed in great detail here.

Time of flight

There are two forms of time of flight: two dimensional (2D ToF) and three dimensional (3D ToF). In time of flight or inflow imaging, the background protons are suppressed and the inflowing protons with full longitudinal magnetisation enter the excitation volume and generate a strong signal. The difference in longitudinal magnetisation between the stationary saturated background tissue and unsaturated incoming blood generates high intensity within vessels, a phenomenon known as flow-related enhancement[12,13]. In 2D ToF, protons are excited slice by slice and with 3D ToF, a large volume is imaged. 2D ToF is most commonly used for carotid neck imaging due to its superior flow-related enhancement.

Phased contrast (PC) angiography

In phased contrast angiography, a magnetic field is applied to create a phase shift that is proportional to the velocity of flow. The magnitude of the phase shift is used to create an image with high signal representing flowing protons. The second step background suppression is accomplished mathematically using pixel by pixel subtraction of the flow-compensated mask. PC angiography requires the use and choice of a velocity encoding factor (VENC) which is usually selected to correspond to the maximum velocity through a region. Incorrect choice of VENC can lead to errors, particularly aliasing where areas of signal dropout can be mistaken for stenosis or occlusion (flow aliasing).

ToF imaging is acquired in a much shorter time than PC imaging, allowing more time for acquisitions and better resolution. PC imaging can have better background suppression, allowing better depiction of slower flow and smaller vessels[14,15]. We routinely use 2D ToF for carotid imaging. The final data are presented as a MIP which looks like a conventional angiogram. The brightest pixels are selected by computer and displayed. The data can be further manipulated to show both carotids and vertebrals or each individual vessel. It is, of course, essential, both in imaging vessels in the neck and in the head, to review the MIP imaging with source images otherwise errors can be made, particularly in distinguishing occlusion from near occlusion.

Contrast-enhanced MRA

Traditional ToF MRA cannot yet completely replace catheter angiography. Two non-invasive tests are needed, and conventional angiography is required in a number of cases. Gadolinium-enhanced MRA is a new technique available on the latest generation of MR scanners. This may be the leap forward in eliminating the use of conventional angiography. The technique is practical and straightforward to use, even in busy units[16]. Remonda et al have described the technique and compared it with conventional DSA in patients with carotid stenosis[16]. The images are acquired without a breath hold and with manual injection of contrast. The 3D images obtained during the arterial phase of the bolus passage are identified by means of visual inspection and the data set subtracted from the pre-contrast data set after the background signal of fat is eliminated. MIP images are then generated. Grading of stenoses in their study of

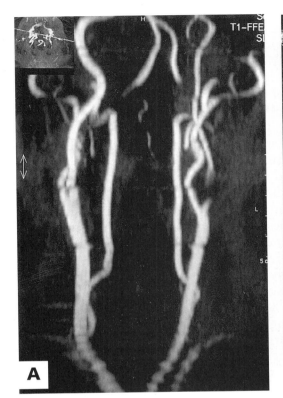
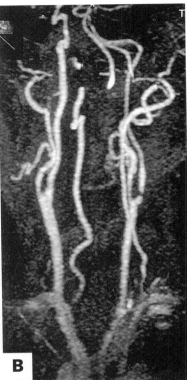

Fig. 1 (**A**) Maximum intensity projection MRA 2D time of flight, showing the aortic arch, carotid vessels in the neck and both vertebral arteries. On the left, a flow gap of about 1 cm is seen, perhaps indicating a long stenosis. On the right, there are 'steps' in the internal and external common carotid arteries due to swallowing artefact. Definition through the aortic arch is also poor with artefact. (**B**) Contrast enhanced (Gadolinium fast gradient echo) 3D time of flight imaging performed on the same patient at the same examination. This shows much better definition. The swallowing artefact on the right is eliminated, showing a normal bifurcation. On the left, the true extent of the stenosis is seen, with a very tight focal stenosis about 1 cm from the origin of the left internal carotid artery.

MRA agreed with DSA in 92% of 44 cases. All occlusions were accurately detected with MRA.

Timing from the start of the acquisition to the arrival of the contrast bolus is critical in contrast MRA. It can be acquired using a timing bolus[17] or alternatively using an automated bolus detection and scan-triggering scheme such as SMARTPREP (GE Medical Systems, Milwaukee, WI, USA)[18]. Similar systems are available from other manufacturers.

Figure 1A,B is a comparison, in the same patient, of 2D ToF and contrast enhanced 3D ToF, showing much better demonstration of carotid stenosis and less artefact with contrast enhanced 3D ToF than 2D ToF.

Vertebral artery stenosis

One-tenth of all ischaemic strokes occur in the posterior circulation[19] of which 20% are thought to be cardio-embolic in origin, with a further 20% due to intra-arterial embolism usually from the vertebral artery[20]. Imaging of the arteries of the posterior circulation is often not considered because of the perception that it will not alter patient management. However, Crawley *et al*[21] looked at 53 patients with conventional vertebral angiography and this was significantly abnormal in 60% of patients, 16 of whom had vertebral artery stenoses, and 12 of whom were considered suitable for percutaneous transluminal angioplasty (PTA). The results indicated that using vertebral angiography to investigate posterior circulation ischaemia will identify a significant number of potentially treatable lesions. Vertebral angiography is not, however, without risk. It is invasive and is expensive. A good non-invasive technique is needed. MRA has been reported to be highly sensitive and specific (97% and 98.9%, respectively) compared with catheter angiography in identifying stenoses and occlusions in the posterior circulation. The sensitivity of ultrasound is less (76.4%). My own view is that Gadolinium-enhanced MRA will be the imaging technique of choice, but this will initially have to be validated by comparison with conventional angiography. Our own experience is that neither MRA nor duplex ultrasound is sufficiently sensitive to stenosis at the origin of the vertebral artery (the commonest site to find lesions suitable for PTA) to be used for screening at the present.

Other non-atheromatous vascular diseases in the neck

Dissection

This is an increasingly recognised condition, particularly with the advent of MR. It causes approximately 2% of all strokes but up to 20% of strokes in younger patients[22]. Dissection may be post traumatic, spontaneous or secondary to conditions such as fibromuscular dysplasia. Dissection is best detected with fat suppressed T1 and T2 axial images rather than MRA. MRA can elegantly show the length of the stenosis but does not necessarily aid the diagnosis of dissection. Duplex ultrasonography may be helpful. The primary investigation in a patient suspected of having distal carotid dissection is thus conventional spin echo MR. (Fig. 2A,B)

Fibromuscular dysplasia

MR can identify severe lesions but is much less sensitive than catheter angiography, which is the imaging method of choice. MR artefacts may also mimic lesions[23].

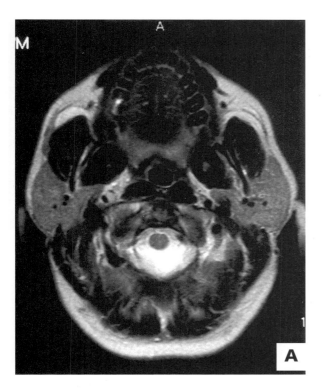

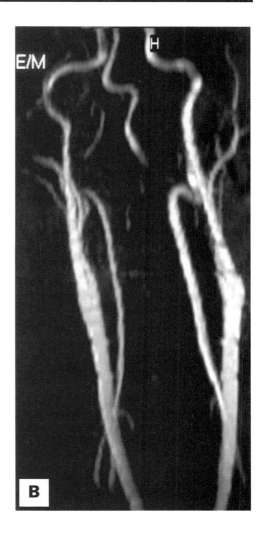

Fig. 2 (**A**) Axial T2 weighted image through the skull base, showing narrowing of the lumen of the right internal carotid artery with a surrounding crescent of high signal, consistent with intramural haematoma, secondary to carotid dissection. (**B**) The MRA sequence shows narrowing of the right distal cervical carotid at this level compared to the left.

Intracranial MRA

Screening for intracranial aneurysms

The gold standard for detection of intracranial aneurysms is intra-arterial digital subtraction angiography but, as discussed above, this is invasive and has morbidity. Recent papers, however, show a lower rate of rupture of coincidental aneurysms and question whether screening is indicated even in patients with two or three first degree relatives with subarachnoid haemorrhage[24,25].

Detection of aneurysms in patients with subarachnoid haemorrhage

Obviously, if a non-invasive test could detect an aneurysm with 100% sensitivity and specificity, this would be a major advance. However, as

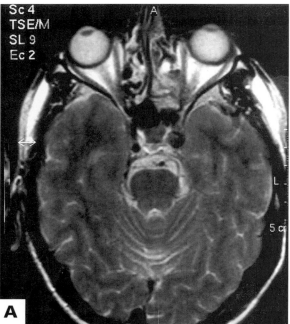

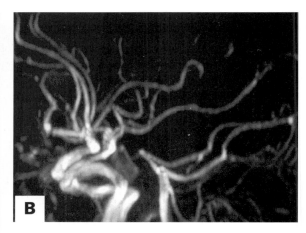

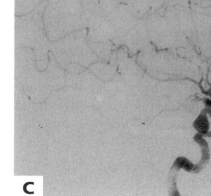

Fig. 3 (**A**) Axial T2 weighted MR scan showing flow void from a left carotid aneurysm, in the left supracavernous region. (**B**) Maximum intensity projection of the circle of Willis, MRA showing the aneurysm. (**C**) Left internal carotid digital subtraction angiography with selective injection into the left internal carotid artery, showing clear delineation of the left posterior communicating artery aneurysm pointing caudally.

yet, MRA is only approximately 90% sensitive and specific[24,26], and thus cannot yet be recommended for first line imaging of ruptured aneurysms.

At present, formal angiography is required to accurately delineate the anatomy of the aneurysm neck and the surrounding vessels. Digital subtraction angiography with 3D acquisition and post processing is also being increasingly used, particularly when endovascular treatment is contemplated.

Figure 3A–C shows a large posterior communicating artery aneurysm demonstrated on spin echo MR, MRA and conventional angiography.

Arteriovenous malformations

Straightforward spin echo imaging in multiple planes is the most accurate method of detecting arteriovenous malformations (AVMs) with magnetic resonance; MRA does not really provide any more useful information. Catheter angiography is still necessary for accurate anatomical delineation of the AVM, its architecture and feeders prior to consideration for possible embolic, surgical or radiosurgical therapy. If a patient has had an intracranial haemorrhage, even if MR is negative, conventional angiography is mandatory if an AVM is suspected radiologically and clinically from the pattern of haemorrhage. Delayed angiography may also be indicated to allow for resolution of the mass effect. Small AVMs and fistulas can be invisible on MR.

New techniques such as MR digital subtraction angiography, however, do show promise in replacing catheter angiography, particularly in the work up for therapies such as radiosurgery[27].

Dural sinus thrombosis

Dural sinus thrombosis[28,29] accounts for approximately 1–2% of strokes in young adults. It may be idiopathic but is often associated with local and systemic diseases, being particularly common in pregnancy, the puerperium and in patients on the oral contraceptive pill.

On conventional MR, in dural sinus thrombosis, the normal flow void in the sinus is lost. Care must be taken in particular when looking at the transverse and sigmoid sinuses, as slow flow may mimic thrombosis. One or other transverse sinus may be small or atretic and lack of clear visualisation of a transverse sinus may not necessarily mean thrombosis. The right sinus is usually the largest. T2 spin echo imaging is the most useful and coronal images perpendicular to the dural sinus are particularly helpful.

MR venography provides an overall global view of the sinuses and helps non-neuroradiologists appreciate the extent of a thrombosis. However, as far as aiding the diagnosis, MR venography does not add very much to the standard spin echo sequences.

Routine MR also enables detection of any venous infarction or underlying causes of thrombosis such as infection or tumour[28].

Key points for clinical practice

- Non-invasive techniques should replace invasive catheter angiography in the detection of carotid artery stenosis in the neck

- Either ultrasound followed by MRA or MRA followed by ultrasound, if the first test is positive, should be performed. The combination of both studies shows sensitivities of 100% and specificities between 90–98%

- Conventional angiography should be performed if the results are discordant.

- *Carotid dissection*: this is best detected with standard spin echo angiography, particularly using T2 and fat suppressed T2 images through the neck

- *Intracranial aneurysms*: MRA has as yet only 90% sensitivity and specificity. Catheter angiography is the gold standard and should be used in ruptured aneurysms. The role of screening for unruptured aneurysms is very debatable

- *Dural sinus thrombosis*: spin echo imaging, particularly perpendicular to the sinuses, is the most sensitive test. This can be supplemented by MR venography

References

1 Foulkes MA, Wolf PA, Price TR *et al*. The stroke data bank, design, methods and baseline characteristics. *Stroke* 1998; **19**: 547–54

2 Executive Committee for the Asymptomatic Carotid Atherosclerosis Study. Endarterectomy for asymptomatic carotid artery stenosis. *JAMA* 1995; **273**: 1421–8

3 Prior JC, Setton A, Nelson PK *et al*. Complications of diagnostic cerebral angiography and tips on its avoidance. *Neuroimaging Clin North Am* 1996; **6**: 756

4 De Marco JK, Schonfield S, Wesbey G. Can non-invasive studies replace conventional angiography in the pre-operative evaluation of carotid stenosis? Neuroimaging Clin North Am 1996; **6**: 914

5 Patel MR, Kuntz KM, Klufas RA *et al*. Pre-operative assessment of the carotid bifurcation. Can magnetic resonance angiography and duplex ultrasonography replace contrast arteriography? *Stroke* 1995; **26**: 1753–8

6 Nicholas GG, Osborne AM, Jaffe JW *et al*. Carotid artery stenosis: pre-operative non-invasive evaluation in a community hospital. *J Vasc Surg* 1995; **22**: 9–16

7 Kent KC, Kuntz KM, Patel MR *et al*. Peri-operative imaging strategies for carotid endarterectomy; an analysis of morbidity and cost effectiveness in symptomatic patients. *JAMA* 1995; **274**; 888–93

8 Currie IC, Murphy KP, Jones AJ *et al*. Magnetic resonance angiography of IADSA for diagnosis of carotid pseudo-occlusion. *Eur J Vasc Surg* 1994; **8**: 562–6

9 Brant-Zawadzki M, Heiserman JE. The roles of MR angiography, CT angiography and sonography in vascular imaging of the head and neck. *AJNR Am J Neuroradiol* 1997; **18**: 1820–5

10 Keller PJ. Magnetic resonance angiography of the neck: technical issues. *Neuroimaging Clin North Am* 1996; **6**: 853–61

11 Rosovsky MA, Litt AW, Krinsky MD. Magnetic resonance carotid angiography of the neck (clinical implications). *Neuroimaging Clin North Am* 1996; **6**: 863–74

12 Bradley WG, Waluch V. Blood flow: magnetic resonance imaging. *Radiology* 1985; **154**: 443–50

13 Bradley WG, Waluch V, Lai K *et al*. Appearance of rapidly flowing blood on MRI. *AJR Am J Roentgenol* 1984; **143**: 1167–74

14 Enzmann DR, Ross MR, Marks M *et al*. Blood flow in major cerebral arteries measured by phase contrast angiography. *AJNR Am J Neuroradiol* 1994; **15**: 123–9

15 Atlas SW. MR angiography in neurologic disease. *Radiology* 1994; **193**: 1–16

16 Remonda L, Head O, Silroth G. Carotid artery stenosis, occlusion and pseudo-occlusion: first-pass Gadolinium-enhanced, three dimensional MR angiography – preliminary study. *Radiology* 1998; **209**: 95–102

17 Kim JK, Farb R, Wright GA. Test bolus examination in the carotid artery at dynamic Gadolinium-enhanced MR angiography. *Radiology* 1998: **206**: 283–9

18 Foo TKF, Saranathan M, Prince MK *et al*. Automated detection of bolus arrival and initiation of data acquisition in fast, three dimensional, Gadolinium-enhanced angiography. *Radiology* 1997; **203**: 275–80

19 Bamford J, Sandercock P, Dennis M *et al*. Classification and natural history of clinically identifiable subtypes of cerebral infarction. *Lancet* 1991; **337**: 1521–6

20 Caplan LR. Brain embolism revisited. *Neurology* 1993; **43**: 1281–7

21 Crawley F, Clifton A, Brown MM. Treatable lesions demonstrated on vertebral angiography for posterior circulation ischaemic events. *Br J Radiol* 1998; **71**: 1266–70

22 Provenzale JM. Dissection of the internal carotid and vertebral arteries: imaging features. *AJR Am J Roentgenol* 1995; **165**: 1099–104

23 Heiserman JE, Drayer BP, Frake EK *et al*. MR angiography of cervical fibromuscular dysplasia. *AJNR Am J Neuroradiol* 1992; **13**: 1451–4

24 Crawley F, Clifton A, Brown M. Should we screen for intracranial aneurysms? *Stroke* 1999; **30**: 312–6

25 The International Study of Unruptured Intracranial Aneurysms Investigators. Unruptured intracranial aneurysms – risk of rupture and risks of surgical intervention. *N Engl J Med* 1998; **339**: 1725–33

26 Wardlaw JM, White PM. The detection and management of unruptured intracranial aneurysm. [Review]. *Brain* 2000; **123**: 205–21

27 Aoki S, Nanbu A, Yoshiskawa T, Hori M, Kumagai H, Araki T. 2D in thick-slice MR digital subtraction angiography with one second temporal resolution: assessment of cerebrovascular disorders. *Proceedings of the American Society of Neuroradiology*, May 1999; **110**: 122

28 Bogousslavsky J, Pierre P. Ischaemic stroke in patients under the age of 45. *Neurol Clin* 1992; **10**: 113–24

29 Amoli SR, Turski PA. The role of MR angiography in the evaluation of acute stroke. *Neuroimaging Clin North Am* 1999; **9**: 430–7

Transcranial Doppler ultrasound

Hugh S Markus

Department of Clinical Neurosciences, Guy's Kings and St Thomas' School of Medicine and Institute of Psychiatry, London, UK

Transcranial Doppler ultrasound allows measurements of blood flow velocity to be made from the basal intracerebral vessels. The major advantages of transcranial Doppler ultrasound are that it is non-invasive, relatively cheap, can be performed with portable machines, allows monitoring for prolonged periods, and has a high temporal resolution making it ideal for studying dynamic cerebrovascular responses. In addition it has recently been demonstrated that it can be used to detect circulating cerebral emboli; these cannot be detected by any other currently available imaging modality.

Transcranial Doppler ultrasound (TCD) allows measurements of blood flow velocity to be made from the basal intracerebral vessels. Although Doppler ultrasound was first applied to patients in the 1960s,[1] it was not appreciated for many years that sufficient ultrasound could pass through the skull to allow recording from intracerebral vessels. It was only in the 1980s that successful insonation of the middle cerebral artery was described by Aaslid *et al*[2]. To enable sufficient transmission of ultrasound through the skull, a low frequency transducer (usually 2 MHz) is used. This has the consequence that the spatial resolution is poor and, therefore, the technique is primarily useful for giving Doppler information on blood flow velocity. Duplex machines, which provide a two dimensional B-mode image of the intracranial structures, have been developed more recently, but the spatial resolution is of low quality and provides limited clinically useful information. Even using state-of-the-art TCD ultrasound equipment, it is impossible to successfully insonate the intracerebral vessels in approximately 10% of individuals due to the lack of an acoustic window; this proportion is increased in black individuals and with increasing age. A number of acoustic windows are used to provide access to different intracerebral vessels[3]. Most commonly, a temporal window above the zygomatic arch is used, through which the terminal internal carotid artery, middle cerebral artery, anterior cerebral artery, and proximal posterior cerebral artery can be insonated. The distal vertebral arteries and basilar artery can be insonated via an occipital window. Access can be obtained to the distal internal carotid artery and the ophthalmic artery via the orbit.

Correspondence to:
Prof. H S Markus,
Department of Clinical Neuroscience, St George's Hospital Medical School, Cranmer Terrace, London SW17 0RE, UK

Table 1 Major uses of transcranial Doppler ultrasound

Detection of intra-cranial stenosis

    Atheromatous stenosis

    Acute stroke

    Sickle cell disease

    Subarachnoid haemorrhage

Evaluation of the presence or absence of collateral flow channels

Measurement of dynamic cerebrovascular responses

    Carbon dioxide reactivity

    Dynamic autoregulation

    Vasoneuronal coupling

Intra-operative monitoring

    Carotid endarterectomy

    Cardiopulmonary bypass

    Interventional neuroradiological procedures

Embolic signal detection

Major advantages of TCD are that it is non-invasive, relatively cheap, can be performed with portable machines, allows monitoring for prolonged periods, and has a high temporal resolution making it ideal for studying dynamic cerebrovascular responses. In addition, it has recently been demonstrated that it can be used to detect circulating cerebral emboli; these cannot be detected by any other currently available imaging modality. The major uses of TCD are shown in Table 1.

Detection of intracranial stenosis

TCD is widely used in many countries for detection of intracranial stenoses usually caused by atheromatous disease. Stenosis can be identified by the presence of a high velocity jet and is most commonly detected in the middle cerebral artery[4]. One difficulty with using conventional TCD ultrasound is that one cannot correct for the angle between the ultrasound beam and the direction of flow. This is less of a problem for the middle cerebral artery where the angle is usually less than 20°, but it means that the sensitivity for detecting middle cerebral artery stenoses is reduced, particularly in subjects in whom the angle is at the upper end of the normal range. Using duplex TCD systems it is possible to determine and correct for this angle[5]. Intracranial stenoses can be detected in a number of patients with acute stroke, but it has been argued that the finding does not alter management and, therefore, in many countries TCD is not routinely used in acute stroke. There is some evidence that intracranial stenoses may be better treated with warfarin than aspirin[6], and, if this is confirmed, the importance of detecting such stenoses will be increased. Recently, this use of TCD has been challenged by magnetic resonance angiography. Both have potential advantages, but a major use of TCD is in ill patients with acute stroke or where serial monitoring is required. It has also been shown in an elegant study that, in patients with acute stroke, the presence of both middle cerebral artery occlusion and the subsequent time course of its recanalisation can be monitored using TCD[7]. Using TCD to identify individuals with acute stroke who have persisting middle cerebral artery occlusion, and who, therefore, might be particularly suitable for thrombolysis, is attractive. However, no large thrombolysis studies using it as a screening tool have yet been performed.

TCD is ideally suited to situations where repeated measurements are required. This potential use is illustrated by a recent stroke prevention study in sickle cell disease study[8]. Children with sickle cell disease are at markedly increased risk of stroke, which frequently occurs secondary to intra-cranial stenosis. TCD was used to identify children with sickle cell disease who had middle cerebral artery stenoses, and in a prospective study it was shown that these individuals were at markedly increased stroke risk[8]. In a follow on study, sickle cell children with intracranial stenoses, as detected by TCD, were randomised to either exchange transfusion or no additional treatment[9]. There was a very marked reduction in strokes during follow-up in the actively treated group.

Subarachnoid haemorrhage is another situation where the ability to perform repeated measurements is useful, primarily for the detection of vasospasm, which can be identified by TCD[10].

Evaluation of the presence or absence of collateral flow channels

TCD ultrasound can be used to identify the directionality of flow within collateral pathways[3] and provides useful information about whether collateral supply is adequate in cases of arterial occlusion. For example, in carotid artery occlusion the directionality of ophthalmic artery flow will indicate whether blood is being shunted from the extracranial circulation into the intracranial circulation. The technique can also be used to demonstrate the integrity of the circle of Willis. In practice, dynamic techniques such as carbon dioxide reactivity (as discussed below) may give a better global estimate of the adequacy of collateral supply.

Measurement of dynamic cerebrovascular responses

A major advantage of TCD is its very high temporal resolution. This makes it ideal to study rapid changes in cerebral haemodynamics. This has led to its use in the measurement of cerebral autoregulation. One potential problem in this setting is that TCD measures blood flow velocity and not absolute blood flow. Therefore, it is only a valid method to estimate changes in cerebral blood flow if the vessel diameter does not change during the intervention. It has been demonstrated using angiography that there is very little or no change in the middle cerebral artery diameter during carbon dioxide inhalation at the concentrations used during carbon dioxide reactivity measurements[11]. Therefore, in this setting, it appears a valid technique. Similarly, the middle cerebral artery does not change in diameter following certain drugs. However, some drugs, particularly those affecting the nitric oxide system, can cause marked changes in middle cerebral artery diameter. For example, nitric oxide synthase inhibition in man resulted in a 30% reduction in cerebral blood flow, as determined by absolute carotid artery volume flow. In contrast, there was no change in middle cerebral artery blood flow[12]. This is consistent with vasoconstriction in the middle cerebral artery, and similar studies using nitric oxide donors have suggested that marked vasodilation can occur[13].

Carbon dioxide reactivity has been widely used as a surrogate measure of autoregulation, particularly in patients with carotid stenosis, as a way to determine the adequacy of collateral supply. Middle cerebral artery blood flow velocity is measured while the patient breathes air, and then while they breathe a mixture of 5–8% carbon dioxide in air. The percentage change in blood flow velocity is then calculated[14]. If a concentration of carbon dioxide is used which does not maximally vasodilate (i.e. 5 or 6%), the change in blood flow velocity is divided by the change in end tidal carbon dioxide, an estimate of the partial pressure of carbon dioxide in the blood. A proportion of patients with carotid stenosis and occlusion have impaired carbon dioxide reactivity, and this is primarily seen in individuals with poor collateral supply[14]. An improvement is seen after carotid endarterectomy[15]. Studies have demonstrated that, in patients with carotid occlusion, impaired reactivity identifies individuals at particularly high risk of future stroke or TIA[16]. There is less firm data as to whether the same technique identifies individuals with carotid stenosis who are at high risk. If so, it may be a useful technique to identify high-risk asymptomatic patients with carotid stenosis for endarterectomy. One potential problem with the technique is that high doses of carbon dioxide can result in hypertension and, in some patients, this results in a 'passive' rise in cerebral artery blood flow velocity. This can sometimes obscure impaired autoregulation[17]. For this reason, it is recommended that a non-invasive technique such as a Finapres is used to monitor blood pressure during the procedure. An alternative vasodilatory stimulus which is frequently used is acetazolamide, a carbonic anhydrase inhibitor[18]. However, some studies have suggested that the results are less reproducible than those obtained using carbon dioxide as a vasodilator[19].

Carbon dioxide reactivity is an indirect measure of autoregulation. More recently, a direct measure of cerebral autoregulation has been developed by Aaslid et al[20]. Following a sudden stepwise drop in blood pressure, cerebral blood flow drops suddenly and then returns to normal. The rate of rise of blood flow is greater than that of systemic blood pressure, and this difference is caused by the cerebral autoregulatory response. A sudden stepwise blood pressure drop can be induced by inflating leg cuffs, and then suddenly deflating them, resulting in a reactive hyperaemia. Middle cerebral artery blood flow velocity can be recorded by TCD and blood pressure non-invasively monitored at the same time by a Finapres or other similar method. The rate of rise of the two parameters can then be compared to derive an autoregulatory index[20]. There has been concern that the stepwise drop in blood pressure might alter middle cerebral artery diameter. However, validation studies have shown that an autoregulatory index measured in this way correlates well with that measured using carotid artery flow monitoring, which provides an absolute measure of blood flow[21]. A good correlation has been found between dynamic autoregulation, estimated using this method, and estimates of static autoregulation[22]. Therefore, the technique does appear to be valid, and impaired autoregulation has been found both in patients with head injury[21] and in a subgroup of patients with carotid artery stenosis[23]. This technique may be useful at identifying those individuals at high risk who may benefit from revascularisation. It may also allow identification of individuals with carotid stenosis or occlusion who have a particularly poor collateral supply, and in whom lowering of blood pressure to the normal range could precipitate cerebral ischaemia.

Vasoneuronal coupling describes the increase in regional blood flow seen in response to neuronal activity. An estimate of this can also be obtained using TCD. Using the high temporal resolution of TCD, the rise in cerebral blood flow velocity in the artery supplying a particular brain region can be determined while that brain region is activated. Most commonly the occipital cortex is activated, using a flashing visual stimulus, while posterior artery blood flow velocity is recorded[24]. By averaging over a number of stimuli, a reliable measurement can be obtained. Using a language activation task, and recording from both middle cerebral arteries, the technique may allow hemispheric dominance for language to be determined[25,26]. Using other activation tasks, the technique has also been used to study mechanisms of recovery following stroke[27]. However, the application of TCD here is limited by its poor spatial resolution, and the mechanisms of neural recovery following stroke may be better answered using positron emission tomography or functional magnetic resonance imaging.

Intra-operative monitoring

The non-invasive nature of TCD and its high temporal resolution make it ideally suited to intra-operative monitoring. In this context, it is most used during carotid endarterectomy[28]. In a proportion of patients during cross clamping, if collateral supply is inadequate, middle cerebral artery blood flow can drop dramatically and there is a danger of cerebral ischaemia. In such patients, it is necessary to insert a shunt. One method of identifying individuals who require shunt insertion is to continuously monitor middle cerebral artery blood flow velocity during the operation, and only insert a shunt in individuals in whom it falls below a particular threshold on cross-clamping. Monitoring can also identify individuals in whom the potential problems arise such as shunt kinking. The technique is also used to monitor for embolisation occurring during both carotid endarterectomy and cardiopulmonary bypass as discussed below.

Embolic signal detection

Doppler ultrasound has the unique ability to detect emboli as they pass through the circulation. Due to increased scattering and reflection of ultrasound from the embolus, compared with the surrounding red blood cells, an embolus appears as a short duration high intensity signal within the Doppler flow spectrum. It has been appreciated since the 1960s that gas bubbles can be detected using ultrasound[29], and the technique has been applied to both decompression sickness and cardiopulmonary bypass to detect gaseous emboli[30,31]. However, it was only in 1990 that it was appreciated that solid emboli, composed of thrombus or platelet aggregates, could also be detected. While recording during carotid endarterectomy for air emboli introduced during the operation, Spencer and colleagues noted that similar embolic signals occurred prior to arterial opening, *i.e.* before any air could be introduced into the system[32]. They deduced these must be solid emboli dislodged from the carotid plaque during surgical manipulation. Although there was initial scepticism, subsequent *in vitro* and *in vivo* studies have demonstrated that the technique is highly sensitive and specific[33–35]. Embolic signals have been detected in patients with a wide variety of potential embolic sources including carotid artery stenosis, atrial fibrillation, and valvular heart disease[36]. Conventionally, recordings are made from the middle cerebral artery. The low frequency transducer used for TCD increases the embolic-to-background blood signal ratio and, therefore, makes them easier to detect[37]. In addition, prolonged recording can be performed using simple headpieces. Good interobserver reproducibility in identifying embolic signals has been reported[38] and recent consensus criteria have been developed for applying this technique in clinical practice[39].

Most work has been performed in carotid artery stenosis. Asymptomatic embolic signals are surprisingly frequent and are usually detected in 20–50% of patients with symptomatic carotid stenosis if recordings are performed for an hour[40–45]. Their presence has been shown to correlate with known markers of increased risk including symptomatic status[40,41], time since last symptoms[45–47], and plaque ulceration determined either histo-logically[48] or on angiography[43,44]. Recently, small studies have suggested that asymptomatic embolisation may be an independent predictor of future stroke risk[49–51] and this is being tested in larger multicentre studies.

Asymptomatic embolic signal detection has a number of potential uses. It may allow identification of individuals at high risk of stroke for targeted pharmacological or surgical therapy. For example, operating on an asymptomatic carotid stenosis has a poor risk-benefit ratio. Eighty-five patients have to be operated on to prevent one stroke over a one-year period[52]. Identifying a high-risk group of individuals would improve both cost-benefit and risk-benefit ratios. Embolic signal detection may also be useful in monitoring the effectiveness of antithrombotic therapy in individuals. It may also be useful in monitoring during interventional procedures. For example, it has been demonstrated that embolic signals during the dissection phase of carotid endarterectomy (before arterial opening) correlate with both new peri-operative MRI infarcts[53] and neuropsychological decline[54]. Intra-operative use of the technique may aid the surgeon in reducing embolisation. Furthermore, embolisation in the postoperative period has been associated with early postoperative stroke and TIA risk[55]. It has been suggested that the technique may allow the identification of individuals in this setting who require more aggressive postoperative antithrombotic measures such as a Dextran infusion[56].

Embolic signal detection may also prove useful in evaluating new antithrombotic and antiplatelet therapies. Currently, these are evaluated in large expensive clinical trials with an endpoint of stroke. For example, the recent CAPRIE trial recruited approximately 20,000 patients and only just achieved a significant result[57]. There is a wide gulf between *ex vivo* assessment of platelet function and clinical effectiveness, and animal models are not always truly representative of the situation occurring in man. Because asymptomatic embolic signals are much more frequent than stroke and TIA, they provide a surrogate endpoint which can be used to test the effectiveness of novel therapies. For this application, a situation is required where embolisation is frequent, and asymptomatic emboli have clinical significance. The setting of the postoperative period following carotid endarterectomy has been used. It was possible to show the highly significant antithromboembolic effect of a novel and potentially platelet-specific nitric oxide donor, S-nitrosothiol, in only 12 cases and 12 controls using this technique[58].

Asymptomatic embolic signal detection may also be useful in patients with acute stroke both in identifying the stroke subtype and mechanism, in localising the embolic source by recording from multiple sites along the arterial tree simultaneously, and possibly in identifying individuals at high risk of recurrent stroke[59]. Particularly in patients with carotid artery stenosis and acute stroke, continued embolisation is frequent even at 2 weeks post-stroke[59,60].

Other recent advances

Recently, duplex ultrasound machines have been adapted for transcranial imaging. The B-mode modality does allow some delineation of structure, and lesions such as intracranial haemorrhage and mid-line shift have been identified; however, the spatial resolution is much inferior to computed tomography or magnetic resonance imaging. Nevertheless, this imaging modality does have advantages for studying intracerebral vessels, primarily due to the use of the colour coded modality. It can be easier to identify certain intracranial arteries, and this can help in determining whether they are absent or merely difficult to identify due to a poor acoustic window. It allows the sample volume to be placed in the vessel of interest and the Doppler angle to be adjusted manually so that angle corrected flow velocity can be determined[61]. The technique has also been used to study other intracranial vascular structures such as the pulsatility of intracranial aneurysms[62].

A major problem with TCD remains the lack of an acoustic window in approximately 10% of individuals. The use of ultrasonic contrast agents can overcome this problem[63]. An intravenous injection is given of an agent containing stabilised microbubbles. This passes into the intracranial arterial circulation, and results in increased back-scattering and signal intensity. Using this technique in combination with colour flow duplex imaging the anatomy of the complete circle of Willis can be visualised.

Conclusions

In its early days, TCD ultrasound was primarily used to identify intra-cranial stenoses. With the advent of magnetic resonance angiography,

TCD is less used for this indication by many units. However, its non-invasive nature and high temporal resolution make it ideal to for the study of cerebral hemodynamics, to monitor during interventional procedures, or where repeated measurements are required particularly in sick patients. It also offers the only technique by which asymptomatic emboli can be detected non-invasively.

References

1   Satomura S, Kaneko Z. Ultrasonic blood rheograph. Proceedings of the 3rd International Conference on Medical Electronics. 1960; 254–8

2   Aaslid R, Markwalder T-M, Nornes H. Noninvasive transcranial Doppler ultrasound recording of flow velocity in basal cerebral arteries. *J Neurosurg* 1982; **50**: 570–7

3   Fujioka KA, Douville CM. Anatomy and freehand examination techniques. In: Newell DW, Aaslid R. (eds) *Transcranial Doppler*. New York: Raven, 1992

4   Ley-Pozo J, Ringlestein EB. Noninvasive detection of occlusive disease of the carotid siphon and middle cerebral artery. Ann Neurol 1990; **28**: 640–7

5   Baumgartner RW, Arnold M, Gonner F et al. Contrast-enhanced transcranial color-coded duplex sonography in ischemic cerebrovascular disease. *Stroke* 1977; **28**: 2473–8

6   The Warfarin-Aspirin Symptomatic Intracranial Disease (WASID) Study Group. Prognosis of patients with symptomatic vertebral or basilar artery stenosis. *Stroke* 1998; **29**: 1389–92

7   Ringlestein EB, Biniek R, Weiller C, Ammeling B, Nolte PN, Thron A. Type and extent of hemispheric brain infarctions and clinical outcome in early and delayed middle cerebral artery recanalization. *Neurology* 1992; **42**: 289–98

8   Adams RJ, McKie VC, Carl EM et al. Long-term stroke risk in children with sickle cell disease screened with transcranial Doppler. *Ann Neurol* 1997; **42**: 699–704

9   Adams RJ, McKie VC, Hsu L et al. Prevention of first stroke by transfusions in children with sickle cell anaemia and abnormal results on transcranial Doppler ultrasonography. *N Engl J Med* 1998; **339**: 5–11

10 Sloan MA. Transcranial Doppler monitoring of vasospasm after subarachnoid haemorrhage. In: Tegeler CH, Babikian VL, Gomez CR (eds) *Neurosonology*. St Louis: Mosby, 1995; 156–71

11 Huber P, Handa J. Effect of contrast material, hypercapnia, hyperventilation, hypertonic glucose and papaverine on the diameter of cerebral arteries. *Invest Radiol* 1967; **2**: 17–32

12 White RP, Deane C, Vallance P, Markus HS. Nitric oxide synthase inhibition in humans reduces cerebral blood flow but not the hyperaemic response to hypercapnia. *Stroke* 1998; **29**: 467–72

13 Dahl A, Russell D, Nyberg Hansen R, Rootwelt K. Effect of nitroglycerin on cerebral circulation measured by transcranial Doppler and SPECT. *Stroke* 1989; **20**: 1733–6

14 Ringelstein EB, Sievers C, Ecker S, Schneider PA, Otis SM: Noninvasive assessment of CO_2-induced cerebral vasomotor response in normal individuals and patients with internal carotid artery occlusions. *Stroke* 1988; **19**: 963–9

15 Hartl WH, Janssen I, Furst H. Effect of carotid endarterectomy on patterns of cerebrovascular reactivity in patients with unilateral carotid artery stenosis. *Stroke* 1994; **25**: 1952–7

16 Kleiser B, Widder B. Course of carotid artery occlusions with impaired carbon dioxide reactivity. *Stroke* 1992; **23**: 171–4

17 Dumville J, Panerai RB, Lennard NS, Naylor AR, Evans DH. Can cerebrovascular reactivity be assessed without measuring blood pressure in patients with carotid artery disease? *Stroke* 1998; **29**: 968–74

18 Piepgras A, Schmiedek P, Leinsinger G, Haberl RL, Kirsch CM, Einhaupl KM. A simple test to assess cerebrovascular reserve capacity using transcranial Doppler sonography and acetazolamide. *Stroke* 1990; **21**: 1306–11

19 Keliser B, Scholl D, Widder B. Assessment of cerebrovascular reactivity by Doppler CO_2 and diamox testing – which is the appropriate method. *Cerebrovasc Dis* 1994; **4**: 134–8

20 Aaslid R, Lindegaard KF, Sorteberg W, Nornes H. Cerebral autoregulation dynamics in humans. *Stroke* 1989; **20** :45–52

21 Newell DW, Aaslid R, Lam AM, Mayberg TS, Winn R. Comparison of flow and velocity during dynamic autoregulation testing in humans. *Stroke* 1994; **25**: 793–7

22 Tiecks FP, Lam AM, Aaslid R, Newell DW. Comparison of static and dynamic cerebral autoregulation measurements. *Stroke* 1995; **26**: 1014-9

23 White RP, Markus HS. Non-invasive determination of impaired dynamic cerebral autoregulation in carotid artery stenosis. *Stroke* 1997; **28**: 1340–4

24 Panczel G. Daffertshofer M. Ries S. Spiegel D. Hennerici M. Age and stimulus dependency of visually evoked cerebral blood flow responses. *Stroke* 1999; **30**: 619–23

25 Markus HS, Boland M. Cognitive activity monitored by non-invasive measurement of cerebral blood flow velocity and its application to the investigation of cerebral dominance. *Cortex* 1992; **28**: 575–81

26 Klingelhofer J, Matzander G, Sander D, Schwarze J, Boecker H, Bischoff C. Assessment of functional hemispheric asymmetry by bilateral simultaneous cerebral blood flow velocity monitoring. *J Cereb Blood Flow Metab* 1997; **17**: 577–85

27 Silvestrini M, Cupini LM, Placidi F, Diomedi M, Bernardi G. Bilateral hemispheric activation in the early recovery of motor function after stroke. *Stroke* 1998; **29**: 1305–10

28 Gaunt ME. Transcranial Doppler: preventing stroke during carotid endarterectomy. *Ann R Coll Surg Engl* 1988; **80**: 377–87

29 Austen WG, Howry D. Ultrasound as a method to detect bubbles or particulate matter in the arterial line during cardiopulmonary bypass. *J Surg Res* 1965; **5**: 283–4

30 Spencer MP. Decompression limits for compressed air determined by ultrasonically detected blood bubbles. *J Appl Physiol* 1976; **2**: 229–35

31 Padayachee TS, Parsons S, Theobold R, Linley J, Gosling RG, Deverall PB. The detection of microemboli in the middle cerebral artery during cardiopulmonary bypass: a transcranial Doppler ultrasound investigation using membrane and bubble oxygenators. *Ann Thorac Surg* 1987; **44**: 298–302

32 Spencer MP, Thomas GI, Nicholls SC, Sauvage LR. Detection of middle cerebral artery emboli during carotid endarterectomy using transcranial Doppler ultrasonography. *Stroke* 1990; **21**: 415–23

33 Russell D, Madden KP, Clark WM, Sandset PM, Zivin JA. Detection of arterial emboli using Doppler ultrasound in rabbits. *Stroke* 1991; **22**: 253–8

34 Markus HS, Brown MM. Differentiation between different pathological cerebral embolic materials using transcranial Doppler in an in vitro model. *Stroke* 1993; **24**: 1–5

35 Markus H, Loh A, Brown MM. Detection of circulating cerebral emboli using Doppler ultrasound in a sheep model. *J Neurol Sci* 1994; **122**: 117–24

36 Markus HS. Transcranial Doppler detection of circulating cerebral emboli: a review. *Stroke* 1993; **24**: 1246–50

37 Spencer M, Granado L. Ultrasonic frequency and Doppler sensitivity to arterial microemboli [abstract]. *Stroke* 1993; **24**: 510

38 Markus HS, Ackerstaff R, Babikian V et al. Inter-centre agreement in reading Doppler embolic signals: a multicentre international study. *Stroke* 1997; **28**: 1307–10

39 Ringlestein EB, Droste DW, Babikian VL et al and the International Consensus Group on Microembolus Detection. Consensus on microembolus detection by TCD. *Stroke* 1998; **29**: 725–9

40 Siebler M, Nachtmann A, Sitzer M et al. Cerebral microembolism and the risk of ischaemia in asymptomatic high-grade internal carotid artery ischaemia. *Stroke* 1995; **26**: 2184–6

41 Markus HS, Thomson N, Brown MM, Thomson ND. Asymptomatic cerebral embolic signals in symptomatic and asymptomatic carotid artery disease. *Brain* 1995; **118**: 1005–11

42 Georgiadis D, Lindner A, Manz M et al. Intracranial microembolic signals in 500 patients with potential cardiac or carotid embolic source and in normal controls. Stroke 1997; **28**: 1203–7

43 Orlandi G, Parenti G, Bertolucci A, Puglioli M, Collavoli P, Murri L. Carotid plaque features on angiography and asymptomatic cerebral microembolism. *Acta Neurol Scand* 1997; **96**: 183–6

44 Valton L, Larrue V, Arrue P, Geraud G, Bes A. Asymptomatic cerebral embolic signals in patients with carotid stenosis : correlation with the appearance of plaque ulceration on angiography. *Stroke* 1995; **26**: 813–5

45   Molloy J, Khan N, Markus HS. Temporal variability of asymptomatic embolisation in carotid artery stenosis, *Stroke* 1998; **29**: 1129–32

46   Van Zuilen EV, Moll FL, Vermeulen FE, Mauser HW, van Gijn J, Ackerstaff RG. Detection of cerebral microemboli by means of transcranial Doppler monitoring before and after carotid endarterectomy. *Stroke* 1995; **26**: 210–3

47   Siebler M, Sitzer M, Rose G, Bendfeldt D, Steinmetz H. Silent cerebral embolism caused by neurologically symptomatic high-grade carotid stenosis. Event rates before and after carotid endarterectomy. *Brain* 1993; **116**: 1005–15

48   Sitzer M, Muller W, Siebler M et al. Plaque ulceration and lumen thrombus are the main sources of cerebral microemboli in high-grade internal carotid artery stenosis. *Stroke* 1995; **26**: 1231–3

49   Siebler M, Nachtmann A, Sitzer M et al. Cerebral microembolism and the risk of ischaemia in asymptomatic high-grade internal carotid artery ischaemia. *Stroke* 1995; **26**: 2184–6

50   Valton L, Larrue V, Le Traon AP, Massabuau P, Gerard G. Microembolic signals and risk of early recurrence in patients with stroke or transient ischaemic attack. Stroke 1998; **29**: 2125–8

51   Molloy J, Markus HS. Asymptomatic embolisation predicts stroke and TIA risk in patients with carotid artery stenosis. *Stroke* 1999; **30**: 1440–3

52   Warlow C. Endarterectomy for asymptomatic carotid stenosis? *Lancet* 1995; **345**: 1254

53   Jansen C, Ramos LM, Van Heesewijk JP, Moll FL, van Gijn J, Ackerstaff RG. Impact of microembolism and haemodynamic changes in the brain during carotid endarterectomy. *Stroke* 1994; **25**: 992–7

54   Gaunt ME, Martin PJ, Smith JL et al. Clinical relevance of intraoperative embolisation detected by transcranial Doppler ultrasonography during carotid endarterectomy: a prospective study of 100 patients. *Br J Surg* 1994; **81**: 1435–9

55   Levi CR, O'Malley HM, Fell G et al. Transcranial Doppler-detected cerebral microembolism following carotid endarterectomy: high microembolic signal loads predict post-operative cerebral ischaemia. *Brain* 1997; **120**: 621–9

56   Lennard N, Smith J, Dumville J et al. Prevention of postoperative thrombotic stroke after carotid endarterectomy; the role of transcranial Doppler ultrasound. *J Vasc Surg* 1997; **26**: 579–84

57   CAPRIE Steering Committee. A randomised, blinded, trial of clopidogrel versus aspirin in patients at risk of ischaemic events (CAPRIE). *Lancet* 1996; **348**: 1329–39

58   Molloy J, Martin JF, Baskerville PA, Fraser SCA, Markus HS. S-nitrosoglutathione reduces the rate of embolisation in humans. Circulation 1998; **98**: 1372–5

59   Kapostza Z, Young E, Bath PMW, Markus HS. The clinical application of asymptomatic embolic signal detection in acute stroke: a prospective study. *Stroke* 1999; **30**: 1814–8

60   Konnecke H, Mast H, Trocio SH et al. Frequency and determinants of microembolic signals on transcranial Doppler in unselected patients with acute carotid territory ischaemic: a prospective study. Cerebrovasc Dis 1998; **8**: 107–12

61   Bartels E. Transcranial color-coded ultrasonography. In: Babikian V, Weschsler LR. (eds) *Transcranial Doppler Ultrasonography*, 2nd edn. Boston: Butterworth Heineman, 1999; 271–83

62   Wardlaw JM, Cannon JC. Color transcranial 'power' Doppler ultrasound of intracranial aneurysms. *J Neurosurg* 1996; **84**: 459–61

63   Baumgartner RW, Mattle HP. Contrast-enhanced transcranial ultrasonography. In: Babikian V, Weschsler LR. (eds) *Transcranial Doppler Ultrasonography*, 2nd edn. Boston: Butterworth Heineman, 1999; 389–97

Thrombolysis

Kennedy R Lees

University Department of Medicine and Therapeutics, Gardiner Institute, Western Infirmary, Glasgow, UK

The most widely studied thrombolytic drugs in stroke have been streptokinase (SK) and alteplase. The three large trials with streptokinase were terminated prematurely. The combined results reveal an early increased risk of cerebral haemorrhage and death, with no net benefit at final follow-up, even in subgroups. Some controversy persists, however. The dose may have been inappropriately high, very early treatment has not been fully tested, and concomitant use of aspirin or heparin may have contributed to the deleterious effect. Even so, there is no evidence to guide the choice of a lower dose, streptokinase predisposes to a prolonged anticoagulant effect, and is associated with hypotension which may offset any benefit. The four large alteplase trials in acute stroke were more encouraging. The NINDS study was clearly positive and supporting evidence comes from the two ECASS trials when subjected to meta-analysis. The trials have shown additional functional recovery in 0.6% of patients receiving SK within 6 h and in 7.6% with alteplase, at the expense of excess mortality of 1.1% for alteplase and 11.7% for SK. There was an absolute cerebral haemorrhage excess of 10.7% with SK and 8% for alteplase. If alteplase use is restricted to < 3 h from stroke onset, the NNT is 10.7 with no excess mortality; later treatment (3–6 h) gives an NNT of 26 and absolute mortality of 3.4%. Finally, early fibrinogen depletion with ancrod also appears to have beneficial effects when treatment is started within 3 h of stroke onset.

Further trials are still required to establish, *inter alia*, the outer limit of the therapeutic window, to identify sub-groups of patients in whom clear benefit (or harm) exists and to establish appropriate management protocols for concomitant treatment. Thrombolysis with alteplase within 3 h of stroke onset may be considered for patients in whom haemorrhage and established infarction have been excluded. Trained assessment is essential, since there is an increased risk of haemorrhagic conversion that may be fatal. Patients considering thrombolytic treatment should appreciate that 1 in 10 patients have improved outcome, 1 in 20 suffer haemorrhagic conversion and 1 in 100 may die as a result of treatment. Treatment much later than 3 h from stroke onset in unselected patients is as likely to kill as to cure.

Correspondence to:
Prof. Kennedy R Lees,
University Dept of
Medicine and
Therapeutics,
Gardiner Institute,
Western Infirmary,
Glasgow G11 6NT, UK

Vascular occlusion can be demonstrated in most patients with early ischaemic stroke. Relief of the obstruction leads to reperfusion and possibly, through reduction of infarct size, to improved outcome[1]. Experimental evidence suggests that reperfusion should take place within a few hours of stroke onset in order to produce benefit. There are three potential concerns over the use of thrombolysis in acute stroke. First, haemorrhagic stroke must be excluded before treatment is given. Second, restoration of blood flow to damaged tissue may increase cerebral oedema, thereby increasing intracranial pressure and possibly causing further damage. Third, some spontaneous bleeding into infarcted tissue is often seen, but haemorrhage may be precipitated or exacerbated by thrombolysis with potentially fatal effects. It is several decades since thrombolytic agents were first tried for the treatment of stroke, but it is only within the last few years that adequately designed and powered studies have been undertaken.

Drugs available

The most widely studied thrombolytic drugs in stroke have been streptokinase and alteplase. Urokinase, pro-urokinase and ancrod have also been used. Streptokinase is prepared by filtration of β-haemolytic streptococci cultures, and is thus weakly antigenic. By activating the fibrinolytic system, streptokinase induces dissolution of intravascular thrombi and emboli. Plasminogen and fibrinogen levels decrease and fibrin degradation products increase. The biological and elimination half-life of streptokinase is around 80 min but the fibrin and fibrin degradation fragments following fibrinolysis have an additional anticoagulant effect and the thrombin time may be prolonged for 4 h or more.

Urokinase is an active protease isolated from urine or from human fetal renal cell culture. It converts plasminogen to plasmin and has a half-life of approximately 2.5 h. Compared with streptokinase, it has greater specificity for fibrin and less systemic effects, and is not antigenic.

Alteplase is a tissue plasminogen activator produced by recombinant DNA technology. It acts as a serine protease which has the property of fibrin-enhanced conversion of plasminogen to plasmin. In the absence of fibrin, there is little conversion of plasminogen and this promotes local fibrinolysis with limited systemic proteolysis. Fibrinogen levels are reduced. Alteplase is cleared from the plasma with an initial half-life of less than 5 min.

Ancrod, which is a purified extract of venom from the Malayan pit viper, induces defibrinogenation by splitting fibrinopeptide A from fibrinogen. The reduction in fibrinogen reduces blood viscosity, and produces anticoagulation by depleting the substrates required for thrombus formation. Some local thrombolysis may occur via stimulation of endogenous plasminogen activators, and platelet activation by fibrinogen is secondarily reduced, but ancrod is not a true thrombolytic drug.

Trials

Three urokinase trials were conducted in the 1980s. These were relatively small and have wide confidence intervals[2]. The more recent thrombolysis trials[3–11] have a number of points in common. All had mandatory CT scanning prior to treatment, to exclude primary haemorrhage. A restricted time interval from stroke onset to treatment was stipulated (3, 4, 5 or 6 h according to the trial). Outcome was assessed according to a combined endpoint: death and disability were considered as poor outcome and recovery to functional independence was considered favourable, though the definition of independence varied amongst trials. Outcome was assessed 3–6 months after treatment.

There were three large trials with streptokinase[5,8,11] and all of these were terminated prematurely after MAST-Europe demonstrated a deleterious effect of streptokinase[6]. Meta-analysis of the results[12] shows an early increased risk of cerebral haemorrhage and death, with no net benefit at final follow-up (Figs 1–3). No subgroup of patients could be identified in whom the risk/benefit ratio was improved, though some controversy persists. All of these trials had used a fixed dose of 1.5 MU of streptokinase; patient weight was recorded only within the MAST-Europe trial and retrospective analysis suggests that the outcome was less favourable in lighter patients. Thus, the dose may have been inappro-

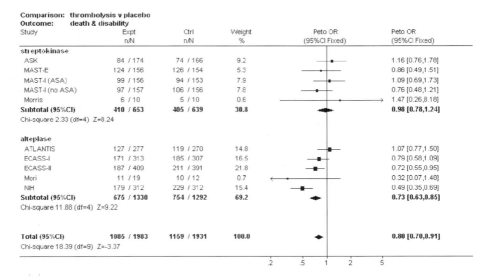

Comparison: thrombolysis v placebo
Outcome: death & disability

Study	Expt n/N	Ctrl n/N	Weight %	Peto OR (95%CI Fixed)	Peto OR (95%CI Fixed)
streptokinase					
ASK	84 / 174	74 / 166	9.2		1.16 [0.76,1.78]
MAST-E	124 / 156	126 / 154	5.3		0.86 [0.49,1.51]
MAST-I (ASA)	99 / 156	94 / 153	7.9		1.09 [0.69,1.73]
MAST-I (no ASA)	97 / 157	106 / 156	7.8		0.76 [0.48,1.21]
Morris	6 / 10	5 / 10	0.6		1.47 [0.26,8.18]
Subtotal (95%CI)	410 / 653	405 / 639	30.8		0.98 [0.78,1.24]
Chi-square 2.33 (df=4) Z=8.24					
alteplase					
ATLANTIS	127 / 277	119 / 270	14.8		1.07 [0.77,1.50]
ECASS-I	171 / 313	185 / 307	16.5		0.79 [0.58,1.09]
ECASS-II	187 / 409	211 / 391	21.8		0.72 [0.55,0.95]
Mori	11 / 19	10 / 12	0.7		0.32 [0.07,1.48]
NIH	179 / 312	229 / 312	15.4		0.49 [0.35,0.69]
Subtotal (95%CI)	675 / 1330	754 / 1292	69.2		0.73 [0.63,0.85]
Chi-square 11.88 (df=4) Z=9.22					
Total (95%CI)	1085 / 1983	1159 / 1931	100.0		0.80 [0.70,0.91]
Chi-square 18.39 (df=9) Z=-3.37					

.2   .5   1   2   5

Fig. 1 Meta-analysis of intravenous thrombolysis trials in which treatment commenced within 6 h of stroke onset. Outcome is based on death and disability, with disability defined according to Barthel score of < 60, modified Rankin of > 2 or the nearest equivalent (Rankin >1 for ATLANTIS trial). There is heterogeneity amongst the alteplase trials ($P < 0.02$), and between the streptokinase and alteplase trials ($P < 0.04$), but not within the streptokinase trials.

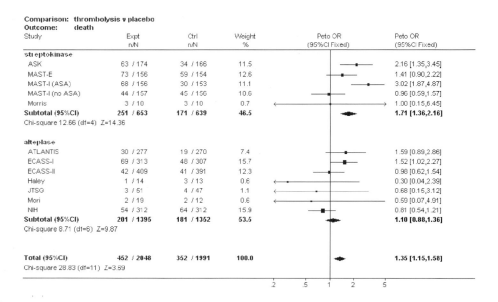

Fig. 2 Meta-analysis of intravenous thrombolysis trials in which treatment commenced within 6 h of stroke onset. Outcome is based on mortality. There is heterogeneity amongst the streptokinase trials (*P* < 0.02), and between the streptokinase and alteplase trials (*P* < 0.01), but not within the alteplase trials.

Comparison: thrombolysis v placebo
Outcome: cerebral haemorrhage

Study	Expt n/N	Ctrl n/N	Weight %	Peto OR (95%CI Fixed)	Peto OR (95%CI Fixed)
streptokinase					
ASK	22 / 174	4 / 166	9.0		4.24 [1.91,9.43]
MAST-E	33 / 156	4 / 154	12.2		5.81 [2.93,11.53]
MAST-I (ASA)	15 / 156	3 / 153	6.4		4.02 [1.55,10.40]
MAST-I (no ASA)	10 / 157	1 / 156	4.0		5.39 [1.62,17.91]
Morris	2 / 10	0 / 10	0.7		8.26 [0.48,142.44]
Subtotal (95%CI)	82 / 653	12 / 639	32.3		4.94 [3.24,7.53]
Chi-square 0.68 (df=4) Z=22.95					
alteplase					
ATLANTIS	20 / 277	2 / 270	7.9		5.34 [2.28,12.53]
ECASS-I	62 / 313	20 / 307	26.7		3.18 [2.00,5.06]
ECASS-II	48 / 407	12 / 386	20.8		3.46 [2.04,5.85]
Haley	0 / 14	1 / 13	0.4		0.13 [0.00,6.33]
JTSG	4 / 51	5 / 47	3.1		0.72 [0.18,2.81]
Mori	2 / 19	1 / 12	1.0		1.27 [0.12,14.12]
NIH	20 / 312	2 / 312	8.0		5.44 [2.32,12.73]
Subtotal (95%CI)	156 / 1393	43 / 1347	67.7		3.34 [2.50,4.47]
Chi-square 10.67 (df=6) Z=22.49					
Total (95%CI)	238 / 2046	55 / 1986	100.0		3.79 [2.98,4.82]
Chi-square 13.58 (df=11) Z=10.90					

.1   .2   1   5   10

Fig. 3 Meta-analysis of intravenous thrombolysis trials in which treatment commenced within 6 h of stroke onset. Outcome is based on symptomatic cerebral haemorrhage. There is no significant heterogeneity either between the streptokinase and alteplase trials, or within either set of trials.

priately high. A limited number of patients were treated at less than 3 h since symptom onset[11], prompting claims that efficacy with early treatment remains untested. Third, heparin and aspirin were widely administered to patients in MAST-Europe, and aspirin was used in all patients in ASK and in half of patients in MAST-Italy. These concomitant treatments may have contributed to the deleterious effect of streptokinase.

These doubts and the relatively low cost of streptokinase lend support to calls for further trials with lower doses of streptokinase. Counter arguments include a lack of evidence to guide the choice of lower dose and critical consideration of the pharmacological properties of streptokinase. The prolonged fibrin degradation inevitably predisposes to an anticoagulant effect for several hours after administration, potentially extending the period of risk for haemorrhagic conversion without necessarily enhancing the chance of useful reperfusion. Second, streptokinase is associated with hypotension in up to 10% of patients treated and some blood pressure reduction may occur in many more[13]. Blood pressure reduction early after cerebral infarction is undesirable and this general effect may offset the potential benefit of reperfusion. Thus, whilst there are unresolved issues in relation to the use of strepto-kinase for acute stroke, further trials could only be justified in the absence of a suitable alternative.

Alteplase may be that suitable alternative. There have now been four large trials in acute stroke, with generally consistent results[3,4,9,14]. Only the NINDS study had clearly positive results according to the pre-specified hypothesis but strong supporting evidence comes from the two European trials (ECASS I and ECASS II) which used a later time window to treatment and which showed positive trends, with an overall benefit when subjected to meta-analysis (Fig. 1).

The NINDS trial was conducted in two parts, both of which were individually positive. On both functional and neurological outcome meas-ures, alteplase increased the proportion of patients with favourable out-come by 12%, or a relative increase of approximately 30%, without adversely affecting mortality. The first ECASS study failed to reach statistical significance on intention to treat analysis, though there was significant benefit within the predefined target population of patients. The unfortunately large number of patients entered to ECASS-I who were ineligible for the target population analysis prompted increased training of investigators involved in ECASS-II. The second trial had a reduced rate of haemorrhagic conversion in both the placebo and active groups but narrowly missed statistical significance for efficacy. The primary endpoint for ECASS II was chosen to match that of the successful NINDS trial; had an alternative endpoint been used, which included mild to moderate disability within the favourable outcome group, ECASS-II would have had a significantly positive result. This difference is almost certainly due

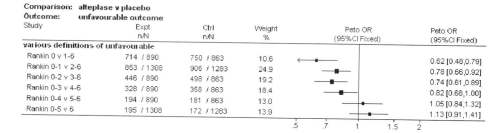

Fig. 4 Meta-analysis of intravenous alteplase trials in which treatment commenced within 6 h of stroke onset. Outcome is based on the Rankin score, showing the effect of varying the definition of 'favourable outcome' between the extremes of no disability (Rankin score 0) to survival regardless of disability (Rankin 0–5).

to the play of chance: when meta-analysis on a series of potential definitions of favourable outcome is undertaken, thrombolysis with alteplase appears to produce benefit, irrespective of the definition of favourable outcome across the higher grades of Rankin handicap scale (Fig. 4). This meta-analysis also reveals a net increase in mortality associated with thrombolysis which is fortunately outweighed by the overall benefit.

Controversies

These meta-analyses fail to consider a point of major controversy. The time window within which treatment is effective has not yet been clearly established. The NINDS trial treated only up to 3 h from stroke onset, with half of patients being treated within 90 min; the ECASS trials treated few patients within 3 h[15] and allowed treatment up to 6 h. The ATLANTIS trial concentrated on patients treated between 3 and 5 h from stroke onset and failed to demonstrate benefit[14]. Meta-analysis confirms the benefit of thrombolysis with alteplase at 3 h or less from stroke onset but between 3–6 h the situation is less clear (Fig. 5). The relationship between time and outcome was explored in a *post hoc* analysis of the NINDS study and after adjustment for co-variates there is evidence that net benefit diminishes with time[16]. However, in highly selected patients, treatment later than 3 h may still be beneficial, as suggested by the PROACT study in which pro-urokinase was administered intra-arterially up to 6 h after stroke onset[17]. Although there are theoretical reasons for anticipating a greater risk of haemorrhagic conversion and consequent death with late treatment, this is not borne out by meta-analysis (Fig 6 & 7): instead, there appears to be a constant risk that must be balanced against a diminishing benefit.

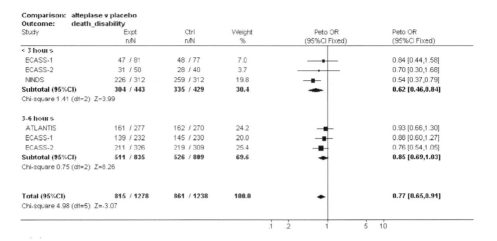

Comparison: alteplase v placebo
Outcome: death_disability

Study	Expt n/N	Ctrl n/N	Weight %	Peto OR (95%CI Fixed)	Peto OR (95%CI Fixed)
< 3 hours					
ECASS-1	47 / 81	48 / 77	7.0		0.84 [0.44,1.58]
ECASS-2	31 / 50	28 / 40	3.7		0.70 [0.30,1.68]
NINDS	226 / 312	259 / 312	19.8		0.54 [0.37,0.79]
Subtotal (95%CI)	**304 / 443**	**335 / 429**	**30.4**		**0.62 [0.46,0.84]**
Chi-square 1.41 (df=2) Z=3.99					
3-6 hours					
ATLANTIS	161 / 277	162 / 270	24.2		0.93 [0.66,1.30]
ECASS-1	139 / 232	145 / 230	20.0		0.88 [0.60,1.27]
ECASS-2	211 / 326	219 / 309	25.4		0.76 [0.54,1.05]
Subtotal (95%CI)	**511 / 835**	**526 / 809**	**69.6**		**0.85 [0.69,1.03]**
Chi-square 0.75 (df=2) Z=8.26					
Total (95%CI)	**815 / 1278**	**861 / 1238**	**100.0**		**0.77 [0.65,0.91]**
Chi-square 4.98 (df=5) Z=-3.07					

Fig. 5 Meta-analysis of intravenous alteplase trials comparing treatment < 3 h with treatment 3–6 h from stroke onset. The ATLANTIS and NINDS protocols were very similar; the ECASS trials included patients in both groups. Outcome is based on death and disability, *i.e.* Rankin grades 2–6. There is no significant heterogeneity amongst the trials.

Early fibrinogen depletion with ancrod also appears to assist recovery. A small randomised trial showed a trend towards benefit of ancrod within 6 h of stroke onset[18] and the recent STAT trial showed efficacy on functional outcome at 3 months when treatment was started within 3 h of stroke onset[19]. An additional 8% of patients had a favourable functional outcome (22% relative increase) without any difference in mortality and with a 3% increase in symptomatic intracranial haemorrhage.

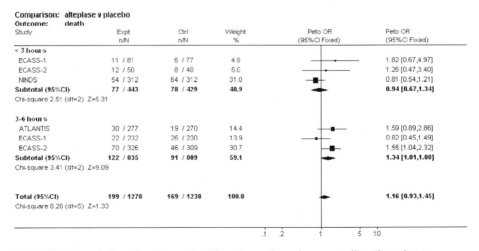

Comparison: alteplase v placebo
Outcome: death

Study	Expt n/N	Ctrl n/N	Weight %	Peto OR (95%CI Fixed)	Peto OR (95%CI Fixed)
< 3 hours					
ECASS-1	11 / 81	6 / 77	4.9		1.82 [0.67,4.97]
ECASS-2	12 / 50	8 / 40	5.0		1.26 [0.47,3.40]
NINDS	54 / 312	64 / 312	31.0		0.81 [0.54,1.21]
Subtotal (95%CI)	**77 / 443**	**78 / 429**	**40.9**		**0.94 [0.67,1.34]**
Chi-square 2.51 (df=2) Z=5.31					
3-6 hours					
ATLANTIS	30 / 277	19 / 270	14.4		1.59 [0.89,2.86]
ECASS-1	22 / 232	26 / 230	13.9		0.82 [0.45,1.49]
ECASS-2	70 / 326	46 / 309	30.7		1.55 [1.04,2.32]
Subtotal (95%CI)	**122 / 835**	**91 / 809**	**59.1**		**1.34 [1.01,1.80]**
Chi-square 3.41 (df=2) Z=9.09					
Total (95%CI)	**199 / 1278**	**169 / 1238**	**100.0**		**1.16 [0.93,1.45]**
Chi-square 8.26 (df=5) Z=1.33					

Fig. 6 Meta-analysis as for Figure 5, with outcome based on mortality. There is no significant heterogeneity amongst the trials.

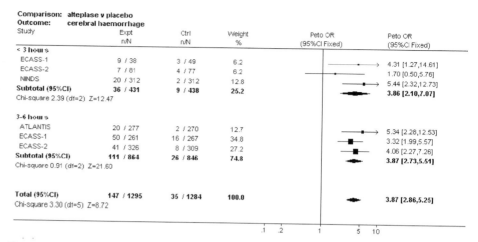

Fig. 7 Meta-analysis as for Figure 5, with outcome based on cerebral haemorrhage. There is no significant heterogeneity amongst the trials.

Taken together, several conclusions can be drawn. First, thrombolysis and related strategies to improve perfusion enhance favourable outcome when administered within 3 h of acute ischaemic stroke. Second, use of these drugs is associated with an increased risk of haemorrhagic conversion that in some cases may be fatal. Third, the randomised trials to date have demonstrated success only within carefully controlled conditions in specialist centres; fears that widespread unselected use, concomitant treatment with aspirin or heparin, and treatment beyond 3 h lead to risks that outweigh the benefit, may be justified. Only a small proportion of patients, probably around 1%, were eligible for the successful trials. With local patient education and suitable service provision some urban areas are now treating 15–20% of patients with alteplase, but there remains a need for treatment that can be safely administered to a wider population.

Unanswered questions

Further trials are still required to establish the outer limit of the therapeutic window, to identify subgroups of patients in whom clear benefit (or harm) exists and to establish appropriate management protocols for concomitant treatment. Thus, whilst there is a *prima facie* case for treatment between 3–6 h from stroke onset, it is likely that the infarct is already established in most patients. Selection for treatment using MRI may be a possible strategy since a diffusion/perfusion mismatch may represent salvageable penumbra. The numbers of patients treated so far are too limited to guide strategies for blood pressure control, antiplatelet therapy or anticoagulation. The possibility of neuroprotection combined with thrombolysis remains an experimental approach. Alteplase use outside specialist centres has not been tested. Optimal methods need to be found for educating the public and the emergency services to facilitate rapid presentation at suitably equipped hospitals. The challenge will be to fund and recruit to future thrombolysis trials in stroke without compromising either patient safety or the new-found status of this effective treatment.

Conclusions

Odds ratios help with trial interpretation but should not determine clinical practice: for this, absolute risk reductions, or numbers needed to treat (NNT) merit consideration. Thus, a treatment associated with an odds ratio for unfavourable outcome of 0.7 is useful if the population treated has an underlying risk for poor outcome of 50%, since the true benefit will be 50% – (0.7 x 50%) = 15%; but if the underlying rate of poor outcome is only 5% then universal application of the treatment will only be of benefit to 1.5%. The NNT is the reciprocal of the absolute benefit: in the latter case, only one patient would benefit out of every 67 treated. Taking the trial data from Figures 1–3 and 4–6, absolute risk changes and associated NNT can be calculated for various strategies.

Streptokinase within 6 h of stroke cannot be justified: mortality was 38.4% with streptokinase *versus* 26.8% with placebo, the cerebral haemorrhage rates were 12.6% *versus* 1.9%, and the final outcome was unfavourable in 62.8% *versus* 63.4%. Thus, the NNT was 167 for streptokinase under the circumstances of the trials, at the expense of 18–20 significant brain haemorrhages and 19–20 deaths.

By contrast, alteplase within 6 h of stroke has an NNT of 13, at the expense of one cerebral haemorrhage and rare mortality (0.14 deaths for every favourable outcome). Even this is misleading, in view of the time-dependency of results. Assuming that alteplase use is restricted to < 3 h from stroke onset, the benefit is more convincing. A conservative estimate of the NNT is 10.7 without a net increase in mortality, even after accounting for the 6.3% absolute risk of cerebral haemorrhage; with alternative definitions of disability smaller NNTs should be achieved. In contrast, treatment between 3–6 h from stroke onset gives an NNT of 26 and absolute mortality approaching one – a true 'kill or cure' situation.

Patients who present early to hospital with suspected stroke should be assessed urgently. If the time of stroke onset can be clearly established and

Table 1 An example of a screening protocol for considering thrombolysis with alteplase after acute ischaemic stroke, modified from entry criteria used in the NINDS trial[4]

The following should be answered YES:

Does the patient have symptoms of acute stroke?
Is there a measurable deficit on the NIH stroke scale?
Was the patient previously independent?
Is there a clear time of onset within the last 180 min?
Has a CT brain scan since stroke onset excluded haemorrhage?
Have you personally looked at the CT film?

The following should be answered NO:

Are there early signs of infarction on the CT scan, affecting more than a third of
    the MCA territory?
Has the patient suffered head trauma or stroke within the last 3 months?
Has the patient undergone major surgery within the last 2 weeks?
Is there a history of intracranial haemorrhage?
Is the history suggestive of subarachnoid haemorrhage?
Is the systolic BP > 185 mmHg?
Is the diastolic BP > 110 mmHg?
Has any hypertensive treatment been used to attain the above limits?
Are the symptoms/signs minor or rapidly improving?
Has there been gastrointestinal or urinary tract haemorrhage within the last 21 days?
Has there been an arterial puncture at a non-compressible site within the last 7 days?
Was there a seizure at the time of stroke onset?
Has the patient taken anticoagulants or heparin within the last 48 h, with an increased PTT?

And if available:

Is the prothrombin time > 15 s?
Is the platelet count < 100,000?
Is the plasma glucose < 2.7 mmol/l or > 22.2 mmol/l?

a good quality CT brain scan has excluded evidence of intracranial haemorrhage or of a cause for the neurological symptoms other than ischaemic stroke, then the patient should be considered for thrombolysis with alteplase. Eligibility criteria as used by NINDS (Table 1) should be confirmed[4], but additional CT criteria may be justified: if early infarction already involves more than a third of the relevant middle cerebral artery territory, then thrombolysis may be unsafe. These CT changes can be subtle, and both training and experience are necessary to interpret the scan reliably. With modern electronic data transfer facilities, regional centres could be established to assist in on-line CT scan interpretation; video links could even be used to confirm clinical details.

Where possible, the potential risks and benefits should be explained to the patient, important points being improved likelihood of recovery from disability (1 in 10 patients benefit), a 6–10-fold increased risk of haemorrhagic conversion (approximately 1 in 20 patients) and little change in the risk of death (at worst, 1 in 100 patients). The opportunity cost of treatment is probably greatly outweighed by the reduction in long-term disability. A strategy of reserving thrombolysis for patients with severe stroke is probably counter productive, since the risk:benefit ratio may be greater within that group than in patients with mild stroke; conversely, patients who have an insignificant neurological deficit 3 h after stroke onset are unlikely to derive benefit. Alteplase should not be used beyond 3 h from stroke onset unless the patient accepts that this strategy is as likely to kill as to cure. Heparin, warfarin or further doses of aspirin should be withheld until 24 h from time of alteplase treatment.

New centres proposing to offer a thrombolysis service should carefully consider the training issues, the need for 24 h staffing and the obligation to audit their results. There is scope for nationally organised approaches to these issues.

References

1   Barber PA, Davis SM, Infeld B *et al*. Spontaneous reperfusion after ischemic stroke is associated with improved outcome. *Stroke* 1998; **29**: 2522–8

2   Wardlaw JM, Warlow CP, Counsell C. Systematic review of evidence on thrombolytic therapy for acute ischaemic stroke. *Lancet* 1997; **350**: 607–14

3   The European Cooperative Acute Stroke Study (ECASS). Intravenous thrombolysis with recombinant tissue plasminogen activator for acute hemispheric stroke. *JAMA* 1995; **274**: 1017–25

4   The National Institute of Neurological Disorders and Stroke rt-PA Stroke Study Group. Tissue plasminogen activator for acute ischemic stroke. *N Engl J Med* 1995; **333**: 1581–7

5   Multicentre Acute Stroke Trial–Italy (MAST-I) Group. Randomised controlled trial of streptokinase, aspirin, and combination of both in treatment of acute ischaemic stroke. *Lancet* 1995; **346**: 1509–14

6   Hommel M, Boissel J, for the MAST Group. Trials of streptokinase in severe acute ischaemic stroke. *Lancet* 1995; **345**: 578

7   Hommel M, Boissel JP, Cornu C *et al*. Termination of trial of streptokinase in severe acute ischaemic stroke. *Lancet* 1995; **345**: 57

8   The Multicenter Acute Stroke Trial – Europe Study Group. Thrombolytic therapy with streptokinase in acute ischemic stroke. *N Engl J Med* 1996; **335**: 145–50

9   Hacke W, Kaste M, Fieschi C *et al*. Randomised double-blind placebo-controlled trial of thrombolytic therapy with intravenous alteplase in acute ischemic stroke (ECASS II). *Lancet* 1998; **652**: 1245–51

10   Donnan GA, Davis SM, Chambers BR *et al*. Trials of streptokinase in severe acute ischaemic stroke (The Australian Streptokinase Trial). *Lancet* 1995; **345**: 578–9

11   Donnan GA, Davis SM, Chambers BR *et al*. Streptokinase for acute ischemic stroke with relationship to time of administration: Australian Streptokinase (ASK) Trial Study Group. *JAMA* 1996; **276**: 961–6

12   Cornu F, Boutitie F, Candelise, et al. Streptokinase in acute ischemic stroke: An individual patient data meta-analysis: The thrombolysis in Acute Stroke Pooling Project. *Stroke* 2000; **31**: 1555–60

13   ISIS-2 (Second International Study of Infarct Survival) Collaborative Group. Randomised trial of intravenous streptokinase, oral aspirin, both, or neither among 17,187 cases of suspected acute myocardial infarction: ISIS2. *Lancet* 1988; **ii**: 349–60

14 Clark WM, Albers GW, for the ATLANTIS Stroke Study Investigators. The ATLANTIS rt-PA (alteplase) Acute Stroke Trial: final results [Abstract]. *Stroke* 1999; **30**; 234

15 Steiner T, Bluhmki E, Kaste M *et al.* The ECASS 3-hour cohort. *Cerebrovasc Dis* 1998; **8**: 198–203

16 Marler JR, Tilley BC, Lu M, *et al.* Earlier treatment associated with better outcome in the NINDS TPA Stroke Study [Abstract]. *Stroke* 1999; **30**: 244

17 Del Zoppo GJ, Higashida RT, Furlan AJ *et al.* PROACT: a phase II randomized trial of recombinant pro-urokinase by direct arterial delivery in acute middle cerebral artery stroke. *Stroke* 1998; **29**: 4–11

18 Olinger CP, Brott TG, Barsan WG *et al.* Use of ancrod in acute or progressing ischemic cerebral infarction. *Ann Emerg Med* 1988; **17**: 1208–9

19 Sherman DG, Atkinson RP, Chippendale T *et al.* Intravenous ancrod for treatment of acute, ischemic stroke: the STAT study: a randomized controlled trial. *JAMA* 2000; 282: 2395–403

Neuroprotection

Kennedy R Lees

University Department of Medicine and Therapeutics, Gardiner Institute, Western Infirmary, Glasgow, UK

Thrombolysis improves stroke outcome, but is applicable to a limited number of patients. Neuroprotection has the prospect to be universally offered, either alone or in combination with thrombolysis. Potential drug targets include elements of the excitotoxic glutamate cascade, calcium entry, intracellular protease activation, free radical damage, the inflammatory response and membrane repair. Clinical trials with many agents have so far been disappointing, but hindsight reveals flaws in the choice of compound, the dose that was administered or trial design. A further crop of trials has recently been initiated or completed, with results expected from 2000 to 2003. More selective, potent or better tolerated neuroprotective strategies are still being developed for clinical use, and approaches to trial conduct are advancing: increased use of computer randomisation algorithms or diffusion-weighted magnetic resonance imaging should improve trial power. The prospects for a safe and effective treatment to improve stroke outcome remain good.

Within the first hours after stroke onset, human brain tissue can be salvaged and functional outcome improved by thrombolysis. Barriers to widespread application of thrombolysis include the short time window, the need for expert assessment and imaging, and the inherent risk of haemorrhagic conversion. Alternative forms of treatment are required that can be given universally. The biochemical and inflammatory cascades that are initiated by ischaemia can be interrupted experimentally to limit infarct size and improve functional outcome. Inevitably, clinical trials lag several years behind experimental research, and often produce less definitive results. The last decade has seen major trials with free radical scavengers and various forms of glutamate antagonist, and preliminary work on the inflammatory response.

Neuroprotective approaches

Cerebral ischaemia triggers excessive presynaptic release of the excitatory neurotransmitter glutamate and the energy uncoupling prevents active removal of glutamate from the synaptic cleft. The excess of

Correspondence to: Prof. Kennedy R Lees, University Department of Medicine and Therapeutics, Gardiner Institute, Western Infirmary, Glasgow G11 6NT, UK

glutamate over-stimulates postsynaptic receptors such as the N-methyl-D-aspartate (NMDA) receptor, thereby opening the associated ion channel and allowing sodium and calcium ions to enter the cell whilst potassium flows outwards. The calcium influx activates intracellular proteases and initiates a cascade of further energy consuming and ultimately lethal processes[1,2]. Glutamate release after human stroke has been confirmed, lasting for hours and possibly days[3–5].

The NMDA receptor-ion channel complex has several ligand binding sites that are amenable to manipulation[6]. Magnesium produces a voltage-dependent block of the NMDA ion channel. Open ion channels can be blocked non-competitively by drugs such as aptiganel. Competitive antagonists act at the glutamate recognition site, e.g. selfotel. Glycine is an essential co-agonist for glutamate, and so glycine antagonists such as GV150526[7,8] indirectly prevent activation of the ion channel. The initial release of glutamate is prevented by sodium channel blockers such as sipatrigine[9,10] and lubeluzole[11]. Calcium-dependent proteolysis and nitric oxide synthesis can be targeted directly. Drugs such as lubeluzole may act at several levels in the cascade[11].

Ischaemia and subsequent reperfusion together create ideal conditions for the generation of highly reactive free radicals which exacerbate membrane damage. Membrane repair may be amenable to improvement by provision of precursor molecules such as citicoline.

From several hours until 5–7 days after the onset of ischaemia, an inflammatory response is generated, with infiltration of neutrophils. Although this is part of the re-organisation process, it also appears to contribute to infarct expansion. In experimental circumstances, treatment after the onset of ischaemia with free radical scavengers, glutamate antagonists or anti-inflammatory strategies can limit infarct size, leading to the conclusion that these strategies may have a clinical role.

Recent clinical trials

Tirilazad mesylate is a lipid peroxidation inhibitor, i.e. free radical scavenger, that has been tested in head injury, subarachnoid haemorrhage and ischaemic stroke. Interim analysis of the initial phase III stroke trials suggested a lack of efficacy[12], and trials were recommenced at higher dosage; the subsequent trials were abandoned when questions over safety emerged from the larger, European trial. Full details have not been published. Trials in head injury were also unsuccessful.

Enlimomab is a monoclonal antibody against the intercellular adhesion molecule, ICAM-1. After a small uncontrolled phase II trial[13], a randomised trial in 625 patients compared enlimomab with placebo, within 6 h of ischaemic stroke onset. The 3 month outcome, deaths and adverse events were worse in the enlimomab group and it appears that there may have been a pro-inflammatory response[14].

The results with glutamate antagonists have so far been similarly disappointing. Selfotel is a competitive glutamate antagonist. Its use was associated with sedation, agitation, confusion and hallucinations. Two phase III trials of selfotel within 6 h of ischaemic stroke were abandoned due to a treatment related increase in early mortality[15]. It was uncertain whether this was a direct toxic effect or if it was secondary to the influence of sedation on management[16].

A smaller study with the non-competitive NMDA antagonist, aptiganel, was terminated early on the grounds of futility (unpublished data).

Lubeluzole is an ion channel and nitric oxide blocker[11] that has been tested in 3 large ischaemic stroke studies. Within a 6 h time window, the European study was neutral[17]. The American study suggested improved functional outcome but not mortality, without raising safety concerns[18]. A third and larger trial, with a longer time window of 8 h, failed to confirm benefit from lubeluzole[19].

Clomethiazole is a GABA agonist that was tested within 12 h of stroke onset in 1360 patients. Functional outcome at 3 months was not improved, except within a sub-group of patients with large middle cerebral artery strokes; here, benefit was seen both 0–6 h and 6–12 h from stroke onset (Fig. 1)[20].

Citicoline is a phosphatidyl choline membrane precursor, with putative effects on membrane repair. Current phase III investigation is supported by encouraging trends from preliminary trials.

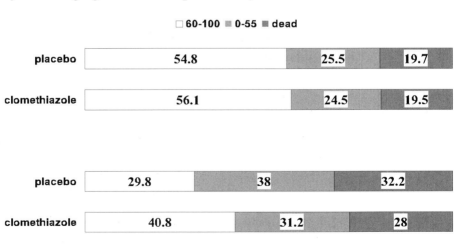

Fig. 1 Results of the CLASS trial of clomethiazole within 12 h of acute ischaemic stroke[20]. The intention-to-treat analysis in all patients was neutral (top bars, *P* = 0.65), but a *post hoc* subgroup analysis was positive (lower bars, *P* = 0.008), suggesting benefit in the patients with large middle cerebral artery strokes ('total anterior circulation syndromes'), possibly because they have a larger volume of penumbral tissue at presentation.

Numerous other potentially neuroprotective compounds have had development abandoned in the light of disappointing clinical experience. Potential reasons for these failures deserve consideration.

Clinical trial design issues

Trial design in stroke is influenced by the high average age of the patients, the many mechanisms and varying severity of the condition, and the interactions between treatment, functional independence and survival.

Endpoints

Reduction of disability is generally perceived as more important than improved survival. Disability is usually determined by stroke severity, whereas age and concomitant disease contribute to mortality. Most stroke trials test for a reduction in the combined endpoint of death and disability. Disability is usually measured according to activities of daily living: the Barthel index records whether the patient requires help from another person for everyday tasks such as feeding, dressing, walking, *etc*. A score of above 60/100 is consistent with life at home in the company of a carer. A score of 95 or higher permits a wholly independent existence[21].

Alternatively, handicap can be recorded using the Rankin scale, with scores of 1 or 0 representing little or no disability, and scores of 3 or higher representing disability that requires considerable support or institutional care[22]. Functional outcome is usually measured at 3 or 6 months after stroke, once recovery is largely complete.

Infarct size from cerebral imaging shows variability and correlates only loosely with function. There is increasing interest in using MRI as a surrogate measure for stroke trials, however. An early diffusion weighted MRI scan can identify tissue 'at risk' of infarction; a perfusion/diffusion mismatch may be used to select patients for intervention trials, or change in infarct volume on a T_2-MRI scan after 1–3 months may be used as a measure of treatment effect[23,24].

Entry criteria

A compromise is necessary, between restrictive measures to maximise success of the trial, and universal applicability of the treatment. A new, measurable neurological deficit on a background of pre-morbid independence is essential where functional independence is the primary outcome measure. Comatose patients are usually excluded on the grounds that they will almost inevitably die. Preclinical data suggest that neuroprotective strategies are unlikely to be effective beyond 6 h from onset of ischaemia, and that detection of benefit clinically will be optimal if treatment is started within about 2 h. It is notable that recent stroke trials have targeted patients within 6 h of symptom onset, but only trials with a 3 h window have been positive[25,26]. The optimal duration of treatment is unknown, but well tolerated drugs are usually administered for up to 72 h to cover the period of continued ischaemia[27].

Prognostic variables

Stratification of patients on the basis of age and stroke severity at entry is justified and early CT scanning is required to detect any confounding imbalance in the numbers of patients with intracerebral haemorrhage. A pretreatment CT scan is essential if thrombolysis is proposed, but neuroprotective drugs that are safe in cerebral haemorrhage can be given prior to the scan. In this case, the target population for the primary analysis ('ischaemic stroke') is defined after objective independent review of the CT scans, undertaken blind to treatment allocation.

General management

The definition of standard treatment varies geographically. Elements of general care that influence outcome include admission to a specialist stroke unit[28,29], measures to avoid aspiration, control of blood sugar, infection, *etc*, and the use of thrombolysis.

Statistical issues

There is continuing debate over the optimal approach to analysis of functional outcome data. Arbitrary division of the Barthel or Rankin scales potentially disregards important information about treatment effects in all but a narrow range of patients whose outcome, if untreated, would have fallen close to the selected cutpoint. In addition, adequate statistical power is only achieved if large numbers of patients (*e.g.* 1500–2000) are recruited. A multicentre approach is essential.

Safety

The value of data monitoring by an independent committee has been demonstrated by several recent stroke trials[15,30–32].

Potential reasons for failure of clinical trials

Failures in drug development are common, particularly in a new therapeutic field. Although superficially discouraging, recent trial results have been informative.

Three primary reasons for trial failure may relate to the concept of salvage-ability, to inappropriate choice of drug or of its dose, or to flawed trial design. With regard to the first of these, the strength of the preclinical evidence for neuroprotective efficacy and the success of post ictus thrombolysis in clinical practice provide proof of concept. By the time patients arrive at hospital, patients will have limited tissue that is amenable to salvage: 70% of the potential infarct volume may be irretrievably damaged, 18% viable but underperfused and 12% is healthy tissue that is fated to be recruited into the infarct, possibly by excitotoxic processes[33].

Choice of drug and/or dose

The issues surrounding preclinical testing of potential neuroprotective compounds have been discussed in a recent consensus statement[34]. Infarct volume reductions seen experimentally may not scale directly to man, and conditions for neuroprotection cannot be optimised in human stroke as they are in the laboratory. Awareness of these issues can lead to more rigorous selection of compounds for clinical trials.

Adverse effects must be considered. Dose-limiting intolerance may prevent attainment of adequate concentrations in humans. There may be species differences in the pharmacokinetics, especially affecting the brain, and the possibility that elderly, ill patients are more sensitive to pharmacodynamic effects such as hypotension than the young, anaesthetised laboratory animal. If adverse effects occur in the laboratory situation, data from the affected animal may be discounted, whereas more rigorous analysis of clinical trials expects the intention-to-treat principle to be applied.

Flaws in trial design

The trial inclusion criteria should define a population in whom the treatment is most likely to produce benefit: the need to 'enrich' the contributing population is increasingly recognised. Patients with subcortical 'lacunar' stroke have largely white matter ischaemic damage that may not be amenable to neuroprotection with glutamate antagonists. Subgroup analysis of the CLASS Study with clomethiazole suggests that

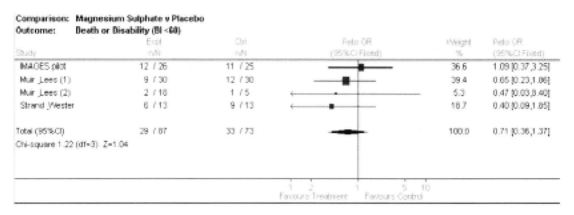

Fig. 2 Meta-analysis of results of pilot trials with intravenous magnesium for the treatment of acute stroke. The primary outcome measure was death or disability, defined as Barthel index < 60/100. The point estimate of the odds ratio for unfavourable outcome (0.71) is similar to that seen with thrombolysis, though with only 160 patients, the confidence intervals remain very wide. The phase 3 trial of magnesium (IMAGES) has now recruited over 900 patients.

patients with large cortical strokes may have derived benefit that was concealed by the inclusion of other groups of patients (Fig. 1)[20]. The first ECASS Study was compromised by the inclusion of many ineligible patients: only 80% of the treated population were eligible for the 'target population' analysis[35]. Although it is reasonable to analyse for treatment effects in a target population, it is crucial to demonstrate that the protocol-recommended inclusion criteria can be applied in practice. The positive target analysis of ECASS-I has been largely discounted since the ineligible patients were inadvertently included in contravention of the protocol, and appeared to experience an adverse outcome with thrombolysis. In contrast, trials such as GAIN and IMAGES are deliberately collecting safety data in patients with haemorrhagic stroke, but should a neutral or deleterious effect be uncovered in this subgroup, any beneficial effect in the ischaemic population will not have been prejudiced.

Choice of trial endpoint may also influence interpretation of the result. Random chance may cause the ideal cutpoint on disability scores to vary from one trial to the next. Underpowered trials such as ECASS appear inconsistent in their effects at different levels of functional outcome, yet meta-analysis reveals consistency across several trials and even suggests that a novel endpoint is optimal (Rankin 0 versus all other patients). Unless a drug is particularly targeted at a mechanism that would affect survival, mortality is an inappropriate primary endpoint for stroke trials: 'survival free from disability' is better.

Preclinical data suggest that the neuroprotective time window is short and that few, if any, drugs are effective beyond 3 h from stroke onset. Conversely, most clinical trials have permitted treatment up to 6, 8 or even 12 h after stroke onset. Whether or not the drugs may have any benefit at this stage, the possibility of detecting neuroprotection diminishes markedly with time.

The duration of neuroprotective therapy must also be considered. Whilst insufficient duration of therapy may simply postpone, rather than prevent, infarction, excessive treatment duration increases the chance of adverse effects and may limit mobilisation and rehabilitation[27]. The optimal approach may be to provide neuroprotection until reperfusion can be achieved with thrombolysis or other means.

Effect of confounding variables

Imbalanced randomisation can lead to substantial variation in risk of poor outcome between groups. Stratification on the major prognostic variables such as age and stroke severity is practical but intracerebral haemorrhage, blood sugar level, temperature, blood pressure and many other variables can influence outcome. Stratification on multiple variables is impractical though adaptive randomisation, sometimes called minimisation, using a computer algorithm can be used to maintain balance[36,37].

Confounding effects of the drug may also interfere with interpretation of trial results. For example, blood pressure reduction even if it appears clinically insignificant, may adversely affect outcome[38]. Raised blood sugar is associated with a substantial reduction in survival and yet the optimal approach to management of hyperglycaemia has yet to be tested within randomised trials[39,40]. The use of concomitant treatment such as aspirin, heparin and sedatives and the threshold for prescription of antibiotics, administration of fluids and supplemental feeding approaches all can influence outcome to a potentially greater extent than drug intervention.

Clinical trials in progress

There is presently no proven neuroprotective drug for clinical use but considerable optimism persists. Several large trials have recently been completed or are in progress, that incorporate some of the above lessons.

GAIN trials

GV150526 is a selective competitive antagonist at the glycine site of the NMDA receptor[7]. It appears to be neuroprotective when administered up to 6 h after onset of ischaemia in the permanent middle cerebral artery occlusion model in the rat[8]. It is well tolerated by patients, with the most notable dose-limiting effect being a transient and asymptomatic rise in bilirubin and liver transaminases[41]. Two phase III multicentre trials have recently completed recruitment. GAIN International randomised 1805 patients within 6 h of stroke onset, of whom approximately 80% had ischaemic stroke. The primary endpoint of the trial is based on reduction in death and disability as defined by a composite endpoint on the Barthel scale. GAIN Americas follows a closely similar design with approximately 1600 patients. Both trials have recently reported, with neutral results[43].

CLASS IHT

CLASS IHT is a group of 3 multicentre trials of clomethiazole administered within 12 h of stroke symptoms, due to complete in 2000. Up to 200 patients with cerebral infarction who are receiving thrombolysis, 200 patients with intracerebral haemorrhage and 1200 patients with large ischaemic cerebral infarctions will be recruited. The primary endpoint is based on functional recovery as defined by the proportion of patients scoring 60 or more on the Barthel index at 3 months.

Citicoline

Citicoline is a phosphatidylcholine precursor and membrane stabiliser that has previously been tested in small phase II/III trials with encouraging but indeterminate results. A phase III trial of citicoline 2000 mg versus placebo for 6 weeks has completed randomisation of approximately 900 patients, with assessment of neurological function after 3 months.

Magnesium

The Intravenous Magnesium Efficacy in Stroke Study (IMAGES) is randomising patients who present within 12 h of stroke onset, who have limb weakness and are conscious. Treatment is with intravenous magnesium 16 mmol over 15 min followed by 65 mmol over 24 h and outcome is assessed by Barthel index at 3 months. 2700 patients will be randomised, with at least 900 treated within 6 h of stroke onset. Results are expected around 2002. Magnesium has the advantages of its known safety profile, simplicity and extremely low cost.

Controversies

Applicability of treatment

The onset time of stroke is unknown in up to half of patients who present to hospital and a low proportion arrive within the first few hours[42]. Recruitment to neuroprotective trials in stroke is generally low, but subject to cost limitations a safe treatment could be administered to many more. As the proven benefits of specialised stroke care are translated into altered provision of services, the prospects for undertaking clinical trials are improving and the practicalities of administering treatment are similarly enhanced. Cerebral imaging is no longer a rarity and selection of patients for trials on the basis of MRI appearances is now a practical possibility. Whether or not the current series of trials produces a successful treatment remains to be seen, but with greater understanding of the mechanisms of ischaemic cell death and new targets for drug treatment, it is only a matter of time before neuroprotection becomes part of standard clinical management.

References

1   Rothman S. Synaptic release of excitatory amino acid neurotransmitter mediates anoxic neuronal death. *J Neurosci* 1984; **4**: 1884–91
2   McCulloch J. Excitatory amino acid antagonists and their potential for the treatment of ischaemic brain damage in man. *Br J Clin Pharmacol* 1992; **34**: 106–14
3   Bullock R, Zauner A, Woodward J, Young HF. Massive persistent release of excitatory amino acids following human occlusive stroke. *Stroke* 1995; **26**: 2187–9
4   Davalos A, Castillo J, Serena J, Noya M. Duration of glutamate release after acute ischemic stroke. *Stroke* 1997; **28**: 708–10
5   Castillo J, Davalos A, Noya M. Progression of ischaemic stroke and excitotoxic aminoacids. *Lancet* 1997; **249**: 79–83
6   Muir KW, Lees KR. Clinical experience with excitatory amino acid antagonist drugs. *Stroke* 1995; **26**: 503–13
7   Fabio RD, Cugola A, Donati D *et al.* Identification and pharmacological characterization of GV150526, a novel glycine antagonist as a potent neuroprotective agent. *Drugs Future* 1998; **23**: 61–9
8   Bordi F, Pietra C, Ziviani L, Reggiani A. The glycine antagonist GV150526 protects somatosensory evoked potentials and reduces the infarct area in the MCAo model of focal ischemia in the rat. *Exp Neurol* 1997; **145**: 425–33
9   Muir KW, Hamilton SJC, Lunnon MW, Hobbiger S, Lees KR. Safety and tolerability of 619C89 after acute stroke. *Cerebrovasc Dis* 1998; **8**: 31–7
10 Muir KW, Lees KR, Holzapfel L. Phase II clinical trial of sipatrigine (619C89) by continuous infusion in acute stroke. *Cerebrovasc Dis* 2000: In press
11 Graul A, Castaner J. Lubeluzole. Neuronal injury inhibitor, glutamate release inhibitor. *Drugs Future* 1997; **22**: 629–33
12 The RANTTAS Investigators. A randomized trial of tirilizad mesylate in patients with acute stroke (RANTTAS). *Stroke* 1996; **27**: 1453–8

13   Schneider D, Berrouschot J, Brandt T *et al.* Safety, pharmacokinetics and biological activity of enlimomab (anti-ICAM-1 antibody): an open-label, dose escalation study in patients hospitalized for acute stroke. *Eur Neurol* 1998; 40: 78–83

14   The Enlimomab Acute Stroke Trial Investigators. The Enlimomab Acute Stroke Trial: Final Results. *Cerebrovasc Dis* 1997; 7(**Suppl 4**): 18 [Abstract]

15   Davis SM, Albers GW, Diener HC, Lees KR, Norris J. Termination of acute stroke studies involving selfotel treatment. *Lancet* 1997; 349: 32

16   Davis SM, Lees KR, Albers GW *et al.* Selfotel in acute ischemic stroke: possible neurotoxic effects of an NMDA antagonist. *Stroke* 2000; 31: 347–354

17   Diener HC, for the European and Australian Lubeluzole Ischaemic Stroke Study Group. Multinational randomised controlled trial of lubeluzole in acute ischaemic stroke. *Cerebrovasc Dis* 1998; 8: 172–81

18   Grotta J, for the US and Canadian Lubeluzole Ischemic Stroke Study Group. Lubeluzole treatment of acute ischemic stroke. *Stroke* 1997; 28: 2338–46

19   Diener HC. Lubeluzole in acute ischemic stroke treatment: lack of efficacy in a large phase III study with an 8-hour window [Abstract]. *Stroke* 1999; 30: 234

20   Wahlgren NG, Ranasinha KW, Rosolacci T *et al.* Clomethiazole Acute Stroke Study (CLASS): results of a randomized, controlled trial of clomethiazole versus placebo in 1360 acute stroke patients. *Stroke* 1999; 30: 21–8

21   Granger CV, Dewis LS, Peters NC, Sherwood CC, Barrett JE. Stroke rehabilitation: analysis of repeated Barthel index measures. *Arch Phys Med Rehabil* 1979; 60: 14–7

22   Rankin J. Cerebral vascular accidents in patients over the age of 60, II: prognosis. *Scot Med J* 1957; 2: 200–15

23   Moseley ME, Kucharczyk J, Mintorovitch J *et al.* Diffusion-weighted MR imaging of acute stroke: correlation with T2-weighted and magnetic susceptibility-enhanced MR imaging in cats. *Am J Neuroradiol* 1990; 11: 423–9

24   Warach S, Boska M, Welch KMA. Pitfalls and potential of clinical diffusion-weighted MR imaging in acute stroke. *Stroke* 1997; 28: 481–2

25   The National Institute of Neurological Disorders and Stroke rt-PA Stroke Study Group. Tissue plasminogen activator for acute ischemic stroke. *N Engl J Med* 1995; 333: 1581–7

26   Sherman DG, Atkinson RP, Chippendale T *et al.* Intravenous ancrod for treatment of acute ischemic stroke: the STAT study: a randomized controlled trial. *JAMA* 2000; 282: 2395–403

27   Dyker AG, Lees KR. Duration of neuroprotective treatment for ischemic stroke. *Stroke* 1998; 29: 535–42

28   Stroke Unit Trialists' Collaboration. Collaborative systematic review of the randomised trials of organised inpatient (stroke unit) care after stroke. *BMJ* 1997; 314: 1151–9

29   Indredavik B, Slordahl SA, Bakke RPT, Rokseth R, Håheim LL. Stroke unit treatment – long term effects. *Stroke* 1997; 28: 1861–6

30   Astrup J, Siesjö BK, Symon L. Thresholds in cerebral ischaemia. The ischaemic penumbra. *Stroke* 1981; 12: 723–5

31   Donnan GA, Davis SM, Chambers BR *et al.* Trials of streptokinase in severe acute ischaemic stroke (The Australian Streptokinase Trial). *Lancet* 1995; 345: 578–9

32   Hommel M, Boissel JP, Cornu C *et al.* Termination of trial of streptokinase in severe acute ischaemic stroke. *Lancet* 1995; 345: 57

33   Heiss WD, Thiel A, Grond M, Graf R. Which targets are relevant for therapy of acute ischemic stroke? *Stroke* 1999; 30: 1486–9

34   Stroke Therapy Academic Industry Roundtable (STAIR). Recommendations for standards regarding preclinical neuroprotective and restorative drug development. *Stroke* 1999; 30: 2752–8

35   The European Cooperative Acute Stroke Study (ECASS). Intravenous thrombolysis with recombinant tissue plasminogen activator for acute hemispheric stroke. *JAMA* 1995; 274: 1017–25

36   Weir CJ, Lees KR. Value of minimisation for treatment allocation in acute stroke trials [Abstract]. *Cerebrovasc Dis* 1998; 8: 32

37   Weir CJ, Lees KR. Power of treatment allocation by adaptive stratification in anacute stroke trial. *Cerebrovasc Dis* 1999; 9: 114 [Abstract]

38 Wahlgren NG, MacMahon DG, De Keyser J, Indredavik B, Ryman T. Intravenous Nimodipine West European Stroke Trial (INWEST) of nimodipine in the treatment of acute ischaemic stroke. *Cerebrovasc Dis* 1994; **4**: 204–10

39 Weir CJ, Murray GD, Dyker AG, Lees KR. Is hyperglycaemia an independent predictor of poor outcome after acute stroke? Results of a long term follow up study. *BMJ* 1997; **314**: 1303–6

40 Scott JF, Robinson GM, French JM, O'Connell JE, Alberti KGMM, Gray CS. Glucose potassium insulin infusions in the treatment of acute stroke patients with mild to moderate hyperclycemia: The Glucose Insulin in Stroke Trial (GIST). *Stroke* 1999; **30**: 793–9

41 Dyker AG, Lees KR. The safety and tolerability of GV150526 (a glycine site antagonist at the NMDA receptor) in patients with acute stroke: Two double blind, randomised, placebo controlled, parallel group, ascending dose studies. *Stroke* 1999; **30**: 986–92

42 Morris AD, Grosset DG, Squire IB, Lees KR, Bone I, Reid JL. The experiences of an acute stroke unit-implications for multicentre acute stroke trials. *J Neurol Neurosurg Psychiatry* 1993; **56**: 352–5

43 Lees KR, Asplund K, Carolei A et al. Glycine antagonist gavestinel in neuroprotection (GAIN international) in patients with acute stroke: a randomised controlled trial. *Lancet* 2000; **355**: 1949–54

Aspirin or heparin in acute stroke

Anthony C Pereira and **Martin M Brown**

Department of Clinical Neurology, Institute of Neurology, University College London, UK

Acute stroke treatment using aspirin and/or heparin was studied in the International Stroke Trial (IST) and Chinese Acute Stroke Trial (CAST) which randomised over 40,000 patients altogether. Combining the results demonstrated that aspirin (150–300 mg) given within 48 h of the onset of stroke produced a small but significant improvement in outcome (death or dependency) 4 weeks to 6 months after stroke of about 1 patient per 100 treated. There was a significant reduction in recurrent ischaemic stroke of similar degree, which was not associated with significant increase in cerebral haemorrhage. Therefore, aspirin should be used as early secondary prevention against recurrent stroke, after excluding cerebral haemorrhage by scanning the patient. Heparin does not improve clinical outcome after stroke even in patients in atrial fibrillation. It decreased recurrent ischaemic stroke significantly in IST, but at the cost of a significant increase in cerebral haemorrhage. Low molecular weight heparins and heparinoids have not proved any more beneficial. Therefore, heparin does not appear to be a useful routine therapy in acute stroke. The use of heparin should, therefore, be limited to patients at high risk of deep vein thrombosis or early recurrence.

Correspondence to:
Prof. Martin M Brown,
Department of Clinical
Neurology, Institute of
Neurology, Queen
Square, London
WC1N 3BG, UK

Antiplatelet and anticoagulation therapy are widely used in the prevention of stroke[1]. In this chapter, the use of aspirin and heparin in the treatment of the acute ischaemic event is discussed. Aspirin, an inhibitor of platelet aggregation, has an antithrombotic effect which has been successfully used to decrease early mortality after myocardial infarction by up to 20%[2]. As 85% of acute strokes are thrombo-embolic in nature, if aspirin had an effect in the cerebral circulation comparable to that in the coronary circulation, it could decrease the number of early deaths from stroke by up to 30,000 per year in Europe and America[3]. Since 1941, heparin has been used to treat thrombosis and stroke[4,5]. Its anticoagulant action may retard the advance of cerebral thrombo-embolism while arterial recanalisation occurs[5,6] and, by preventing deep venous thrombosis, it may decrease the incidence of pulmonary embolism – one of the causes of death following stroke. Accompanying the potential advantages of these two drugs is the risk of haemorrhage: particularly intracerebral haemorrhage. Therefore, the question was where the balance of risk and benefit of these two treatments lay. The answers to these important questions are mainly provided by two very large clinical trials published recently: the International stroke Trial (IST)[7] and the Chinese Acute Stroke Trial (CAST)[8]. The two trials were prospectively designed to allow a meta-analysis of the pooled data[8].

In IST, 19,435 patients were randomised either to receive 300 mg aspirin daily or avoid aspirin and, in a 2 x 2 factorial design, either subcutaneous heparin (low dose [5000 mg b.d.] or medium dose [12,500 mg b.d.]) or avoid heparin. Treatment continued for 14 days in hospital or until earlier discharge. Patients were recruited within 24 h of the onset of symptoms; a CT brain scan was not required prior to randomisation. The primary outcome measures were death within 14 days or death or dependency at 6 months. The trial design allowed all patients receiving either aspirin or heparin to be compared to all those avoiding that drug (provided there was no interaction between aspirin and heparin).

In CAST, 21,106 patients were randomised within 24 h of the onset of symptoms, either to receive 160 mg of aspirin or to avoid it. Treatment continued in hospital for 4 weeks or earlier discharge. The primary outcome measures were death from any cause in the first 4 weeks, and death or dependency at discharge.

Aspirin in acute stroke

In IST, 9.0% died within 14 days in the aspirin-treated group compared to 9.4% in those avoiding aspirin, which was not a significant difference (Table 1). In the aspirin-treated group, 2.8% had recurrent stroke compared to 3.9% of controls ($P < 0.001$) and only 0.9% suffered haemorrhagic stroke compared to 0.8% of controls (non-significant). Overall, therefore, there was a significant reduction in the likelihood of death or

Table 1 Results of IST and CAST

	CAST		IST			
	Aspirin	No aspirin	Aspirin	No aspirin	Heparin	No heparin
Number randomised	10,335	10,320	9,719	9,714	9,717	9,718
Early death	3.3*	3.9*	9.0	9.4	9.0	9.3
Recurrent ischaemic stroke	1.6**	2.1**	2.8***	3.9***	2.9**	3.8**
Haemorrhagic stroke	1.1	0.9	0.9	0.8	1.2****	0.4****
Recurrent stroke or death	5.3*	5.9*	11.3*	12.4*	11.7	12.0
Dead or dependent at discharge/6 months	30.5	31.6	61.2	63.5	62.9	62.9

All the figures except the numbers randomised are percentages.
*$P < 0.05$, **$P < 0.01$, ***$P < 0.001$, ****$P < 0.00001$.

Study	Aspirin n/N	Control n/N	Odds ratio (95% CI)	Odds ratio	(95% CI Fixed)
MAST-I 1995	94/153	106/156		0.75	(0.47,1.20)
CAST 1997	3153/10335	3266/10320		0.95	(0.89,1.01)
IST 1997	6000/9719	6125/9714		0.95	(0.89,1.00)
Total	9247/20207	9497/20190		0.95	(0.91,0.98)

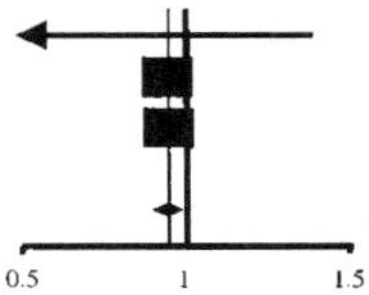

0.5   1   1.5

Fig. 1 Meta-analysis of the benefits of aspirin therapy compared to control in acute stroke: Reduction in death or dependency at end of follow up. n/N, number of events/number of subjects; CI, confidence interval; MAST-I, Multicentre Acute Stroke Study – Italy[9]; CAST, Chinese Acute Stroke Study[8]; IST, International Stroke Study[7].

recurrent stroke (11.3% *versus* 12.4%, $P = 0.02$). This was equivalent to 11 fewer events per 1000 patients treated. At 6 months, 61.2% of the aspirin-treated group were dead or dependent compared to 63.5% of the controls, a non-significant difference.

In CAST, in-hospital mortality was significantly reduced in the aspirin-treated group (3.3% *versus* 3.9%, $P = 0.04$; Table 1). This was equivalent to 5 avoidable deaths for every 1000 treated patients. There was a significant reduction of recurrent ischaemic stroke (1.6% *versus* 2.1%, $P <0.01$), but not in all recurrent strokes (3.2% *versus* 3.4%, $P = $ ns). As in IST, there was a non-significant increase in the risk of haemorrhage (1.1% *versus* 0.9%, $P = $ ns). Therefore, there was a significant reduction in the likelihood of death or recurrent stroke (5.3% *versus* 5.9%, $P = 0.03$): 7 fewer events per 1000 patients treated. At discharge, 30.5% of the aspirin group were dead or dependent compared to 31.6% of controls: a non-significant difference. The reason for the better long-term outcome of patients in CAST compared to IST was probably the result of there being a greater proportion of patients under 70 years of age and patients with milder strokes randomised in CAST.

The meta-analysis of the data from IST, CAST and the small (309 patients) aspirin treatment arm of the Multi-centre Acute Stroke Trial – Italy (MAST-I)[9] showed that the groups randomised to aspirin had fewer recurrent ischaemic strokes (2.5% *versus* 3.2%, $P = 0.00002$) without significantly more haemorrhagic strokes (1.0% *versus* 0.8%, $P = $ ns) and, by the end of follow-up, had fewer dead or dependent (45.8% *versus* 47.0%, $P = 0.007$; Fig. 1)[8]. Thus, one can conclude that early aspirin benefits about 1 per 100 patients treated by preventing death or dependency. It appears that most of this benefit can be explained by the prevention of early recurrence. Although this benefit seems small, it is very cost-effective given the low cost of aspirin and the fact that stroke is common. In the UK alone, 1000 patients would be saved from death and disability if all of the 100,000 strokes per year were treated with aspirin within 48 h of admission.

IST and CAST confirm that the role of aspirin in acute stroke is in very early secondary prevention of further stroke, but not as a specific treatment of the acute infarct, despite the fact that during the first few weeks after stroke, platelet activation[10,11] and thromboxane biosynthesis[12] are increased. Given the level of platelet activation, this conclusion may seem surprising, but it is consistent with other studies. For example, patients taking aspirin prior to suffering a stroke do not have a better outcome compared to patients not on aspirin[13]. It is possible that the dose of aspirin administered in IST and CAST may have been too low. There is evidence that patients who have a stroke in spite of taking aspirin have residual levels of platelet aggregation which can be suppressed by higher doses of aspirin[14]. However, higher doses of aspirin do not necessarily completely suppress platelet aggregation[10,14] or platelet activation[11]. Although smaller doses of aspirin are as good as larger doses for secondary prevention[15], perhaps much larger doses or combinations of antiplatelet agents, would be needed if aspirin is to be a more effective treatment for acute stroke. On the other hand, this would be likely to increase the risk of haemorrhage. Alternatively, there is evidence that a systemic increase of hyper-aggregable platelets and plasma activators of platelet function accompanies thrombotic infarcts but not infarcts secondary to cardiac embolism[16], suggesting that it may be necessary to consider the aetiology of the infarct when deciding treatment. Further trials of more powerful antiplatelet regimens in acute stroke, *e.g.* glycoprotein IIb/IIIa receptor antagonists, in appropriate patients are certainly justified.

The next consideration is whether administration of aspirin should be delayed until after the results of a CT or MRI head scan to exclude haemorrhage are known. The published results of CAST and IST provide some data that can be tentatively used to examine this question. In CAST, 3.7% of aspirin-treated patients, randomised without a CT scan, had an outcome event (death or recurrent stroke) during the follow-up period compared to 5.1% of controls: the corresponding figures are 5.5% and 6.1% in those randomised after a CT scan. Our analysis of these published data indicates that there is no significant difference in the number of outcome events in either aspirin-treated patients versus controls (3.7% *versus* 5.1%, P = ns) nor is there a significant difference in outcome between the 'avoid-aspirin' groups of patients (6.1% *versus* 5.1%, P = ns) randomised with or without a CT scan. In IST, the numbers of actual events are not given. However, in those patients randomised after a CT scan, there was no significant difference in the proportion dead or dependent at 6 months in the aspirin-treated group compared to controls (59.0% *versus* 60.5%, χ^2 = 3.2, P = ns). The corresponding figures in those who did not have a pre-randomisation CT were 68.8% and 69.6%, respectively (χ^2 = 0.48, P = ns). However, in patients treated with aspirin, those with a pre-randomisation CT scan had a significantly better outcome than those without a pre-randomisation CT (59.0% versus 68.8%, χ^2 = 75.3, P <0.0001) and similarly in the control group of patients (60.5% versus 69.6%, χ^2 = 75.3, P <0.0001). These results support the view that it is worth knowing the results of a brain scan before treating the patient. However, the aspirin-avoid group of patients, who did not have a pre-randomisation CT, also fared significantly worse than those who did have a pre-randomisation CT, which makes it difficult to form clear conclusions, but does emphasise the importance of making an accurate diagnosis. Based on the currently available data, we recommend delaying aspirin treatment until after the result of cerebral imaging is known, because the benefit of aspirin is modest and may be decreased if patients who ultimately turn out to have intracerebral haemorrhage are inadvertently given aspirin.

Unfractionated heparin in acute stroke

In IST, 9.0% died within 14 days in the heparin group compared to 9.3% in those avoiding heparin (a non-significant difference). In the heparin-treated group, 2.9% had recurrent stroke compared to 3.8% of controls (P <0.005) but 1.2% suffered haemorrhagic stroke compared to 0.4% of controls (P <0.00001) and 1.3% had major extracranial haemorrhage compared to 0.4% of controls (P <0.00001). Therefore, the benefit of a significant reduction of recurrent stroke was offset by an increase in intracerebral haemorrhage. There was no significant reduction in the likelihood of death or recurrent stroke at 14 days (11.7% versus 12.0%). Heparin did decrease the incidence of pulmonary embolism (0.5% versus 0.8%, P <0.05). At 6 months, 62.9% of both the 'heparin' and 'avoid-heparin' group were dead or dependent. Therefore, in acute stroke, heparin appears to confer no benefit.

In the heparin treated patients, the frequency of any major haemorrhagic complication was 2.5% and of intracerebral haemorrhage was 1.2%. This was comparable to that reported in other series[17,18]. Heparin-related intracerebral haemorrhage is thought to occur early after the onset of infarction[19,20], and to be associated with large infarcts[19-21] and an activated partial thromboplastin time (APTT) greater then two times control[21]. The more frequent presence of intracerebral micro-haemorrhages in patients with ischaemic stroke (26%) compared to patients with myocardial infarction (4%) or peripheral vascular disease (13%), suggests that the cerebral vessels of patients with ischaemic stroke are more prone to rupture than those of other patients with vascular disease[22]. As IST did not require that either the aetiology of stroke was elucidated prior to treatment or that the APTT was monitored, the results cannot exclude that there may be a subset of stroke patients who are not prone to haemorrhagic complications and may benefit from anti-coagulation. In IST itself, there were fewer early deaths or recurrent strokes in those on low dose, compared to medium dose, heparin (10.8% *versus* 12.6%, $P < 0.01$). The main reason for this was fewer haemor-rhagic strokes (0.7% *versus* 1.8%, $P < 0.00001$) in the low dose heparin group. There was no significant benefit in 6 month outcome with either treatment. The early benefits of low dose heparin appear similar to those of 300 mg aspirin in terms of prevention of recurrent stroke without a major increase in haemorrhagic complications. However, the long-term outcome is not significantly better than controls.

There are no large trials of full dose intravenous heparin in acute stroke, but it is unlikely that the overall benefits or risks would be any different to the those found in the higher dose subcutaneous arm of IST. However, it is possible that there might be subgroups of patients at particularly high risk of recurrence who would benefit from early anticoagulation. A particular consideration is in the management of patients who have an obvious and current cardiac source of emboli. The role of anticoagulation for stroke prevention in patients with non-rheumatic mitral valvular atrial fibrillation (AF) is established[23], but the best management in the acute phase of stroke is still very unclear. In the subset of patients in IST in AF, the frequency of recurrent ischaemic stroke was decreased from 4.9% to 2.8% ($P < 0.01$) in patients treated with heparin. This was offset by an increase in haemorrhage from 0.4% to 2.1% ($P < 0.001$). Therefore, there was a non-significant reduction in all recurrent stroke from 5.3% to 4.9% and death and recurrent stroke from 20.7% to 19.1%. Aspirin decreased the frequency of recurrent ischaemic stroke in patients without AF, but had no significant benefit in those patients in AF. This agrees with other data which showed that the frequency of symptomatic intracerebral haemorrhage was 2% and early recurrent cerebral embolism was also 2% in both, those anticoagulated and untreated controls[24]. Therefore, the data currently available suggest that patients in AF should not be treated as a special case and given early heparin. Other data suggest that early intravenous heparin is particularly likely to cause haemorrhage in patients with large cardio-embolic infarcts[23]. Given the overall lack of benefit of subcutaneous heparin in AF in IST, it would seem reasonable to delay anticoagulation in patients with cardio-embolic stroke for 7–14 days after onset, except in those with small infarcts.

One can, therefore, conclude that there is no indication for the routine use of heparin in acute stroke, but its use in patients at particularly high risk of deep vein thrombosis to prevent pulmonary embolus, or in patients at higher than average risk of early recurrence, it is unlikely to be harmful, unless they have a large infarct.

Low molecular weight heparin

Low molecular weight heparins (LMWH) have been shown to have advantages over standard unfractionated heparins in the prevention of pulmonary embolism and, in this context, appear to have a better safety profile. There was, therefore, considerable hope that they would prove more efficacious in the treatment of acute stroke. The first randomised study of a low molecular weight heparin, the Fraxiparin in Stroke Study (FISS) appeared to bear out this hope[25]. The efficacy of nadroparin calcium (Fraxiparine) given subcutaneously within 48 h of acute ischaemic stroke for 10 days, was assessed in a randomised, double-blind placebo-controlled trial in Hong Kong. There appeared to be a significant 31% (95% CI 10–46%) reduction in the relative risk of death or dependency at 6 months in the high dose nadroparin group compared to those receiving placebo, whereas the difference between the low dose and placebo groups did not reach statistical significance. However, the trial was small, with only just over 100 patients in each arm, and it seems likely that the results were a false positive finding occurring by chance, because a much larger trial of nadroparin, known as FISS bis, with 766 patients, did not confirm the findings of the smaller study. The results have only been published in abstract form[26]. Therefore, there is currently insufficient evidence to recommend LMWH as a treatment modality to prevent early recurrent ischaemic stroke, but further studies may be warranted to reassess the effects of LMWHs.

Heparinoids

Heparinoids are thought to have similar advantages to LMWH, but again have not been proven to be of benefit in patients with acute ischaemic stroke. The TOAST study (Trial of ORG 10172 in Acute Stroke Treatment) was a randomised, double-blind placebo-controlled trial of a low molecular weight heparinoid, danaparoid sodium, in patients with acute ischaemic stroke[27]. A total of 1281 patients, 18–85 years of age, received either the active drug or placebo intravenously within 24 h of acute or progressing ischaemic stroke. An intravenous bolus of danaparoid was given and the dose adjusted after 24 h to maintain the antifactor Xa activity at 0.6–0.8 antifactor Xa U/ml; treatment was continued as an infusion for 7 days. There was no significant difference in the primary outcome measure between the two groups. Although significantly more patients in the danaparoid group had a very favourable outcome at 7 days compared to placebo (33.9% *versus* 27.8%, $P = 0.01$), danaparoid was associated with more adverse events (8.5% *versus* 5.4%, $P < 0.05$), an increased risk of major bleeding (3.4% *versus* 1%, $P < 0.005$) and an increased rate of major intracranial haemorrhage within the first 10 days compared to placebo (2.4% *versus* 0.8%, $P < 0.05$). Danaparoid did not reduce the rate of recurrent ischaemic stroke overall, but, intriguingly, patients with stroke secondary to large artery atherosclerosis appeared to benefit from active treatment. In this subgroup, patients treated with danaparoid more commonly had a favourable ($P = 0.04$) or very favourable ($P = 0.02$) outcome at 3 months after stroke compared to placebo. It was postulated that anticoagulation in these patients might help maintain collateral flow or prevent progression of thrombus in a stenosed vessel. However, it was disappointing that danaparoid did not significantly reduce the rate of recurrent stroke in this subgroup and it is possible that the apparent effect on outcome was fortuitous. Therefore, the safety and efficacy profile of danaparoid is unfavourable in patients with acute ischaemic stroke overall, and there is no evidence that treatment significantly reduces early stroke recurrence. However, further large-scale studies are warranted to re-examine the potential benefit of this treatment in patients with carotid stenosis.

Recommendations for clinical practice

Aspirin (150–300 mg) has a small but definite benefit if given within 48 h of the onset of acute ischaemic stroke but it seems prudent to delay administration until intracerebral haemorrhage has been excluded. Patients should be discharged from hospital on a regular antiplatelet agent. Heparin (at least in doses of 12,500 mg b.d. subcutaneously or higher) should be avoided as a routine treatment for acute stroke even in patients with have atrial fibrillation. Further evaluation of low molecular weight heparins and heparinoid is needed. In the meantime, the use of low dose subcutaneous heparin should be limited to patients at high risk of deep vein thrombosis. In patients with an indication for long-term anticoagulation as a result of cardio-embolic stroke or other indicator of higher than average risk of recurrence, anticoagulation should be delayed for 7–14 days, unless the infarct is small.

Acknowledgement

ACP was supported by a grant from The Stroke Association.

References

1 Wolf PA. Prevention of stroke. *Lancet* 1998; **352** (**Suppl 3**): 15–8
2 ISIS-2 Collaborative Group. Randomised trial of intravenous streptokinase, oral aspirin, both or neither among 17187 of acute myocardial infarction. *Lancet* 1988; **91**: 311–22
3 Sandercock PAG, van den Belt AGM, Lindley RI, Slattery J. Antithrombotic therapy in acute ischaemic stroke: an overview of the completed randomised trials. *J Neurol Neurosurg Psychiatry* 1993; **56**: 17–25
4 Hedenius P. The use of heparin in internal disease. *Acta Med Scand* 1941; **107**: 170–82
5 Korczyn AD. Heparin in the treatment of acute stroke. *Neurol Clin* 1992; **10**: 209–17
6 Sherman DG. Heparin and heparinoids in stroke. *Neurology* 1998; **51**: S56–8
7 International Stroke Trial Collaborative Group. The International Stroke Trial (IST): a randomised trial of aspirin, subcutaneous heparin, both, or neither among 19 435 patients with acute ischaemic stroke. *Lancet* 1997; **349**: 1569–81
8 CAST (Chinese Acute Stroke Trial) Collaborative Group. CAST: randomised placebo-controlled trial of early aspirin use in 20 000 patients with acute ischaemic stroke. *Lancet* 1997; **349**: 1641–9
9 Multi-centre Acute Stroke Trial – Italy (MAST-I) Group. Randomised controlled trial of streptokinase, aspirin and combination of both in treatment of acute ischaemic stroke. *Lancet* 1995; **346**: 1509–14
10 Dougherty JHJ, Levy DE, Weksler BB. Platelet activation in acute cerebral ischaemia. Serial measurements of platelet function in cerebrovascular disease. *Lancet* 1977; i: 821–4
11 Grau AJ, Ruf A, Vogt A *et al.* Increased fraction of circulating activated platelets in acute and previous cerebrovascular ischemia. *Thromb Haemost* 1998; **80**: 298–301
12 Koudstaal PJ, Ciabattoni G, van Gijn J *et al.* Increased thromboxane biosynthesis in patients with acute cerebral ischemia. *Stroke* 1993; **24**: 219–23
13 De Keyser J, Herroelen L, De Klippel N. Early outcome in acute ischemic stroke is not influenced by the prophylactic use of low-dose aspirin. *J Neurol Sci* 1997; **145**: 93–6
14 Helgason CM, Tortorise KL, Winkler SR *et al.* Aspirin response and failure in cerebral infarction. *Stroke* 1993; **24**: 345–50
15 van Gijn J. Aspirin: dose and indications in modern stroke prevention. *Neurol Clin* 1992; **10**: 193–207
16 Uchiyama S, Takeuchi M, Osawa M *et al.* Platelet function tests in thrombotic cerebrovascular disorders. *Stroke* 1983; **14**: 511–7
17 Ramirez-Lassepas M, Quinones MR. Heparin therapy for stroke: hemorrhagic complications and risk factors for intracerebral hemorrhage. *Neurology* 1984; **34**: 114–7
18 Albers GW, Bittar N, Young L *et al.* Clinical characteristics and management of acute stroke in patients with atrial fibrillation admitted to US university hospitals. *Neurology* 1997; **48**: 1598–604
19 Cerebral Embolism Study Group. Immediate anticoagulation of embolic stroke: brain hemorrhage and management options. *Stroke* 1984; **15**: 779–89
20 Babikian VL, Kase CS, Pessin MS, Norrving B, Gorelick PB. Intracerebral hemorrhage in stroke patients anticoagulated with heparin. *Stroke* 1989; **20**: 1500–3
21 Chamorro A, Vila N, Saiz A, Alday M, Tolosa E. Early anticoagulation after large cerebral embolic infarction: a safety study. *Neurology* 1995; **45**: 861–5
22 Kwa VIH, Franke CL, Verbeeten B, Stam J, for the Amsterdam Vascular Medicine Group. Silent intracerebral microhaemorrhages in patients with ischaemic stroke. *Ann Neurol* 1998; **44**: 372–7
23 Morley J, Marinchak R, Rials SJ, Kowey P. Atrial fibrillation, anticoagulation and stroke. *Am J Cardiol* 1996; **77**: 38A–44A
24 Rothrock JF, Dittrich HC, McAllen S, Taft BJ, Lyden PD. Acute anticoagulation following cardioembolic stroke. *Stroke* 1989; **20**: 730–4
25 Kay R, Wong KS, Yu YL *et al.* Low-molecular-weight heparin for the treatment of acute ischemic stroke. *N Engl J Med* 1995; **333**:1588–93
26 Hommel M, for the FISS bis Investigators Group. Fraxiparine in Ischaemic Stroke Study (FISS bis). *Cerebrovasc Dis* 1998; **8** (**Suppl 4**): 1–103
27 The Publications Committee for the Trial of ORG 10172 in Acute Stroke Treatment (TOAST) Investigators. Low molecular weight heparinoid, Org 10172 (danaparoid), and outcome after acute ischaemic stroke. A randomised controlled trial. *JAMA* 1998; **279**: 1265–72

Optimising homeostasis

Philip M W Bath

Division of Stroke Medicine, University of Nottingham, City Hospital Campus, Nottingham, UK

There is a wealth of experimental and clinical information showing that hypertension, hyperglycaemia, hyperthermia and intracranial hypertension are each independent indicators of a poor prognosis after stroke, but there is an astonishing lack of evidence from randomised controlled trials to tell us how to manage these problems, bearing in mind their frequency in stroke patients.

The therapeutic options will, in most cases, not involve patented drugs, and financial support for running the necessary randomised controlled trials will have to come from government or charity sponsors rather than from the pharmaceutical industry. It is vital that academic researchers now devise studies of appropriate design and size to answer these important questions. In the absence of randomised data, severe hyperglycaemia and pyrexia should be treated, whilst acute hypertension is probably best left untreated unless very severe or complicated by other medical conditions. The management of cerebral oedema remains an enigma.

Homeostasis can be defined as[1]: 'the various physiologic arrangements which serve to restore the normal state, once it has been disturbed'. Stroke is clearly associated with massive physiological disturbance of both vascular and neuronal function. Rather than attempting to describe all those homeostatic mechanisms relevant to stroke, this chapter focuses on four forms of disequilibrium which complicate stroke[2] and are associated with a poor outcome, namely hypertension, hyperglycaemia, hyperthermia, and intracranial hypertension.

Blood pressure

Correspondence to:
Prof. P M W Bath, Division
of Stroke Medicine,
University of Nottingham,
City Hospital Campus,
Nottingham
NG7 2UH, UK

Both ischaemic stroke and primary intracerebral haemorrhage are associated with acute rises in blood pressure; hypertension is present in three-quarters of stroke patients, irrespective of subtype, and develops rapidly after the onset[3-8]. Blood pressure falls during the first week in most patients with the greatest decline occurring in those with the highest admission values; however, 30% of patients remain hypertensive and are then candidates for secondary prevention. Although the causes

Table 1 Causes of hypertension in acute stroke

Previous hypertension[9,10]
Stress of hospitalisation ('white coat hypertension')
Activation of corticotrophic (ACTH, cortisol) system[11–14]
Activation of sympathetic nervous system[11]
Activation of renin-angiotensin system
Increased cardiac output[15]
Secondary to raised intracranial pressure (Cushing reflex)

Table 2 Relative arguments in favour of, or against, raising or lowering blood pressure

	Arguments in favour	Arguments against
Raise	Cerebral autoregulation[26] is lost after stroke[27]; hence, perfusion may increase as BP is elevated	Hypertension is associated with forced vasodilation, cerebral oedema, capillary vasoconstriction, and ultimately in hypoperfusion, and possible re-infarction or bleeding[30].
	Increase perfusion in the absence of cerebral autoregulation	Acute stroke is associated with a raised cardiac output[15]. Inotropes will exacerbate this, and the risk of cardiac ischaemia and failure. Trials using the NMDA ion channel blocker, aptiganel (which raises BP), were unsuccessful (unpublished data)
	Induced hypertension (triple therapy) improves outcome in subarachnoid haemorrhage. Case series involving levarteronol or phenylephrine[28,29]	
Lower	Case series in intracerebral haemorrhage[31]	Cerebral autoregulation[26] is lost after stroke[27]; hence, perfusion may fall as BP is decreased.
	Observational study in ischaemic stroke[32]	Case studies in ischaemic stroke[36].
	Aggressive BP lowering used in 'positive' alteplase trials[33–35]	Trials of calcium channel blockers were complicated by a worsening in outcome in parallel with BP lowering and a reduction in cerebral blood flow[37–41]
Leave alone	No trials to suggest otherwise[25]	Both hypertension and hypotension are associated with a poor outcome[16]

of acute hypertension are multifactorial (Table 1), half of patients have a past history of hypertension[9,10].

Early hypertension (systolic blood pressure >180 mmHg[16]) is associated with a poor outcome, whether assessed as death, dependency or disability[16–21], although some earlier studies did not find this relationship[22,23]. The mechanisms linking hypertension and outcome are poorly defined but probably include[24]: (i) hypertension promotes early re-infarction; (ii) hypertension promotes symptomatic haemorrhagic transformation; and (iii) hypertension promotes cerebral oedema.

Less recognised is the association between acute hypotension (systolic BP < 140 mmHg) and a poor outcome, as identified in the International Stroke Trial[16]. This finding needs further examination, but two explanations for this observation are plausible: (i) hypotension is a marker for serious comorbid disease (*e.g.* ischaemic heart disease, infection) which may themselves contribute to a poor outcome; and (ii) hypotension (for whatever reason) reduces cerebral perfusion (in the absence of cerebral autoregulation) and, therefore, may extend infarct size.

Lowering blood pressure

No definitive trials have suggested the optimal management of blood pressure during the acute phase of stroke, although a number of small studies have shown that it is possible to therapeutically lower BP[25]. In the case of hypertension, arguments, largely indirect, can be made to both raise or lower BP, or to leave it alone (Table 2).

In the absence of trial evidence, many experts have published guidelines on the treatment of hypertension in acute stroke[30,36,42–46]. In general, these recommend leaving BP alone unless extreme levels (180/120 to 240/130 mmHg in different guidelines) or signs of accelerated hypertension or hypertensive encephalopathy are present, patients are deteriorating (secondary to re-infarction or continued bleeding), or have complicating medical problems such as heart failure, symptomatic ischaemic heart disease, or aortic dissection. Hypertension should also possibly be treated if thrombolytic agents are to be administered since trials of these agents have lowered BP prior to treatment[33–35].

Table 3 Drugs for lowering or elevating blood pressure in acute stroke

Drug	Comments	Effect on outcome in stroke RCTs
Lower BP		
Alpha receptor antagonistsblockers		No trials
Angiotensin II receptor antagonists	One on-going study[48]	No trials
Angiotensin converting enzyme inhibitors	Maintains global CBF[49]	
Beta receptor antagonists		Neutral[50]
Calcium channel blockers	May reduce regional CBF[41]	Neutral[51]
Diuretics	BP lowering associated with a worse outcome[37–40] May cause haemoconcentration and dehydration	No trials
Nitric oxide	Maintains regional CBF[52] Donors may, or may not, have antiplatelet effects[52,53] Used in alteplase trials[33–35]	No trials
Dextrorphan	Adverse central events, *e.g.* stupor, apnoea[54]	
Raise BP		
Corticosteroids	Complicated by hyperglycaemia, infection, gastrointestinal bleeding[55]	Neutral[55]
Haemodilution	Used in SAH[56]	Neutral[57]
Nitric oxide synthase inhibitors	Cerebral vasoconstriction	No trials
Sympathomimetics	Platelet activation may extend thrombosis	No trials

CBF, cerebral blood flow; SAH, subarachnoid haemorrhage; RCT, randomised clinical trial; BP, blood pressure.

The optimum agent to alter BP during the acute phase of stroke is unclear. Indirect evidence suggests that a number of drug classes should be avoided, either because of a lack of efficacy or because of potential complications (Table 3). The duration for which therapy should be given is also unclear, but outcome was not different in a small trial comparing 3 days with longer-term treatment using a variety of agents[47]. With this uncertainty, it is evident that one or more large trials investigating whether blood pressure can be safely and beneficially lowered during the acute phase of stroke are now urgently required.

Other aspects of managing BP also need to be considered. The treatment of hypotension is even less well studied than that for hypertension, but hypovolaemia and dehydration should always be reversed. Increasing numbers of patients are admitted taking antihypertensive medication and there is no consensus on whether these drugs should be continued or withdrawn for the first few days after stroke onset. However, it is important to restart therapy after 1–2 weeks if it is stopped; ideally, drugs should be re-introduced one by one to avoid precipitous falls in BP in patients where poor compliance might have been an issue pre-stroke. The secondary prevention of stroke through lowering BP is currently being studied in a large trial[58], but patients who remain hypertensive after stroke should, in general, be treated.

Glucose

Hyperglycaemia is present in 20–50% of patients with acute stroke[59–66], although less than half of these have a prior history of diabetes mellitus (Table 4)[59–61,63,64]. An elevated glucose may also be secondary to previously unrecognised diabetes mellitus (haemoglobin A_{1c} concentration is elevated) or be transient (HbA_{1c} is normal). Hyperglycaemia may be present in all types of stroke, whether haemorrhagic or ischaemic, cortical, lacunar or brain stem[59,67].

Most studies in animal models of stroke suggest that hyperglycaemia worsens outcome[68-71], although other work has not confirmed this association[72] (Table 5). Similarly, human studies have found that hyperglycaemia (plasma glucose >8 mmol/l), whether secondary to diabetes mellitus or

Table 4 Causes of hyperglycaemia in acute stroke

Previous diabetes mellitus or impaired glucose tolerance
Previously unrecognised (latent) diabetes mellitus or impaired glucose intolerance
Stress/reactive hyperglycaemia
Activation of corticotrophic (ACTH, cortisol) system[11–14]
Activation of sympathetic nervous system[11]

Table 5 Mechanisms by which hyperglycaemia may worsen outcome after stroke

Reduced oxidative metabolism, increased anaerobic glycolysis, increased lactate acidosis[77]
Increased infarct size[69]
Increased haemorrhagic transformation of the infarct[78-80]
Damage blood-brain barrier[81]
Increased cerebral oedema[78]
Reduced regional cerebral blood flow and cerebrovascular reserve[82]

not, is associated with an increased mortality and reduced functional outcome after stroke, irrespective of its subtype[12,61,63,66,73,74]. However, this is not a universal finding[75] and some studies have reported a univariate, but not multivariate, relationship suggesting that glucose is not in the direct causal pathway linking stroke with outcome[76].

Lowering glucose

The most direct and immediate treatment of hyperglycaemia is to administer insulin. Experimental evidence suggests that insulin is directly neuroprotective in addition to its glucose lowering effect[83-85]. Treatment of hyperglycaemia may also reduce rates of infarct haemorrhagic transformation.

No large trials have tested the effect of relatively aggressive normalisation of glucose levels with insulin and several calls have been made for such a study[66,86]. Indirect evidence that insulin therapy might be beneficial in stroke comes from the DIGAMI study of diabetics with acute myocardial infarction where insulin treatment reduced long-term mortality by 29%[87]. In a more recent study, combined insulin, glucose and potassium therapy (GKI) reduced mortality after myocardial infarction in 470 normoglycaemic patients[88,89]. A phase II trial of GKI infusion in 53 patients has shown that it is feasible to reduce glucose levels to below 7 mmol/l in stroke patients with hyperglycaemia without causing significant hypoglycaemia[90]; a relatively large trial of GKI treatment is now testing its effect on mortality and functional outcome[90].

Temperature

Hyperthermia, defined as a temperature above 37.5°C, is a common complication of acute stroke occurring in 25–60% of patients[91–94]. A variety of causes explain pyrexia (Table 6) although infection is present in most cases[93].

Experimental studies in models of focal ischaemia have shown that hyperthermia is a critical factor for determining infarct size. The timing of temperature rise does not appear to be important and delayed hyperthermia by 24 h or more can also worsen neuronal damage[95]. Analogous

Table 6 Causes of high temperature in acute stroke

Co-existing infection, usually urinary or respiratory tract infection
Infarct necrosis
Anterior hypothalamic infarction (thermoregulatory centre)
Pontine haemorrhage

observations have also been made in man where pyrexia is a risk factor for large infarcts, early neurological deterioration, and increased morbidity and mortality after stroke[91–93,96]. However, only early hyperthermia (within 24 h of stroke onset) appears to be prognostically important in man[94].

Hyperthermia, of whatever cause, increases cerebral metabolism thereby increasing oxygen requirements, cerebral blood flow and ICP. Hence, avoiding rises in temperature are important through prevention and early identification of infection. Equally, fever should be aggressively treated, although there are no trial results to guide practice. Readily available interventions should usually prove effective, including the use of active cooling with fans, cooling blankets, or tepid sponging. Although the routine use of aspirin in acute ischaemic stroke may have some antipyretic action, paracetamol should be used for active temperature reduction.

Lowering temperature

If a high temperature worsens infarct size and outcome after stroke, lowering core temperature below 37°C should reduce metabolic rate and have other neuroprotective properties (Table 7).

Experimental studies in animal models of permanent and transient ischaemic stroke have confirmed the hypothesis that inducing hypothermia (down to 24–34°C) reduces stroke lesion size[100–103].

No randomised controlled trials of hypothermia in human stroke have been reported, although evidence from other areas of medicine, *e.g.* during cardiac surgery and after traumatic brain injury[104,105], suggest that lowering systemic temperature to 32–33°C is feasible and might reduce intracranial pressure and brain damage, and improve outcome.

Table 7 Mechanisms by which hypothermia might improve outcome after stroke (reviewed in[97–99])

Reduce cerebral metabolic rate
Reduce levels of excitatory amino acids
Reduce intracranial pressure
Stabilise blood-brain barrier
Reduce oedema formation
Stabilise membranes

Feasibility studies are underway on how best to actively lower temperature. Patients with large hemispheric strokes and evidence of a raised ICP are most likely to benefit. Although internal cooling could be induced using extracorporeal circuits or peritoneal lavage, such invasive methods will increase complexity and the risk of infection. Since external cooling blankets can quickly lower temperature, these would appear to be most appropriate. Patients will need to be anaesthetised since hypothermia induces profound shivering and pain; hence, elective ventilation with neuromuscular blockade and sedation will be required. A major question is the extent to which core temperature should be reduced? Metabolic rate declines by approximately 7% for every degree centigrade below normal. The lower limit of cooling is likely to be around 31°C since cardiac function starts to decline rapidly and metabolic instability becomes problematical with more severe hypothermia. Furthermore, cooling for several days is also associated with an increased risk of infection.

An uncontrolled study of inducing moderate hypothermia in 25 cases of severe middle cerebral artery infarction found that lowering body temperature by 4°C for 48–72 h appeared to reduce mortality from an expected value of 78% to 44%[106]. It is now evident that randomised controlled trials assessing the effect of inducing hypothermia on outcome after ischaemic stroke are required[97,106].

Intracranial pressure

Intracranial hypertension is a common complication of both ischaemic and haemorrhagic stroke, particularly in large middle cerebral artery and cerebellar infarction or haemorrhage, and is usually secondary to cerebral oedema. Stroke is associated with both forms of oedema, cytotoxic and vasogenic. Space-occupying brain oedema typically presents with drowsiness and declining consciousness 1–5 days after stroke onset[107,108]. Subsequent signs include pupillary dilatation and asymmetry, gaze palsy, extensor posturing, periodic breathing, and death. This 'malignant' middle cerebral artery infarction typically follows complete middle cerebral artery territory infarction[108] and is fatal in more than half of cases. Oedema produces brain swelling thereby inducing pressure gradients leading to brain herniation. Typically, herniation after middle cerebral artery infarction occurs horizontally between hemispheres and, if extreme, vertical movement of the brain leads to brainstem coning, loss of brainstem function and death. Local pressure on the vascular supply of other parts of the brain can cause infarct extension, *e.g.* middle cerebral artery infarction can be complicated by secondary anterior and posterior cerebral artery territory infarction.

Table 8 Methods for reducing intracranial pressure in acute ischaemic stroke

Intervention	Mechanism of action	Complications	Effect of outcome in stroke RCTs
Acute stroke unit or general ward			
Head elevation	Improve venous return	Reduces arterial pressure at level of head and potentially perfusion	No trials
Glycerol	Reduce brain water and thence brain volume	Transient fluid overload -> pulmonary oedema; transient hypertension; dehydration; haemolysis and haemoglobinuria[119]	Neutral[119]
Mannitol	Reduce brain water and thence brain volume	Transient fluid overload -> pulmonary oedema; dehydration; fever	No trials
Loop diuretics (e.g. frusemide)	Reduce brain water and thence brain volume	Haemoconcentration and dehydration	No trials
Steroids	Decreases vasogenic, but not cytotoxic, oedema	Hyperglycaemia; infection; gastrointestinal bleeding[55]	Neutral[55]
Intensive therapy unit			
Hyperventilation	Induces cerebral vasoconstriction	Paradoxical intracranial hypertension; vasoconstriction -> reduced perfusion	No trials
Barbiturates	Reduces cerebral vascular volume and brain metabolism	Hypotension and infection	No trials
Muscle relaxants	Prevents stress/strain; increases ICP		No trials
Temperature reduction	Reduces brain metabolism and ICP	Infection	No trials
Decompressive craniectomy	Allow brain expansion	Those of surgery	No trials

ICP, intracranial pressure; RCT, randomised clinical trial.

The management of a raised ICP and cerebral oedema can be largely grouped together since their aims are the same. Practically, it is worth splitting treatment manoeuvres into those that can be performed in a general ward or high dependency nursing environment, and those that require intensive care facilities (Table 8). Unfortunately, the efficacy of most of the techniques is unknown, owing to the absence of satisfactory evidence from randomised trials. Instead, the justifications for these approaches are borrowed from other areas of medicine, especially the management of patients with traumatic brain injury and intracranial tumours[105].

Decompressive craniectomy

The rationale for removing part of the skull overlying the stroke (craniectomy) in patients with, or at risk of developing, cerebral oedema and intracranial hypertension is simply to decompress brain swelling and prevent herniation. Decompressive craniectomy has been assessed in experimental cerebral infarction and was effective in reducing death and neurological impairment whether performed 1 h or 24 h after induction of permanent MCA occlusion[109]. Case reports suggest that hemicraniectomy and dural incision may rescue patients with large supratentorial infarction from inevitable death although many are left in a dependent state after surgery[110,111]. An uncontrolled trial comparing patients treated with hemicraniectomy with historical controls found that mortality rates were significantly reduced from 80% to 35% in the surgical group[112]. However, such non-randomised studies are notoriously subject to bias and the effect on combined death and disability remains unclear. It is vital that properly controlled trials of craniectomy for malignant middle cerebral artery infarction are undertaken as soon as possible.

Thrombolysis

An interesting observation in some trials of alteplase is that rates of fatal oedema are lower in thrombolysed patients than those randomised to placebo. This observation has been reported in the second European Co-operative Acute Stroke trial[35], where oedema rates were reduced from 4.3% to 2.0%. This observation can be explained, in part, by thrombolytics reducing lesion volume[113].

Cerebellar haemorrhage and infarction

Cerebellar stroke typically present with vertigo, nausea and vomiting, gait and truncal ataxia, nystagmus, or dysarthria. Although most patients do well, those with space-occupying cerebellar infarcts or haemorrhages have a poor prognosis due to the development of obstructive hydrocephalus and brainstem compression. Such patients develop cranial nerve palsies, gaze paresis or deviation, and a Horner's syndrome[114]. Finally, they become stuperosed or comatosed, and develop posturing, vascular instability, ataxic breathing and pinpoint pupils.

Although never tested in a randomised trial, the standard management for patients with posterior fossa strokes who deteriorate is to treat hydrocephalus and intracranial hypertension with one or both of external ventricular drainage (ventriculostomy) and surgical evacuation of the lesion[114–118].

References

1 Cannon WB. *The Wisdom of the Body*. Norton, 1932
2 Oppenheimer S, Hachinski V. Complications of acute stroke. *Lancet* 1992; **339**: 721–4

3 Wallace JD, Levy LL. Blood pressure after stroke. *JAMA* 1981; **246**: 2177–80
4 Britton M, Carlsson A, de Faire U. Blood pressure course in patients with acute stroke and matched controls. *Stroke* 1986; **17**: 861–4
5 Carlsson A, Britton M. Blood pressure after stroke. A one-year follow-up study. *Stroke* 1993; **24**: 195–9
6 Broderick J, Brott T, Barsan W et al. Blood pressure during the first minutes of focal cerebral ischemia. *Ann Emerg Med* 1993; **22**: 1438–43
7 Phillips SJ. Pathophysiology and management of hypertension in acute ischemic stroke. *Hypertension* 1994; **23**:131–6
8 Morfis L, Schwartz RS, Poulos R, Howes LG. Blood pressure changes in acute cerebral infarction and hemorrhage. *Stroke* 1997; **28**: 1401–5
9 Carlberg B, Asplund K, Hagg E. Factors influencing admission blood pressure levels in patients with acute stroke. *Stroke* 1991; **4**: 527–30
10 Harper G, Castleden CM, Potter JF. Factors affecting changes in blood pressure after acute stroke. *Stroke* 1994; **25**: 1726–9
11 Feibel JH, Hardy PM, Campbell RG, Goldstein MN, Joynt RJ. Prognostic value of the stress response following stroke. *JAMA* 1977; **238**: 1374–6
12 O'Neill PA, Davies I, Fullerton KJ, Bennett D. Stress hormone and blood glucose response following acute stroke in the elderly. *Stroke* 1991; **22**: 842–7
13 Murros K, Fogelholm R, Kettunen S, Vuorela A-L. Serum cortisol and outcome of ischemic brain infarction. *J Neurol Sci* 1993; **116**: 12–7
14 Fassbender K, Schmidt R, Mobner R, Daffertshofer M, Hennerici M. Pattern of activation of the hypothalamic-pituitary-adrenal axis in acute stroke. *Stroke* 1994; **6**: 1105–8
15 Treib J, Hass A, Krammer L, Stoll M, Grauer MT, Schimrigk K. Cardiac output in patients with acute stroke. *J Neurol* 1996; **243**: 575–8
16 Warlow CP, Dennis MS, van Gijn J et al: Stroke. *A Practical Guide to Management*. Oxford: Blackwell Science, 1996
17 Marshall J, Shaw DA. The natural history of cerebrovascular disease. *BMJ* 1959; i: 1614–7
18 Bourestom NC. Predictors of long term recovery in cerebrovascular disease. *Arch Phys Med Rehabil* 1967; **48**: 415–59
19 Marquarsden J. The natural history of acute cerebrovascular disease: a retrospective study of 769 patients. *Acta Neurol Scand* 1969; **45**: 118–24
20 Carlberg B, Asplund K, Hagg E. The prognostic value of admission blood pressure in patients with acute stroke. *Stroke* 1993; **24**: 1372–5
21 Robinson T, Waddington A, Ward-Close S, Taub N, Potter J. The predictive role of 24-hour compared to casual blood pressure levels on outcome following acute stroke. *Cerebrovasc Dis* 1997; **7**: 264–72
22 Adams GF. Prospects for patients with strokes, with special reference to the hypertensive hemiplegic. *BMJ* 1965; ii: 253–9
23 Droller H. The outlook in hemiplegia. *Geriatrics* 1965; **20**: 630–6
24 Bath FJ, Bath PMW. What is the correct management of blood pressure in acute stroke? The Blood pressure in Acute Stroke Collaboration. *Cerebrovasc Dis* 1997; **7**: 205–13
25 Blood pressure in Acute Stroke Collaboration (BASC). *Interventions for deliberately altering blood pressure in acute stroke*. Oxford: Cochrane Library, 2000
26 Strandgaard S, Olesen J, Skinhoj E, Lassen NA. Autoregulation of brain circulation in severe arterial hypertension. *BMJ* 1973; ii: 507–10
27 Meyer JS, Shimazu K, Fukuuchi Y et al. Impaired neurogenic cerebrovascular control and dysautoregulation after stroke. *Stroke* 1973; **4**: 169–86
28 Wise G, Sutter R, Burkholder J. The treatment of brain ischaemia with vasopressor drug. *Stroke* 1972; **3**: 135–40
29 Rordorf G, Cramer SC, Efird JT, Schwamm LH, Buonanno F, Koroshetz WJ. Pharmacological elevation of blood pressure in acute stroke. Clinical effects and safety. *Stroke* 1997; **28**: 2133–8
30 Spense JD, Del Maestro RF. Hypertension in acute ischaemic strokes – *treat. Arch Neurol* 1985; **42**: 1000–2
31 Dandapani BK, Suzuki S, Kelley RE, Reyes-Iglesias Y, Duncan R. Relation between blood pressure and outcome in intracerebral haemorrhage. *Stroke* 1995; **26**: 21–4

32 Chamorro A, Vila N, Ascaso C, Elices E, Schonewille W, Blanc R. Blood pressure and functional recovery in acute ischemic stroke. *Stroke* 1998; **29**: 1850–3

33 The National Institute of Neurological Disorders and Stroke rt-PA Stroke Study Group. Tissue plasminogen activator for acute stroke. *N Engl J Med* 1995; **333**: 1581–7

34 Brott T, Lu M, Kothari R et al. Hypertension and its treatment in the NINDS rt-PA stroke trial. *Stroke* 1998; **29**: 1504–9

35 Hacke W, Markku K, Fieschi C et al. Randomised double-blind placebo-controlled trial of thrombolytic therapy with intravenous alteplase in acute ischaemic stroke (ECASS II). *Lancet* 1998; **352**: 1245–51

36 Lavin P. Management of hypertension in patients with acute stroke. *Arch Intern Med* 1986; **146**: 66–8

37 Bridgers SL, Koch G, Munera C, Karwon M, Kurtz NM. Intravenous nimodipine in acute stroke: interim analysis of randomized trials [abstract]. *Stroke* 1991; **22**: 153

38 Wahlgren NG, MacMahon DG, de Keyser J, Indredavik B, Ryman T, INWEST Study Group. Intravenous Nimodipine West European Stroke Trial (INWEST) of nimodipine in the treatment of acute ischaemic stroke. *Cerebrovasc Dis* 1994; **4**: 204–10

39 Kaste M, Fogelholm R, Erila T et al. A randomised, double-blind, placebo-controlled trial of nimodipine in acute ischemic hemispheric stroke. *Stroke* 1994; **25**: 1348–53

40 Squire IB, Lees KR, Pryse-Phillips W, Kertesz A, Bamford J. The effects of lifarizine in acute cerebral infarction: a pilot study. *Cerebrovasc Dis* 1996; **6**: 156–60

41 Lisk DR, Grotta JC, Lamki LM et al. Should hypertension be treated after acute stroke? A randomised controlled trial using single photon emission computed tomography. *Arch Neurol* 1993; **50**: 855–62

42 Yatsu FM, Zivin J. Hypertension in acute ischaemic strokes – not to treat. *Arch Neurol* 1985; **42**: 999–1000

43 Hachinski V. Hypertension in acute ischaemic strokes. *Arch Neurol* 1985; **42**: 1002

44 Powers WJ. Acute hypertension after stroke: the scientific basis for treatment decisions. *Neurology* 1993; **43**: 461–7

45 O'Connell JE, Gray GS. Treating hypertension after stroke. *BMJ* 1994; **308**: 1523–4

46 The European Ad Hoc Consensus Group. European strategies for early intervention in stroke. *Cerebrovasc Dis* 1996; **6**: 315–24

47 Popa G, Voiculescu V, Popa C, Stanescu A, Nistorescu A, Jipescu I. Stroke and hypertension. Antihypertensive therapy withdrawal. *J Neurol* 1995; **33**: 29–36

48 Schrader J, Rothmeyer M, Luders S, Kollmann K. Hypertension and stroke – rationale behind the ACCESS trial. *Basic Res Cardiol* 1998; **93 (Suppl 2)**: 69–78

49 Dyker AG, Grosset DG, Lees K. Perindopril reduces blood pressure but not cerebral blood flow in patients with recent cerebral ischemic stroke. Stroke 1997; **28**: 580–3

50 Barer DH, Cruickshank JM, Ebrahim SB, Mitchell JR. Low dose beta blockade in acute stroke ('BEST' trial): an evaluation. *BMJ* 1988; **296**: 737–41

51 Horn J, Limburg L, Orgogozo JM. Calcium antagonists for acute ischemic stroke (Cochrane Review). Oxford: Cochrane Library 2000

52 Butterworth RJ, Cluckie A, Jackson SHD, Buxton-Thomas M, Bath PMW. Pathophysiological assessment of nitric oxide (given as sodium nitroprusside) in acute ischaemic stroke. *Cerebrovasc Dis* 1998; **8**: 158–65

53 Bath PMW, Pathansali R, Iddenden R, Bath FJ. The effect of nitric oxide, given as transdermal glyceryl trinitrate, on blood pressure and platelet function in acute stroke. Cerebrovasc Dis 2000; In press

54 Albers GW, Atkinson RP, Kelley RE, Rosenbaum DM, for the Dextrorphan Study Group. Safety, tolerability, and pharmacokinetics of the N-methyl-D-aspartate antagonist Dextrorphan in patients with acute stroke. *Stroke* 1995; **26**: 254–8

55 Qizilbash N, Lewington SL, Lopez-Arrieta JM. Corticosteroids for acute ischaemic stroke (Cochrane Review). Oxford: Cochrane Library, 1999

56 Feigin VL, Rinkel GJE, Algra A, van Gijn J. Circulatory volume expansion for aneurysmal subarachnoid hemorrhage (Cochrane Review). Oxford: Cochrane Library, 1999

57 Asplund K, Israelsson K, Schampi I. Haemodilution for acute ischaemic stroke (Cochrane Review). Oxford: Cochrane Library, 2000

58 Neal B, Anderson C, Chalmers J, MacMahon S, Rodgers A, The PROGRESS Management Committee. Blood pressure lowering in patients with cerebrovascular disease: results of the PROGRESS (perindopril protection against recurrent stroke study) pilot phase. *Clin Exp Pharm Physiol* 1996; **23**: 444–6

59 Melamed E. Reactive hyperglycaemia in patients with acute stroke. *J Neurol Sci* 1976; **29**: 267–75

60 Gray CS, Taylor R, French JM et al. The prognostic value of stress hyperglycaemia and previously unrecognized diabetes in acute stroke. *Diabet Med* 1987; **4**: 237–40

61 Gray CS, French JM, Bates D, Cartlidge NEF, Venables GS, James OFW. Increasing age, diabetes mellitus and recovery from stroke. *Postgrad Med J* 1989; **65**: 720–4

62 Woo J, Lam CWK, Kay R, Wong AHY, Teoh R, Nicholls MG. The influence of hyperglycemia and diabetes mellitus on immediate and 3-month morbidity and mortality after acute stroke. *Arch Neurol* 1990; **47**: 1174–7

63 Toni D, Sacchetti ML, Agentino C et al. Does hyperglycaemia play a role on the outcome of acute ischaemic stroke patients? *J Neurol* 1992; **239**: 382–6

64 Kooten F, Hoogerbrugge N, Naarding P, Koudstaal J. Hyperglycemia in the acute phase of stroke is not caused by stress. *Stroke* 1993; **24**: 1129–32

65 Jorgensen HS, Nakayama H, Raaschou HO, Olsen TS. Stroke in patients with diabetes. *Stroke* 1994; **25**: 1977–84

66 Weir CJ, Murray GD, Dyker AG, Lees KR. Is hyperglycaemia and independent predictor of poor outcome after acute stroke? Results of a long term follow up study. *BMJ* 1997; **314**: 1303–6

67 Scott JF, Robinson GM, French JM, O'Connell JE, Alberti KGMM, Gray CS. Prevalence of admission hyperglycaemia across clinical subtypes of acute stroke. *Lancet* 1999; **353**: 376–7

68 Siemkowicz E, Hansen AJ. Clinical restitution following cerebral ischemia in hypo-, normo- and hyperglycemic rats. *Acta Neurol Scand* 1978; **58**: 1–8

69 Courten-Myers G, Myers RE, Schoolfield L. Hyperglycemia enlarges infarct size in cerebrovascular occlusion in cats. *Stroke* 1988; **19**: 623–30

70 Nedergaard M, Diemer NH. Focal ischemia of the rat brain, with special reference to the influence of plasma glucose concentration. *Acta Neuropathol (Berl)* 1987; **73**: 131–7

71 Cruz-Vazquez J, Marti-Vilalta JL, Ferrer I, Perez-Gallofre A, Folch J. Progressing cerebral infarction in relation to plasma glucose in gerbils. *Stroke* 1990; **21**: 1621–4

72 Ginsberg MD, Prado R, Dietrich WD, Busto R, Watson BD. Hyperglycemia reduces the extent of cerebral infarction in rats. *Stroke* 1987; **18**: 570–4

73 Pulsinelli WA, Levy DE, Sigsbee B, Scherer P, Plum F. Increased damage after ischemic stroke in patients with hyperglycemia with or without established diabetes mellitus. *Am J Med* 1983; **74**: 540–4

74 Olsson T, Viitanen M, Asplund K, Eriksson S, Hagg E. Prognosis after stroke in diabetic patients. A controlled prospective study. *Diabetologia* 1990; **33**: 244–9

75 Matchar DB, Divine GW, Heyman A, Feussner JR. The influence of hyperglycemia on outcome of cerebral infarction. *Ann Intern Med* 1992; **117**: 449–56

76 Tracey F, Crawford VLS, Lawson JT, Buchanan KD, Stout RW. Hyperglycaemia and mortality from acute stroke. *Q J Med* 1993; **86**: 439–46

77 Siesjo BK, Ekholm A, Katsura K, Theander S. Acid-base changes during complete brain ischemia. *Stroke* 1990; **21 (Suppl III)**: 194–8

78 de Courten-Myers GM, Kleinholz M, Wagner KR, Myers RE. Fatal strokes in hyperglycemic cats. Stroke 1989; **20**: 1707–15

79 Beghi E, Bogliun G, Cavaletti G et al. Hemorrhagic infarction: risk factors, clinical and tomographic features, and outcome. *Acta Neurol Scand* 1989; **80**: 226–31

80 Broderick JP, Hagen T, Brott T, Tomsick T. Hyperglycemia and hemorrhagic transformation of cerebral infarcts. *Stroke* 1995; **26**: 484–7

81 Dietrich WD, Alonso O, Busto R. Moderate hyperglycaemia worsens acute blood-brain barrier injury after forebrain ischemia in rats. *Stroke* 1993; **24**: 111–6

82 De Chiara S, Mancini M, Vaccaro O et al. Cerebrovascular reactivity by transcranial Doppler ultrasonography in insulin dependent diabetic patients. *Cerebrovasc Dis* 1993; **3**: 111–5

83 Strong AJ, Fairfield JE, Monteiro E et al. Insulin protects cognitive function in experimental stroke. *J Neurol Neurosurg Psychiatry* 1990; **53**: 847–53

84 Zhu CZ, Auer RN. Intraventricular administration of insulin and IGF-1 in transient forebrain ischemia. *J Cereb Blood Flow Metab* 1994; **14**: 237–42

85 Hamilton MG, Tranmer BI, Auer RN. Insulin reduction of cerebral infarction due to transient focal ischemia. *J Neurosurg* 1995; **82**: 262–8

86 Scott JF, Gray CS, O'Connell JE, Alberti KGMM. Glucose and insulin therapy in acute stroke; why delay further? *Q J Med* 1998; **91**: 511–5

87 Malmberg K, Ryden L, Efendic S et al. Randomised trial of insulin-glucose infusion followed by subcutaneous insulin treatment in diabetic patients with acute myocardial infarction (DIGAMI study): effects on mortality at 1 year. *J Am Coll Cardiol* 1995; **26**: 57–65

88 Diaz R, Paolasso EC, Piegas LS, ECLA (Estudios cardiologias Lantinoamerica) Collaborative Group. Metabolic modulation of acute myocardial infarction. The ECLA glucose-insulin-potassium pilot trial. *Circulation* 1998; **98**: 2227–34

89 Apstein CS. Glucose-insulin-potassium for acute myocardial infarction. Remarkable results from a new prospective, randomized trial. *Stroke* 1998; **98**: 2223–6

90 Scott JF, Robinson GM, French JM, O'Connell JE, Alberti KGMM, Gray CS. Glucose potassium insulin infusions in the treatment of acute stroke patients with mild to moderate hyperglycemia. *Stroke* 1999; **30**: 793–9

91 Castillo J, Martinez F, Leira R, Prieto JM, Lema M, Noya M. Mortality and morbidity of acute cerebral infarction related to temperature and basal analytic parameters. *Cerebrovasc Dis* 1994; **4**: 66–71

92 Azzimondi G, Bassein L, Nonino F et al. Fever in acute stroke worsens prognosis. *Stroke* 1995; **26**: 2040–3

93 Reith J, Jorgensen S, Pedersen P et al. Body temperature in acute stroke : relation to stroke severity, infarct size, mortality, and outcome. *Lancet* 1996; **347**: 422–5

94 Castillo J, Davalos A, Marrugat J, Noya M. Timing for fever-related brain damage in acute ischemic stroke. *Stroke* 1998; **29**: 2455–60

95 Young K, Busto R, Dietrich WD, Kraydieh S, Ginsberg MD. Delayed postischemic hyperthermia in awake rats worsens the histopathological outcome of transient focal cerebral ischemia. *Stroke* 1996; **27**: 2274–81

96 Davalos A, Castillo J, Pumar JM, Noya M. Body temperature and fibrinogen are related to early neurological deterioration in acute ischemic stroke. *Cerebrovasc Dis* 1997; **7**: 64–9

97 Ginsberg MD, Sternau LL, Globus MY-T, Dietrich WD, Busto R. Therapeutic modulation of brain temperature: relevance to ischemic brain injury. *Cerebrovasc Brain Metab Rev* 1992; **4**: 189–225

98 Maher J, Hachinski V. Hypothermia as a potential treatment for cerebral ischemia. *Cerebrovasc Brain Metab Rev* 1993; **5**: 277–300

99 Nakashima K, Todd MM. Effects of hypothermia on the rate of excitatory amino acid release after ischemic depolarization. *Stroke* 1996; **27**: 913–8

100 Chopp M, Chen H, Dereski MO, Garcia JH. Mild hypothermic intervention after graded ischemic stress in rats. *Stroke* 1991; **22**: 37–43

101 Baker J, Onesti T, Solomon R. Reduction by delayed hypothermia of cerebral infarction following middle cerebral artery occlusion in the rat: a time-course study. *J Neurosurg* 1992; **77**: 438–44

102 Ridenour TR, Warner DS, Todd MM, McAllister AC. Mild hypothermia reduces infarct size resulting from temporary but not permanent focal ischemia in rats. *Stroke* 1992; **23**: 733–8

103 Zhang R-L, Chopp M, Chen H, Garcia JH, Zheng G, Zhang G. Postischemic (1 hour) hypothermia significantly reduces ischemic cell damage in rats subjected to 2 hours of middle cerebral artery occlusion. *Stroke* 1993; **24**: 1235–40

104 Clifton GL, Allen S, Barrodale P et al. A phase II study of moderate hypothermia in severe brain injury. *J Neurotrauma* 1993; **10**: 263–71

105 Marion DW, Penrod LE, Kelsey SF et al. Treatment of traumatic brain injury with moderate hypothermia. *N Engl J Med* 1997; **336**: 540–6

106 Schwab S, Schwarz S, Spranger M, Keller E, Bertram M, Hacke W. Moderate hypothermia in the treatment of patients with severe middle cerebral artery infarction. *Stroke* 1998; **29**: 2461–6

107 Ropper AH, Shafran B. Brain edema after stroke. *Arch Neurol* 1984; **41**: 26–9
108 Hacke W, Schwab S, Horn M, Spranger M, De Georgia M, von Kummer R. 'Malignant' middle cerebral artery territory infarction. *Arch Neurol* 1996; **53**: 309–15
109 Forsting M, Reith W, Schabitz W-R et al. Decompressive craniectomy for cerebral infarction. An experimental study in rats. *Stroke* 1995; **26**: 259–64
110 Rengachary S, Batnitzky S, Morantz A, Arjunan K, Jeffries B. Hemicraniectomy for acute massive cerebral infarction. *Neurosurgery* 1981; **8**: 321–8
111 Delashaw JB, Broaddus WC, Kassell NF et al. Treatment of right hemispheric cerebral infarction by hemicraniectomy. *Stroke* 1990; **21**: 874–81
112 Rieke K, Schwab S, Krieger D et al. Decompressive surgery in space-occupying hemispheric infarction: results of an open, prospective trial. *Crit Care Med* 1995; **23**: 1576–87
113 von Kummer R, del Zoppo G, Frohlich E, John C, Hacke W, ECASS Study Group. Thrombolysis reduces the volume of ischemic lesions in humans [abstract]. *Stroke* 1996; **27**
114 Roberto C, Heros MD. Cerebellar hemorrhage and infarction. *Stroke* 1982; **13**: 106–9
115 Laun A, Busse O, Calatayud V, Klug N. Cerebellar infarcts in the area of supply of the PICA and their surgical treatment. *Acta Neurochir (Wien)* 1984; **71**: 295–306
116 Krieger D, Busse O, Schramm J, Ferbert A. German-Austrian scape occupying cerebellar infarction study (GASCIS): study design, methods, patient characteristics. *J Neurol* 1992; **239**: 183–5
117 Rieke K, Krieger D, Adams HP, Aschoff A, Meyding-Lamade U, Hacke W. Therapeutic strategies in space-occupying cerebellar infarction based on clinical, neuroradiological and neurophysiological data. *Cerebrovasc Dis* 1993; **3**: 45–55
118 Mathew P, Teasdale G, Bannan A, Oluoch-Olunya D. Neurosurgical management of cerebellar haematoma and infarct. *J Neurol Neurosurg Psychiatry* 1995; **59**: 287–92
119 Rogvi-Hansen B, Boysen G. Glycerol for acute ischaemic stroke (Cochrane Review). Oxford: Cochrane Library, 2000

Organisation of acute stroke care

Peter Langhorne

Academic Section of Geriatric Medicine, Royal Infirmary, Glasgow, UK

Information from randomised trials and systematic reviews is used to address issues in the organisation of early stroke care. Specifically, the following areas are discussed: (i) hospital-based care versus home-based care; (ii) organisation of care in hospital; and (iii) discharge and post-discharge care.

The organisation and delivery of acute stroke care represents only one component of a truly comprehensive stroke service (Fig. 1). However, the last 10 years have seen a renewed interest in the management of acute stroke patients, accompanied by an increased awareness that patient

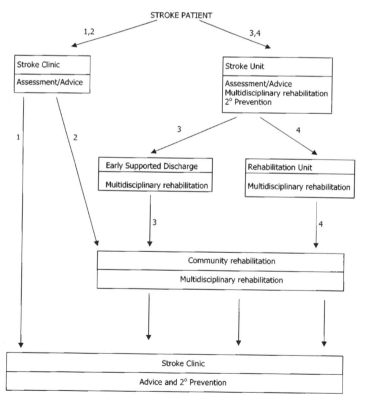

Correspondence to:
Dr Peter Langhorne,
Academic Section of
Geriatric Medicine,
3rd Floor Centre Block,
Royal Infirmary,
Glasgow G4 0SF, UK

Fig. 1 Comprehensive stroke service. Key: 1, very mild or fully resolved symptoms/disability; 2, mild symptoms/disability; 3, moderate symptoms/disability; 4, severe symptoms/disability.

outcomes may be directly influenced by the way services are organised. This chapter will use information from randomised trials and systematic reviews to focus on important issues in the organisation of early stroke care, *i.e.* the structures and processes of care in the first few weeks after stroke.

In addressing the organisation of acute stroke care, the following areas will be discussed: (i) hospital-based care versus home-based care; (ii) organisation of care in hospital; and (iii) discharge and post-discharge care.

Home *versus* hospital

In many countries[1], a great majority of stroke patients are admitted to hospital if only for a short period of time. In contrast, the UK has featured a debate around whether hospital-based or home-based care is the most appropriate for acute stroke patients[2,3]. Most clinicians are comfortable that patients with transient ischaemic attacks can be managed as out-patients, but there has been uncertainty about whether the routine care of stroke patients should be provided in a hospital or home-based setting. The current interest in acute stroke drug therapies has undoubtedly brought this uncertainty into focus.

A recent systematic review[4] has identified three controlled clinical trials which have compared routine processes of care (often involving hospital admission) with a home-based team trying to provide care in the home setting. There was considerable heterogeneity between the different studies with no evidence from either individual studies or combined analyses to support a radical change in stroke care. In fact, there was a trend for greater resource use by those randomised to home-based care. The reviewers concluded that there is currently no evidence to support a radical shift of acute stroke care from hospital-based to home-based services. The picture may be different when considering early discharge services (see below).

Hospital-based care

The majority of stroke patients in the UK are admitted to hospital at least for a short period of time[1]. Recent surveys indicate that stroke patients are often admitted to a variety of different settings and will usually be managed by a general physician or a consultant in geriatric medicine.

The main debate around hospital-based care has been whether a patient should be managed in an organised (stroke unit) setting and if this adds any benefit over conventional care in general wards. There is a long history of research examining this question with 20 controlled clinical trials identified in a recent systematic review[5]. Before proceeding with this discussion we need to define some terms.

Terminology

Stroke unit

The best working definition of a stroke unit is the provision of co-ordinated multidisciplinary care usually provided within a geographically discreet area such as a stroke ward[6]. Typically, these units have a variety of disciplines involved (medical, nursing, physiotherapy, occupational therapy, speech therapy, social work), whose work is co-ordinated through regular (weekly) multidisciplinary meetings.

Type of stroke unit

The stroke units can differ in a variety of ways, for example:
1 *Acute stroke unit* – providing stroke unit care for the first few days after stroke
2 *Rehabilitation stroke unit* – accepting patients 1–2 weeks after stroke and providing rehabilitation care for several weeks if necessary
3 *Comprehensive stroke unit* – combining both acute care and rehabilitation for several weeks if necessary
4 *Dedicated stroke unit* – providing care exclusively for stroke patients
5 *Mixed assessment/rehabilitation unit* – aiming to improve stroke care within a mixed disability setting

Effectiveness of stroke units

A total of 20 controlled clinical trials have compared organised in-patient (stroke unit) care with conventional care usually provided in general wards[5]. Overall, there were significant reductions in the odds of death (odds ratio 0.83: 95% CI 0.71–0.97: $P <0.05$), and the combined adverse outcomes of death or requiring institutional care (odds ratio 0.76; 95% CI 0.65–0.90: $P <0.0001$) and death or dependency (odds ratio 0.75; 95% CI 0.65–0.87; $P <0.0001$). The overall analysis indicated that, for every 100 stroke patients receiving organised (stroke unit) care, 3 additional patients would survive, 3 would avoid long-term institutional care, and an additional 6 would return home, of whom the majority would be physically independent. These apparent benefits were seen in both male and female patients, those aged above or below 75 years, and in those with mild or severe strokes. The benefits were observed in all types of stroke unit which were able to provide a period of care lasting several weeks if necessary (comprehensive stroke units or rehabilitation stroke units). Effective units were housed in a variety of departments including general medicine, geriatric medicine, neurology, and rehabilitation medicine, but all had developed similar processes of care (see below).

There was no systematic increase in the length of hospital stay associated with stroke unit care. This is important because in most Western countries the major healthcare costs of acute stroke are from nursing care and hospital overheads[1] and so relate closely to the length of stay. Costs in the longer term are largely attributable to the care of dependent individuals in hospitals or nursing homes[1] and so are likely to be determined by the number of patients with long-term disability. Therefore, it appears that stroke unit care will be more cost effective than conventional care providing long-term disability is reduced without increasing the cost of an episode of in-patient care or the mean length of stay in a hospital or institution. A recent economic analysis[7] indicates that stroke unit care is likely to save resources or provide improved outcomes for a modest increase in the cost.

Developing stroke unit care

The results of the stroke unit trials indicate that there are ways of improving the quality and outcome of routine stroke patient care in hospital. What lessons can be drawn from the stroke unit trials?

Stroke ward or mobile team?

Most of the stroke unit trials have evaluated a geographically discreet stroke ward with only one small trial specifically evaluating a mobile stroke team. At present, it seems reasonable to focus care within a stroke ward[6]. Firstly, most of the costs of a unit are attributable in the stroke team staff. Secondly, geographically defined units allow nurses to develop skills and act as facilitators for patients' independence and potentially as providers of continued therapy over the full day. Thirdly, stroke units also provide a focus for the development of research, fund-raising, and volunteer support groups. Finally, they can also facilitate the use of clinical guidelines and protocols. In practice, geographically defined units often overspill during busy periods and the staff have to operate as a mobile team to outlying patients.

Acute or rehabilitation unit?

Most of the clinical trial evidence comes from units which have provided a period of care lasting several weeks if necessary. These have included both comprehensive units, which combine acute and rehabilitation care, and rehabilitation units. The former are particularly common in Scandinavia.

Admitting all patients with stroke directly to a unit does allow the introduction of a standardised approach with assessment and treatment protocols, and may result in the early involvement of therapy staff[6]. It can also facilitate research and probably allows skills to be focused. In practice, it is probably important that the process of 'stroke unit' care begins as early as possible and is delivered in a continuous way.

Where should the unit be established?
Whoever is responsible for stroke care should have the necessary knowledge, training, and enthusiasm to take on the task. In the UK, most stroke patients are managed by general physicians and geriatricians, but stroke patient care can often benefit from specialist input of neurologists. Ideally, the development of stroke units and stroke services in general should draw upon the skill of different individuals to provide the best quality patient care.

Stroke unit size and staffing
Most of the stroke units in the systematic review were of moderate size (6–15 beds), although some rehabilitation units were larger. The total number of beds should reflect the local stroke incidence and hospital activity. A major challenge is the ability to cope with large fluctuations in stroke patient numbers[6].

Stroke units require medical, nursing, physiotherapy, occupational therapy, speech and language therapy and social work input as a basic minimum. A number of other professionals will also have a role in the management of some stroke patients[6]. It is difficult to give specific advice on the appropriate staffing levels, but approximate numbers are outlined elsewhere[6].

Patient selection criteria
There appears to be a good case for offering stroke unit care to a wide range of patients extending at least from those who have mild disability (*e.g.* initially requiring assistance with walking) through to those with severe strokes (*e.g.* no sitting balance). The systematic review[5] provides little information to guide the care of patients with very minor stroke or transient ischaemic attacks and those in coma. Where prioritisation is required, it is important to seek local agreement on appropriate triage.

Duration of stay
Some stroke units set a maximum length of stay, although the only real rationale for this is to allow the management of resources and prevent blocking of beds. An appropriately sized unit with flexible operating procedures ought to be able to provide care until discharge home or placement in alternative care. A splitting of acute stroke care and

rehabilitation is common, but it is important to ensure that there is a seamless transition of care as if provided by one single unit.

Practices and procedures

Having focused on aspects of stroke unit structure and policy, what are the important processes of care identified in the systematic review which should be adopted[6]?

Communication

All stroke units had a formal multidisciplinary team meeting at least once per week, lasting between 1–3 h, which was chaired by a senior staff member. These meetings provided a forum for multidisciplinary assessment, identification of problems and for the setting of short and long-term recovery goals. Many units also held less formal meetings on other occasions to ensure effective multidisciplinary working and involvement of carers[6]. A distinctive feature of stroke unit care was the early active involvement of carers in the rehabilitation process, including the provision of appropriate information about stroke disease and its management.

Care pathways

The following care pathways are typical of most stroke units[6].

1 *Assessment*: each patient would have a full medical assessment, including examination to establish the neurological impairment, routine blood chemistry and haematology and cranial CT scan. Other investigations such as MRI scanning, carotid Doppler ultrasound, and echocardiography were usually reserved for selected patients. Nursing and therapy assessments included the general care needs of the patient, identification of swallowing problems, and an assessment of the risk of developing pressure sores plus an evaluation of impairment and disability.

2 *Management*: stroke units which provided care in the acute phase have typically included the use of intravenous fluids to prevent and treat dehydration, early use of antibiotics for suspected infections, and measures to prevent DVT and other complications of immobility. These measures include compression stockings, early mobilisation, careful positioning and turning. Nursing management includes careful attention to posture and positioning, appropriate lifting and handling, and regular observation of key variables, *e.g.* swallowing problems, nutritional status, continence and skin integrity. Therapy input usually begins early, with nurses having a key role in the link between therapy staff and patients, incorporating recommended practices into the everyday handling of the patient. Standardised protocols were often used to detect swallowing problems and prevent aspiration. The routine use of intravenous fluids and nasogastric supplements were often considered in those with impaired swallowing.

The subsequent management of the rehabilitation process involved the regular reassessment of impairments and disabilities, multidisciplinary goal setting (involving patients and carers), and the monitoring of the patient's progress against these goals[6].

Discharge planning and post-discharge support

In the UK, the conventional approach to stroke patient care is to have a period in hospital with discharge planning at the time when the patient has made sufficient functional recovery to have a reasonable prospect of returning home alone or with the support of a carer. A recent development has been the promotion of an earlier discharge from hospital with increased support and rehabilitation input in the home setting. This has been termed 'early supported discharge' and has been tested in a number of randomised controlled trials. A recent systematic review of the four trials currently available[8] has indicated that these systems of care can shorten the length of hospital stay (by approximately 9 days) and there is a trend towards improved functional outcomes in the longer term. The two trials which have undergone economic analysis[9–11] have indicated that there is a marginal balance in favour of early discharge services. A number of trials are currently underway and more information is likely to become available in the future.

Conclusions

The current evidence on the organisation of acute stroke care suggests the following:

- There is no evidence to support a radical shift from hospital-based care to home-based care for the acute stage of stroke
- Within hospital stroke care should be provided in an organised (stroke unit) setting
- Processes of care within the stroke unit should reflect those of the randomised trials
- There may be a future role for early supported discharge services with post-discharge rehabilitation and support.

References

1   Warlow CP, Bamford J, Dennis MS *et al. Stroke: A Practical Guide to Management*. Oxford: Blackwell Science, 1996
2   Young J. Is stroke better managed in the community? Community care allows patients to reach their full potential. *BMJ* 1994; **309**: 1356–7

3   Lincoln NB. Only hospitals can provide the required skills. *BMJ* 1994; **309**:1357–8
4   Langhorne P, Dennis MS, Kalra L, Shepperd S, Wade DT, Wolfe CDA. Services for helping acute stroke patients avoid hospital admission. Oxford: Cochrane Library, 1999
5   Stroke Unit Trialists' Collaboration. Organised in-patient (stroke unit) care for stroke. Oxford: Cochrane Library, 1999
6   Langhorne P, Dennis M. *Stroke Units: An Evidence Based Approach*. London: BMJ Books, 1998
7   Major K, Walker A. Economics of stroke unit care. In: Langhorne P, Dennis M. (eds) *Stroke Units: An Evidence Based Approach*. London: BMJ Books, 1998, 56–65
8   Early Supported Discharge Trialists'. Services for reducing duration of hospital care for acute stroke patients. Oxford: Cochrane Library, 1999
9   Rudd AG, Wolfe CDA, Filling K, Beech R. Randomised controlled trial to evaluate early discharge scheme for patients with stroke. *BMJ* 1997; **315**: 1039–44
10 Rodgers H, Soutter J, Kaiser W *et al*. Early supported hospital discharge following acute stroke: pilot study results. *Clin Rehabil* 1997; **11**: 280–7
11 McNamee P, Rodgers RH, Craig N, Pearson P, Bond J. Cost analysis of early supported hospital discharge for stroke. *Age Ageing* 1998; **27**: 345–51

Surgical treatment of intracerebral haemorrhage

M Shahid Siddique and **A David Mendelow**

Department of Surgery (Neurosurgery), University of Newcastle upon Tyne, Newcastle upon Tyne, UK

There is at present no clear indication for surgical removal of intracerebral haemorrhage (ICH) in the majority of patients. With deterioration from an initially good level of consciousness, many surgeons would agree that removal is life saving. The question is whether or not surgical removal of clot improves the ultimate outcome in patients who are stable or even improving. Improvement in function is based on the concept of a penumbra around an ICH. There is now mounting evidence that there is a penumbra of functionally impaired, but potentially reversible, neuronal injury surrounding a haematoma. A pro-active approach must, therefore, be maintained in the management of these patients to salvage as much of this brain as possible. Alert patients with small (<2 cm) haematomas and moribund patients with extensive haemorrhage may not require surgical evacuation. Indications for clot removal in patients between these extremes are controversial. Current practice favours surgical intervention in the following situations: (i) superficial haemorrhage; (ii) clot volume between 20–80 ml; (iii) worsening neurological status; (iv) relatively young patients; (v) haemorrhage causing midline shift/raised ICP; and (vi) cerebellar haematomas >3 cm or causing hydrocephalus. A large multicentre prospective randomised controlled trial (International Surgical Trial in Intracerebral Haemorrhage) is currently underway to determine if early clot evacuation will lead to a better neurological outcome in patients with spontaneous supratentorial, non-aneurysmal ICH.

Spontaneous intracerebral haemorrhage (ICH) is common and has devastating consequences[1,2], affects a younger age group compared to other forms of stroke and has the highest mortality of all stroke subtypes. More than 50% of patients die and half of the survivors are left severely disabled[1,3], with significant personal, social and health service costs.

The treatment of intracerebral haemorrhage remains anecdotal and inconsistent[4,5]. There is no convincing evidence of benefit from any medical treatment, and the role of surgery remains controversial. There are two reasons for this: (i) the mechanism of neurological damage is poorly understood; and (ii) the prospective randomized controlled clinical trials comparing surgical and medical treatment of ICH have been small and inconclusive[6].

*Correspondence to:
Prof. A D Mendelow,
Department of
Neurosurgery,
Newcastle General
Hospital, Westgate Road,
Newcastle-upon-Tyne
NE4 6BE, UK*

Epidemiology

Accurate epidemiological data on ICH is not available, but various reports put the incidence between 10–44% of all strokes[1,2]. The incidence is highest in Asians, intermediate in blacks and lowest in whites[7] (120 per 100 000 in Japan, 17.5 per 100 000 for blacks, and 13.5 per 100 000 for whites). Risk factors include age, hypertension, history of coronary artery disease, previous stroke or TIA, cigarette smoking, alcohol consumption, low serum cholesterol, low dose aspirin and oral contraception[7]. Because ICH generally occurs without warning and as there is little potential to ameliorate the damage after a haemorrhage has occurred, prevention is of great importance. The decrease in incidence of ICH in the 1970s has been attributed, at least in part, to increased detection and treatment of hypertension[8].

Aetiology and pathophysiology

Intracerebral haemorrhage due to chronic hypertension accounts for about one-half of the cases. The underlying pathology is haemodynamic injury to perforating arteries, 100–400 μm in diameter, which arise directly from much larger trunks to enter the brain at right angles and are end arteries. Whereas the cortical vessels are protected by a thicker smooth muscle layer in the media, a series of bifurcations and collateral vessels, the perforating arteries are subjected directly to changes in blood pressure. The arteries in question include the lenticulostriate arteries, the thalamoperforating arteries, the paramedian branches of the basilar artery and the superior and anterior inferior cerebellar arteries. The pathological lesions may take the form of hyalinosis, lipohyalinosis or focal necrosis and Charcot-Bouchard/miliary aneurysm formation. In a series reported by Wiener[9], the locations of hypertensive ICH were as follows: 65% were in the basal ganglia, 15% were in the subcortical white matter, 10% were cerebellar and 10% were pontine. A number of other conditions are known to cause ICH. Coagulopathies are responsible for a significant proportion of cases. These may be congenital or acquired disorders of platelets, congenital clotting factor deficiencies or administration of anticoagulants and thrombolytic agents. Amongst the vasculopathies, cerebral amyloid angiopathy (CAA) is becoming an increasingly frequent cause due to the increase in the ageing population. Abuse of illicit drugs, which cause acute hypertension, is another cause of brain haemorrhage. Amphetamine, cocaine, phencyclidine and phenylpropanolamine are the drugs commonly responsible[10]. Rarely, ICH can occur following carotid

Table 1 Aetiology of spontaneous ICH

Hypertension	Chronic hypertension is responsible for over 50% of spontaneous cases. Incidence decreasing with better detection and effective treatment of hypertension Acute hypertension – as may occur in eclampsia (ICH is the most frequent direct cause of death[41])
Coagulopathies	Reported incidence 10–26%[42]. Includes congenital and acquired platelet disorders, congenital clotting factor deficiencies and administration of anticoagulants and thrombolytic agents
Arteriovenous malformation	Can occur anywhere in the brain
Aneurysms	Haemorrhage usually located in the Sylvian or the interhemispheric fissures
Vasculopathies	Cerebral amyloid angiopathy is the most common. The incidence is reported to be 10% in people in their 70s and over 60% in those in their 90s.
Recreational drugs	Including cocaine and amphetamines. They can cause an abrupt and often severe increase in systemic blood pressure
Post-operative	Rarely, carotid endarterectomy and cardiac surgery can be complicated by ICH Following craniotomy for excision of AVM, there may be ICH due to 'normal perfusion pressure breakthrough' Cerebellar haemorrhages have been reported following pterional craniotomy and temporal lobectomy[43,44]
Tumours	More commonly metastatic and pituitary tumours
CNS infection	Fungal bacterial and viral infections may be complicated by ICH
Venous or dural sinus thrombosis	Can lead to ICH because of venous hypertension
Miscellaneous	ICH has been reported following a migraine attack, strenuous physical exertion and exposure to cold possibly due to a sudden increase in cerebral blood flow

endarterectomy or cardiac surgery (Table 1). Any ICH may be due to a ruptured arteriovenous malformation. Aneurysms produce ICH in the Sylvian or interhemispheric fissures (Fig. 1). In addition, metastatic and pituitary tumours may present with ICH.

Although it was originally believed that intracerebral haemorrhage is largely a monophasic event[11], a number of investigators over the recent years have shown that early haemorrhage growth in patients with intracerebral haemorrhage is common[12–14]. Serial CT scans obtained at different intervals post ictus have shown an increase in haematoma volume in a varying proportion of patients (3–40%). Factors that have been seen to be associated with haemorrhage growth in the initial post ictus period include a previous history of brain infarction, liver disease, uncontrolled diabetes, elevated systolic blood pressure on admission (195 mmHg), a history of alcohol abuse, coagulation abnormalities (low level of fibrinogen), a large haematoma on initial CT scan, irregular shape of the haematoma, a high peripheral white cell count and elevated

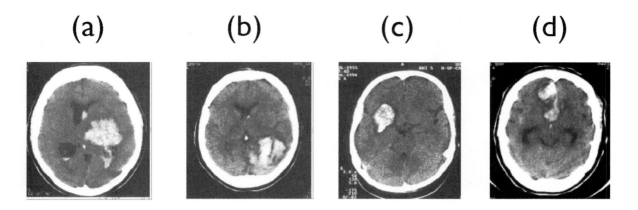

Fig. 1 Typical locations of (**a**) hypertensive basal ganglia bleed, (**b**) haemorrhage due to cerebral amyloid angiopathy and (**c, d**) aneurysmal bleed in the Sylvian and interhemispheric fissures, respectively.

body temperature on admission[13-16]. Murai *et al*[17] have shown that persistent haemorrhage may be detected in patients with acute ICH if CT angiography, performed within 12 h of ictus, shows extravasation of contrast.

Zone of reversible injury surrounding an ICH

Adjacent brain tissue is displaced and compressed by the extravasated blood. Animal models have shown that blood is irritating to the parenchyma, and that there is an area of oedema, ischaemia and haemorrhagic necrosis at the margin of the clot (ischaemic penumbra)[18]. The volume of this ischaemic brain may exceed the volume of the haemorrhage several times. Cerebral blood flow studies with single photon emission computed tomography (SPECT) in patients with ICH have been analyzed by the difference based region growing method[19] and have confirmed the presence of a zone of reversible ischaemia around the haematoma in man (Fig. 2). Kano and Nonomura were able to reverse some of the neurological disability in patients with ICH by giving hyperbaric oxygen[20]. This is strong evidence for the presence of a zone of reversible neuronal injury. Experimental studies in animals have suggested that early removal of the mass lesion can reduce the ischaemic damage[21]. SPECT studies in a series of 14 patients in our department showed greater recovery in the 'ischaemic penumbra' in patients undergoing surgery for evacuation of the haematoma compared with those managed conservatively[22]. In experimental animals, pre-treatment with the calcium channel blocker nimodipine resulted in a significant

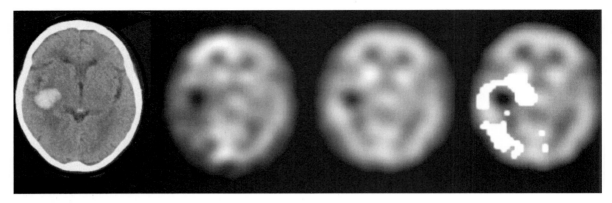

Fig. 2 Zone of reversible ischaemia around an intracerebral haematoma. Spontaneous ICH in a 69-year-old lady. (a) CT scan on day 1 following ictus. (b) SPECT study on day 1. (c) SPECT study on day 28. (d) Analysis of the day 28 SPECT study by the difference based region growing method defines 64.6 cm³ of peri-lesional brain that is absorbing at least more than 15% isotope compared to the same region on the day 1 study.

reduction in the histologically determined volume of ischaemia[23]. Similarly, pre-treatment with the N-methyl-D-aspartate (NMDA) receptor antagonist D-(E)-4-(3-phodphonoprop-2-enyl) piperazine-2-carboxylic acid (D-CPP-ene) reduced the amount of oedema at 24 h post ictus[23]. In addition, the magnitude of oedema was significantly less in leucopaenic animals exposed to irradiation prior to the experimental ictus[23]. This evidence suggests that there are significant therapeutic possibilities in the form of early evacuation of the haematoma and pharmacological neuroprotection that need further investigation.

It is possible that part of the neuronal loss in the penumbra surrounding an ICH is effected by apoptosis. Apoptosis has been shown to be active in neurones in the human brain following cerebral contusion[24]. This finding has also been reported from Pittsburgh[25]. It is now widely believed that it is responsible for some cell death in stroke[26]. In a study that is currently underway, we have seen markers of apoptosis in peri-lesional brain from patients with ICH. Substantial work has already taken place on the development of anti-apoptotic substances[26] and these may have a role to play in the treatment of ICH in the future.

The size of the haemorrhage determines the magnitude of rise in the intracranial pressure and the spectrum of clinical consequences ranges from headache through coma and herniation syndromes to death. The site of the bleed determines the type of neurological deficit produced. The deficit can progress over the course of a few hours following the ictus. Epilepsy is a known complication of ICH. Posterior fossa and third ventricular haematomas may obstruct the CSF pathways and produce hydrocephalus.

Management

It is important to determine the underlying aetiology rapidly. A history of hypertension, drug abuse and anticoagulant treatment is important. If a history of hypertension is not available, it may be difficult in the acute state in a patient with high blood pressure to decide whether it is due to previously undetected hypertension or secondary to raised intracranial pressure (ICP) with a Cushing response. Signs of end organ damage (brain, retina, heart and kidneys) can help differentiate the two. CT scanning is rapid and easily demonstrates blood as high density immediately after haemorrhage. Clot volume can be approximated by a modified ellipsoid volume (a x b x c)/2, where a, b and c are the diameters of the clot in the three dimensions[27]. MRI scanning takes longer, patient monitoring and ventilation are difficult during the study and appearance of ICH is complicated and highly dependent on the age of the clot[28]. It is, therefore, not the procedure of choice for the initial study. MRI scanning, however, is invaluable for identifying an underlying neoplastic lesion or an AVM if there are grounds for suspecting such a pathology following the initial CT scan. Routine laboratory evaluation should include coagulation studies. Screening for haematological abnormalities, infectious processes and vasculitides may be necessary in some cases. Angiography should be performed if there is any suspicion of an underlying vascular lesion, particularly if the appearances suggest an aneurysmal bleed, for example in the Sylvian or interhemispheric fissures (Fig. 1c,d).

Medical treatment

As there is reversibly injured brain around the haematoma at the time of the ictus, a pro-active and aggressive approach must be maintained in the management of these patients in the hope of salvaging as much of this brain as possible. Severely affected patients will need comprehensive management in an intensive care or high dependency unit. Intracranial pressure (ICP) may be raised as a result of the presence of a mass lesion, surrounding oedema, the strategic location of the haematoma causing hydrocephalus or due to hypertension. Hypoxia and hypercapnia, very common accompaniments of an impaired conscious level, may exacerbate brain swelling. Hydrocephalus will require treatment with ventriculostomy. Mannitol is helpful in reducing brain oedema in some patients. Very high blood pressure may contribute to haemorrhage growth in the initial phase and needs to be treated but over-treatment can compromise the cerebral perfusion pressure (CPP = BP – ICP). It has

Table 2 A spectrum of ICH patients

1	Alert patients with subtle neurological signs and small (< 2 cm) haematomas. Surgery not indicated
2	Indications for surgery between 1 and 3 are controversial. The following patients are more likely to be operated upon: (i) clot volumes between 20–80 ml; (ii) superficial/lobar haemorrhages; and (iii) worsening conscious level/neurological deficit
3	Large haemorrhage with significant neuronal destruction and poor neurological status (GCS < 5) Surgery not indicated

been suggested that the mean arterial pressure should be reduced to pre-morbid level if known or by approximately 20% if unknown[29]. The value of intracranial pressure monitoring has not yet been established[30]. In the few reported studies, an elevated ICP was statistically linked with a poor outcome but some patients with ICP in the normal range had a poor outcome. For clinical decision making, ICP monitoring should be considered in patients who are likely to run into problems from suspected elevation of ICP. Some authors recommend the use of prophylactic anticonvulsants for lobar haemorrhages. No benefit has been demonstrated from the use of steroids in ICH[31]. Nevertheless, some surgeons use them if there is significant peri-haemorrhage oedema.

Surgical treatment

There is a wide spectrum of clinical presentation with intracerebral haemorrhage and this determines surgical decision making (Table 2). On the one hand there are patients who present with large haematomas, coma with poor motor responses and unreactive pupils. At the other extreme are those who are orientated with minimal focal deficit and who have small haematomas. It is generally agreed that surgical evacuation is not needed for either of these two extremes. There is little agreement amongst surgeons on the merit of surgical evacuation in patients between these two extremes. Practice is haphazard and inconsistent. The cause for this inconsistency is a lack of objective evidence.

Attempts to evaluate the role of surgery in ICH began with McKissock's trial[32], published in 1961, which showed no benefit from operative treatment, but the study was undertaken prior to the advent of CT and randomization was not concealed. More recent observational studies have had variable results[33,34]. In the largest observational study, Kanaya and Kuroda[35] claimed that surgical treatment was beneficial for haematomas between 25–80 ml in volume, when the patients were stuporose. Six other randomized trials have been reported between

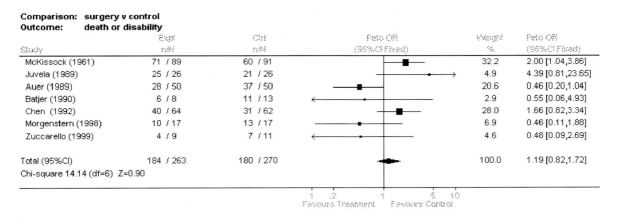

Fig. 3 Meta-analysis of trials comparing surgery with conservative management (from Fernandes *et al*[6] with permission). Odds ratio of being dead or dependent 6 months after surgical treatment for supratentorial primary intracerebral haemorrhage compared with conservative management (control) The odds ration of being disabled or dead after 6 months of ictus is 1.19, favouring conservative treatment. The difference is non-significant. This meta-analysis is based on all the reported prospective randomised controlled trials comparing surgery with conservative management for spontaneous supratentorial intracerebral haemorrhage. The seven trials included are McKissock *et al*[32], Juvela *et al*[45], Auer *et al*[46], Batjer *et al*[47], Chen *et al*[48], Morgenstern *et al*[49] and Zuccarello *et al*[50].

1989–1999. None of these trials was large enough individually to have the statistical power to quantify the risks and benefits of surgery. Meta-analysis of the seven prospective randomized controlled trials shows no significant advantage for either surgical or conservative management (Fig. 3)[6].

Under these circumstances, most therapeutic decisions have to be individualized, taking into consideration variables such as age, site, side and size of the haematoma, the mechanism of ICH and the presence of accompanying systemic complications. Currently, most neurosurgeons in the UK would operate on patients with a deteriorating conscious level and a worsening neurological deficit. In addition, haematomas between 20–80 ml in volume are more likely to be operated upon as are lobar/superficial haematomas[4]. With cerebellar haemorrhage, although there are again no randomized controlled trials comparing surgical and conservative treatment, there seems to be greater agreement that haematomas greater than 3–4 cm should be operated upon, especially when there is concomitant clinical deterioration or hydrocephalus[36,37].

Surgical options consist of: (i) conventional craniotomy and evacuation of the clot under direct vision, with or without the microscope; (ii) stereotactic aspiration through a burr hole – aspiration of a dense clot can be facilitated either by instillation of fibrinolytic agents or by fragmenting it by means of an ultrasonic device[38]; and (iii) endoscopic surgery[39]. There is as yet no evidence to suggest the superiority of one method over another in terms of patient outcome. The haematoma and its wall should be biopsied to rule out tumour, AVM, amyloid angiopathy or other pathology[40].

International Surgical Trial in Intracerebral Haemorrhage (ISTICH)

The uncertainty in clinical practice and the magnitude of this controversy are the ideal platforms from which to launch a randomized trial to identify the risks and benefits of surgery. There is global consensus amongst neurologists/neurosurgeons about the need for such a trial.

Following a successful pilot phase, a prospective randomized controlled trial is currently underway. The study aims to determine whether a policy of early surgical evacuation of the haematoma in patients with spontaneous supratentorial ICH, will improve outcome compared to a policy of initial conservative treatment. Patients are randomized to 'early surgical evacuation' or 'initial conservative treatment' within 72 h of ictus. Patient selection is based on the 'clinical uncertainty principle' (*i.e.* those in whom the surgeon is uncertain about the possible benefits and risks of operation). This includes those in whom the haemorrhage volume is 20–80 ml with a Glasgow Coma Score of 5–15. Survival and functional outcome will be assessed at 6 months by postal questionnaire. The power calculations based on a 10% improvement in favourable outcomes (from 35%) indicate that 1000 patients will be required to complete the study. Because a number of patients cross over (mainly from initial conservative treatment to surgery), this figure allows for subgroup analysis of the non-crossover patients. It is anticipated that recruitment will continue into the year 2000. At the time of publication 400 patients have been randomized.

Key points for clinical practice

There is mounting evidence that there is a zone of reversible neuronal injury surrounding a haematoma at the time of ictus. A pro-active approach must be maintained in the management of these patients in the hope of salvaging as much of this brain as possible.

Evaluation

- Urgent CT scan. (Ensure stability of vital functions prior to scanning)
- Clot volume (a x b x c)/2, where a, b and c are the three diameters of the clot

Table 3 Surgical treatment versus medical therapy

Factors that favour surgical removal of the haematoma	Factors that favour medical therapy
Superficial haemorrhage	Large haemorrhage with moribund patient (GCS < 5)
Clot volume between 20–80 ml	Orientated patient with small haematoma (< 2 cm)
Worsening neurological status	
Relatively young patients	
Haemorrhage causing midline shift/raised ICP	
Cerebellar haematomas > 3 cm or causing hydrocephalus	

- Consider contrast infusion in the following situations:
  * Young patient (< 40 years)
  * Worsening neurological signs
  * Non-hypertensive bleed
  * Atypical appearance/location of the clot
  * Accompanying subarachnoid haemorrhage

Initial management

- Support vital functions in severely ill patients

- Monitor and treat severe elevations of arterial blood pressure

- Administer anti-epileptic medication if indicated

- Check coagulation status. Correct/reverse abnormalities as indicated

- If mass effect is suspected from CT administer mannitol if not contra-indicated and consider ICP monitoring

- Consider angiography/MRI scanning if there is suspicion of underlying vascular abnormality or tumour

Surgical treatment

In the absence of objective evidence, Table 3 offers a guide. Decisions need to be individualized, based on the patient's neurological status, the size and location of the bleed, the age and state of health of the patient and the wishes of the patient/family. Consider the ISTICH trial if uncertain. At surgery, haematoma/wall biopsies should be taken.

Follow-up

Consider late (3–4 months) MRI/angiogram if there was suspicion of underlying vascular/neoplastic abnormality and initial investigations were negative

Acknowledgements

Any centres interested in the ISTICH trial can obtain further information from the following address: ISTICH Office, Ward 31, North Wing, Newcastle General Hospital, Westgate Road, Newcastle-upon-Tyne, NE4 6BE, UK. Tel: +44 (0) 191 219 5000; Fax: +44 (0) 191 256 3268; E-mail: stich@ncl.ac.uk.

Shahid Siddique is supported by grants from the Stroke Association and the UK Medical Research Council.

References

1   Bamford J, Sandercock P, Dennis M, Burn J, Warlow C. A prospective study of acute cerebrovascular disease in the community: the Oxfordshire Community Stroke Project – 1981–86. 2. Incidence, case fatality rates and overall outcome at one year of cerebral infarction, primary intracerebral and subarachnoid haemorrhage. *J Neurol Neurosurg Psychiatry* 1990; **53**: 16–22

2   Li SC, Schoenberg BS, Wang CC, Cheng XM, Bolis CL, Wang KJ. Cerebrovascular disease in the People's Republic of China: epidemiologic and clinical features. *Neurology* 1985; **35**: 1708–13

3   Fogelholm R, Nuutila M, Vuorela AL. Primary intracerebral haemorrhage in the Jyvaskyla region, central Finland, 1985–89: incidence, case fatality rate, and functional outcome. *J Neurol Neurosurg Psychiatry* 1992; **55**: 546–52

4   Fernandes HM, Mendelow AD. Spontaneous intracerebral haemorrhage: a surgical dilemma. *Br J Neurosurg* 1999; **13**: 389–94

5   Masdeu JC, Rubino FA. Management of lobar intracerebral haemorrhage: Medical or surgical. *Neurology* 1984; **34**: 381–3

6   Fernandes HF, Gregson BG, Siddique MS, Mendelow AD. Surgery in intracerebral haemorrhage: the uncertainty continues. Personal communication

7   Wolf PA. Epidemiology of intracerebral haemorrhage. In: Kase CS, Caplan LR. (eds) *Intracerebral Haemorrhage*. Boston: Butterworth-Heinemann, 1994; 21

8   Kaufman HH. *Spontaneous Intraparenchymal Brain Hemorrhage. Neurosurgery*, vol I: 2nd edn. New York: McGraw-Hill, 1996; 2567

9   Wiener H, Cooper P. The management of spontaneous intracerebral haemorrhage. *Contemp Neurosurg* 1992; **14**: 1–8

10 Caplan LR. Intracerebral hematomas. In: H Kaufmann, ed. New York: Raven Press, 1992; 34

11 Herbstein DJ, Schaumburg HH. Hypertensive intracerebral haematoma; an investigation of the initial haemorrhage and rebleeding using chromium Cr 51 labeled erythrocytes. *Arch Neurol* 1974; **30**: 412–4

12 Brot T, Broderick J, Kothari R *et al.* Early haemorrhage growth in patients with intracerebral hemorrhage. *Stroke* 1997; **28**: 1–5

13 Fujii Y, Takeuchi S, Sasaki O, Minakawa T, Tanaka R. Multivariate analysis of predictors of hematoma enlargement in spontaneous intracerebral hemorrhage. *Stroke* 1998; **29**: 1160–6

14 Fujii Y, Tanaka R, Takeuchi S, Koike T, Minakawa T, Sasaki O. Hematoma enlargement in spontaneous intracerebral hemorrhage [see comments]. *J Neurosurg* 1994; **80**: 51–7

15 Kazui S, Minematsu K, Yamamoto H, Sawada T, Yamaguchi T. Predisposing factors to enlargement of spontaneous intracerebral hematoma. *Stroke* 1997; **28**: 2370–5

16 Suzuki S, Kelley RE, Dandapani BK, Reyes-Iglesias Y, Dietrich WD, Duncan RC. Acute leukocyte and temperature response in hypertensive intracerebral hemorrhage. *Stroke* 1995; **26**: 1020–3

17 Murai Y, Takagi R, Ikeda Y, Yamamoto Y, Teramoto A. Three-dimensional computerised tomography angiography in patients with hyperacute intracerebral haemorrhage. *J Neurosurg* 1999; **91**: 424–31

18 Bullock R, Mendelow AD, Teasdale GM, Graham DI. Intracranial haemorrhage induced at arterial pressure in the rat. Part 1: Description of technique, ICP changes and neuropathological findings. *Neurol Res* 1984; **6**: 184–8

19 Zifko UA, Slomka PJ, Young GB, Reid RH, Bolton CF. Brain mapping of median nerve somatosensory evoked potentials with combined 99mTc-ECD single-photon emission tomography and magnetic resonance imaging. *Eur J Nuclear Med* 1996; **23**: 579–82

20 Kanno T, Nonomura K. Hyperbaric oxygen therapy to determine the surgical indication of moderate hypertensive intracerebral hemorrhage. *Minim Invasive Neurosurg* 1996; **39**: 56–9

21 Nehls DG, Mendelow AD, Graham DI, Teasdale GM. Experimental intracerebral hemorrhage: early removal of a spontaneous mass lesion improves late outcome. *Neurosurgery* 1990; **27**: 674–82

22 Siddique MS, Fernandes HF, Arene N U, Wooldridge TD, Fenwick JD, Mendelow AD. Changes in cerebral blood flow as measured by HMPAO SPECT in patients following spontaneous intracerebral haemorrhage. *Acta Neurochirurg* 2000; In press

23 Mendelow AD. Mechanisms of ischaemic brain damage with Intracerebral haemorrhage. *Stroke* 1993; **24 (suppl)**: 115–7

24 Siddique MS, Oakley A, Kalaria RN, Mendelow AD. Activation of caspase-3 in human brain after cerebral contusion. *Br J Neurosurg* 2000; **14**: 164–74

25 Clark RS, Kochanek PM, Chen M *et al*. Increases in Bcl-2 and cleavage of caspase-1 and caspase-3 in human brain after head injury. *FASEB J* 1999; **13**: 813–21

26 Barinaga M. Stroke-damaged neurons may commit cellular suicide. *Science* 1998; **281**: 1302–3

27 Broderick JP, Brott TG, Grotta JC. Intracerebral hemorrhage volume measurement [letter]. *Stroke* 1994; **25**: 1081

28 Bradley Jr WG. MR appearance of haemorrhage in the brain. *Radiology* 1993; **189**: 15–26

29 Kaneko T, Sawada T, Niimi T. Lower limit of blood pressure in treatment of acute hypertensive intracranial haemorrhage. *J Cereb Blood Flow Metab* 1983; **351**: S51–2

30 Janny P, Papo I, Chazal J, Colnet G, Barretto LC. Intracranial hypertension and prognosis of spontaneous intracerebral haematomas. A correlative study of 60 patients. *Acta Neurochirurg* 1982; **61**: 181–6

31 Poungvarin N, Bhoopat W, Viriyavejakul A *et al*. Effects of dexamethasone in primary supratentorial intracerebral hemorrhage. *N Engl J Med* 1987; **316**: 1229–33

32 McKissock W, Richardson A, Taylor J. Primary intracerebral haemorrhage; a controlled trial of surgical and conservative treatment in 180 unselected cases. *Lancet* 1961; **ii**: 221–6

33 Kanno T, Sano H, Shinomiya Y *et al*. Role of surgery in hypertensive intracerebral hematoma. A comparative study of 305 nonsurgical and 154 surgical cases. *J Neurosurg* 1984; **61**: 1091–9

34 Volpin L, Cervellini P, Colombo F, Zanusso M, Benedetti A. Spontaneous intracerebral hematomas: a new proposal about the usefulness and limits of surgical treatment. *Neurosurgery* 1984; **15**: 663–6

35 Kanaya H, Kuroda K. Development in neurosurgical approaches to hypertensive intracerebral haemorrhage in Japan. In: Kaufman HH. (ed) *Intracerebral Hematomas*. New York: Raven, 1992; 197–209

36 Kobayashi S, Sato A, Kageyama Y, Nakamura H, Watanabe Y, Yamaura A. Treatment of hypertensive cerebellar hemorrhage – surgical or conservative management? [see comment in: *Neurosurgery* 1995; **37**: 552–3]. *Neurosurgery* 1994; **34**: 246–51

37 Mathew P, Teasdale G, Bannan A, Oluoch-Olunya D. Neurosurgical management of cerebellar haematoma and infarct. *J Neurol Neurosurg Psychiatry* 1995; **59**: 287–92

38 Hondo H, Uno M, Sasaki K *et al*. Computed tomography controlled aspiration surgery for hypertensive intracerebral hemorrhage. Experience of more than 400 cases. *Stereotact Funct Neurosurg* 1990; **54**: 432–7

39 Auer LM. Endoscopic evacuation of intracerebral haemorrhage. High-tec-surgical treatment – a new approach to the problem? *Acta Neurochirurg* 1985; **74**: 124–8

40 Hinton DR, Dolan E, Sima AF. The value of histopathological examination of surgically removed blood clot in determining the etiology of spontaneous intracerebral haemorrhage. *Stroke* 1984; **15**: 517–20

41 Salerni A, Wald S, Flanagan M. Relationships among cortical ischemia, infarction, and hemorrhage in eclampsia. *Neurosurgery* 1988; **22**: 408–10

42 Tao HJ. *Manual of Neurosurgery. Non Aneurysmal Intracerebral Haematoma.* Edinburgh: Churchill Livingstone, 1996; 486

43 Toczek MT, Morrell MJ, Silverberg GA, Lowe GM. Cerebellar hemorrhage complicating temporal lobectomy. Report of four cases [see comment in *J Neurosurg* 1997; **86**: 916–7]. *J Neurosurg* 1996; **85**: 718–22

44 Papanastassiou V, Kerr R, Adams C. Contralateral cerebellar hemorrhagic infarction after pterional craniotomy: report of five cases and review of the literature. *Neurosurgery* 1996; **39**: 841–52

45 Juvela S, Heiskanen O, Poranen A *et al.* The treatment of spontaneous intracerebral hemorrhage. A prospective randomized trial of surgical and conservative treatment [see comment in *J Neurosurg* 1990; **72**: 152–5]. *J Neurosurg* 1989; **70**: 755–8

46 Auer LM, Deinsberger W, Niederkorn K *et al.* Endoscopic surgery versus medical treatment for spontaneous intracerebral hematoma: a randomized study. *J Neurosurg* 1989; **70**: 530–5

47 Batjer HH, Reisch JS, Allen BC, Plaizier LJ, Su CJ. Failure of surgery to improve outcome in hypertensive putaminal hemorrhage. A prospective randomized trial. *Arch Neurol* 1990; **47**: 1103–6

48 Chen X, Yang H, Cheng Z. Comparative study of the internal medical and surgical treatment of hypertensive intracranial haemorrhage. *Acta Acad Med Shanghai* 1992; **19**: 237–40

49 Morgenstern L B, Frankowski R F, Shedden P, Pasteur W, Grotta J C. Surgical treatment for intracerebral hemorrhage (STICH). A single-center, randomized clinical trial. *Neurology* 1998; **51**: 1359–63

50 Zuccarello M, Brott T, Derex L *et al.* Early surgical treatment for supratentorial intracerebral haemorrhage: a randomized feasibility study. *Stroke* 1999; **30**: 1833–9

Swallowing and prevention of complications

Paul A O'Neill

Department of Geriatric Medicine, University of Manchester, Manchester, UK

Dysphagia occurs in up to half of patients following a stroke. In most, it is transient with only about 1 in 10 of patients having any swallowing problems at 6 months. Persistent dysphagia may be due to lack of bilateral cerebral hemisphere representation of the oral and pharyngeal musculature involved in swallowing. Thus, the unaffected hemisphere is unable to take over the function of the damaged side. Bedside assessment is not a good predictor of aspiration on videofluoroscopy, but measurement of oxygen saturation may improve this. Nevertheless, clinical detection of dysphagia may be the more powerful predictor of an increased mortality and morbidity, including pneumonia, water depletion and poor nutrition. Dysphagia is also closely related to poor nutrition following stroke, but we do not know whether feeding support will improve outcome. Major trials are on-going.

Over the last decade, there has been a great interest in the effect of stroke on swallowing. The historical view was that dysphagia only occurred in patients with brainstem strokes, but it is now clear that many patients with hemispheric stroke also have swallowing difficulties. The dysphagia is often transient following an acute stroke[1], but is a sign indicating a poor prognosis[2], and an increased risk of complications including pneumonia[3], water depletion[4] and malnutrition[2].

Current work is focused on whether any specific therapy might improve the recovery of dysphagia[5] and whether supportive interventions such as percutaneous endoscopic gastrostomy (PEG) feeding might reduce the risk of complications, particularly poor nutrition and possibly pneumonia[6].

This review will begin by looking at the neurological control of swallowing and how this might be affected by stroke, together with the reported incidence of dysphagia in stroke. Following on from this background, the questions that are addressed are whether swallowing problems are of any consequence or are they simply a marker for stroke severity. Finally, the review will look at how complications of dysphagia might be prevented or treated to improve the overall outlook from stroke.

Control of swallowing

Swallowing is the act of moving food from the oral cavity to the stomach. It is usually considered to be 'voluntary', but most swallows occur

Correspondence to:
Dr Paul A O'Neill,
Department of Geriatric
Medicine, Research &
Teaching Building,
Withington Hospital,
Nell Lane, Manchester
M20 2LR, UK

involuntarily in response to saliva production. This link with salivation, rather than solely with the presence of food, is important when considering the risk of aspiration pneumonia.

Swallowing is a complex act that utilises 31 paired striated muscles. Rapid and fine neuromuscular control leads to mastication of food to a consistency appropriate for swallowing and moving the bolus from the oral cavity to the pharynx, oesophagus and finally the stomach. During swallowing, respiration ceases momentarily, which, again, is important when considering aspiration pneumonia.

There are three anatomically and temporally distinct phases: (i) oral, including preparatory and propulsion; (ii) pharyngeal; and (iii) oesophageal.

Oral

Preparatory

Teeth, tongue, lips and cheeks respond to the sensation of taste by forming the food into a bolus. This is then held by the tip of the tongue against the alveolar ridge or superior incisors, which traps the food bolus against the hard palate.

Propulsive

The tongue lifts and presses the bolus against the roof of the mouth and sends it into the oropharynx using a sequential squeezing action. When the bolus reaches the faucial arches, sensory receptors trigger the pharyngeal stage, starting with descent of the tongue base and elevation of the uvula to create a pathway for the bolus that will be helped by gravity.

Pharyngeal

The start of the pharyngeal phase is defined as when the bolus passes the tonsillar pillars and finishes when it enters the oesophagus. A number of mechanisms protect the nasopharynx and airway. The soft palate approximates to the pharyngeal walls to prevent nasal regurgitation. The larynx and hyoid move upwards and anteriorly, and the larynx is closed from the vocal cords to the false cords. The laryngeal entrance is also protected by the epiglottis and aryepiglottic folds.

Pressure from the tongue base moves the bolus from the valleculae to the oesophageal inlet. Waves of pharyngeal peristalsis generate progressive contractile waves. Relaxation of the cricopharyngeal muscle leads to opening of the upper oesophageal sphincter. As the food moves into the oesophagus, the sphincter closes and the larynx and palate open so that respiration can restart. In total, like the oral phase, the pharyngeal phase lasts approximately 1 s.

Oesophageal

A disordered oesophageal phase is not usually a major cause of dysphagia following a stroke. Sequential peristaltic waves move the bolus down the oesophagus and the phase usually lasts 8–20 s.

Innervation and control

In an elegant series of experiments using transcranial magnetic stimulation, Hamdy et al[7] showed that the muscles involved in swallowing are discretely represented on the motor and premotor cerebral cortex with the topography of the oral, pharynx and oesophagus being arranged in set areas. Furthermore, there was marked asymmetry of representation in the two hemispheres, which was independent of handedness. This has major implications in predicting the occurrence of dysphagia following a stroke and also its recovery[8,9]. Others have suggested that there may not be discrete cortex 'swallowing' centres, but a distributed neural network involving both hemispheres[10].

The basic swallowing mechanism starts with trains of impulses from the cortices[7] that produce a temporal summation on the brainstem swallowing centre to trigger a swallow via the cranial nerves directly controlling the muscles involved. If there is residual material in the pharynx, sensory receptors detect this and initiate a second swallow to clear the material. If food goes 'the wrong way', then sensory mechanisms will elicit a cough reflex to protect the airway from aspiration and to clear the pharynx. It is very unusual for a fit person to aspirate or to have detectable pharyngeal foodstuffs after swallowing.

Dysphagia and stroke

Assessment

In dysphagia research, it is important to separate out studies that have used bedside (clinical) assessment tools to determine the presence of swallowing problems (e.g. Gordon et al[11] and Wade & Hewer[12]) and those that have used videofluoroscopy (VF; e.g. Splaingard et al[13]). Research carried out using VF has mainly used aspiration or penetration of food into the larynx as outcome measures, which may or may not have reflected the clinical presence of dysphagia. One blinded study[13] found that a standardised assessment of swallowing by speech and language therapists (SLTs) identified only 42% of patients who were aspirating on VF. Similarly, Smithard et al[14] found that the bedside assessment by a SLT gave a sensitivity of only 47% and a positive predictive value of 50% for the presence of aspiration in acute stroke. It is possible that measurement of oxygen desaturation alone or combined with bedside assessment will improve the clinical detection of aspiration[15], though others have found it to be unhelpful[16].

The other factor is whether VF should be regarded as the gold standard. The imaging is carried out in a controlled environment with good positioning of the patient and filming time of less than 3 min. This probably does not reflect swallowing function whilst feeding on a ward or at home, so the false negative rate may be high.

Given these concerns about the usefulness of very detailed bedside assessments, the most useful factors[14,17-19] in pointing towards the presence of a high risk of aspiration are: (i) any disturbance of conscious level; (ii) 'wet voice'; (iii) weak voluntary cough; (iv) cough on drinking small volumes of water' and (v) a timed water swallowing test. Despite the general moderate results from screening instruments, work continues on trying to delineate a good screening procedure using multiple items[20].

Epidemiology

Many studies have highlighted the high prevalence of swallowing problems following stroke, depending on the phase and type of assessment. In acute stroke, between one-quarter and a half of patients have dysphagia[2,4,11]. One important factor is the timing of the assessment; dysphagia is transient in many patients, resolving in the first couple of days[11].

Following the acute phase of stroke, many studies have used VF to determine the presence of swallowing difficulties. Prevalence rates of a half to two-thirds of patients[21-23] have been found, but the studies have been conducted months to years after a stroke on patients referred to specialist centres. In an unselected stroke population, Smithard et al[1] found that the initial prevalence of 51% had decreased to 11% at 6 months. However, more recently, Mann et al[24] showed that, in many dysphagic patients, the swallowing problems were still present at 6 months, particularly in elderly male patients with initial laryngeal penetration.

Prognosis

Dysphagia has been found in several studies to be associated with excess morbidity and increased mortality rates compared to stroke patients without swallowing difficulties[2,4,17]. When combined with other accepted indicators of poor prognosis (weakness, neglect, hemianopia, incontinence, apraxia, age and sex) in a multivariate logistic regression analysis, the presence of an unsafe swallow, but not aspiration on VF, remained a significant predictor of mortality[2]. Patients with reduced level of consciousness had already been excluded from the study population. Similarly, almost one-third of alert patients with dysphagia were dead by 6 months following their stroke compared to less than 10% of those with a normal swallow[4].

Swallowing difficulties are also an indicator of a worse functional outcome. Barer[4], Wade and Hewer[12], and Smithard et al[2] all reported that patients with dysphagia were more disabled as assessed by the Barthel index score. In addition, stroke patients with dysphagia were more likely to remain in institutionalised care[2,25].

Complications

Dysphagia is associated with: (i) aspiration and associated broncho-pulmonary infections; (ii) fluid depletion; and (iii) malnutrition. Aspiration pneumonia may account for about 1 in 20 deaths following stroke[26]. Gordon et al[11] found that 1 in 5 patients with dysphagia developed pneumonia compared with 1 in 12 without swallowing problems following stroke. In a case-matched study, Schmidt et al[27] reported that aspiration predicted the development of pneumonia with an odds ratio of over 5 in those patients who aspirated on thickened fluids. Although aspiration on VF is a predictor for pneumonia[28], it is likely that dysphagia detected at the bedside is a more powerful pointer to an increased risk: both Smithard et al[2] and Kidd et al[3] found that the risk of pneumonia remained whether or not aspiration was present on VF.

A number of studies have suggested that dehydration is associated with dysphagia following a stroke[4,11,13], but the differences compared with the non-dysphagic group did not reach statistical significance. Neither Schmidt et al[27] nor Smithard et al[2] found any links between swallowing problems and dehydration; the latter authors ascribed this to an active unit policy of fluid support as judged by the use of parenteral fluids.

Elsewhere in this issue, the relationship between stroke and mal-nutrition are reviewed. Axelsonn et al[29,30] noted a gradual deterioration in nutritional status with time following stroke, but considered this to be a function of the severity of brain damage and age of the patient rather than the ability to swallow. Davalos et al[31] also reported a worsening of nutritional indices after admission and also an increased risk of death. Smithard et al[2] found that the risk of malnutrition in the first month following stroke was associated with dysphagia, and suggested that this was due to poor food intake consequent upon the swallowing impairment.

Prevention and management of complications

Although the management of a dysphagic patient by a multidisciplinary team including a trained SLT is regarded as being a marker of good quality of care[32], there is limited evidence for this. Lucas and Rodgers did report a trend towards better outcome measures when an SLT was involved[33] and Jacobsson et al[34] suggested that outcomes were improved with individualised interventions in patients with severe eating problems.

The management of dysphagia and the prevention of complications can be considered in terms of: (i) specific therapies to improve recovery from dysphagia; and (ii) supportive measures to reduce the consequences of dysphagia. Many different therapies have been described in the literature for swallowing difficulties following a stroke and there is not a clear evidence base for selecting one of these to use in a patient with particular characteristics[32]. Some authors suggest that a therapy should be selected on the basis of bedside assessment[35], whilst others argue that such decisions should be determined by VF findings[36,37].

Logemann (38) put forward a framework consisting of 3 categories of therapies:

1 Compensatory: in which the aim is to eliminate the symptoms of dysphagia through altering the direction of food flow. An example is by paying careful attention to the position of the head and body during feeding[21].

2 Indirect: in which the aim is to improve neuromuscular control without giving the patient any food/fluid or causing him/her to swallow. An example is getting the patient to move their tongue or jaw against resistance[39].

3 Direct: in which the aim is to directly improve the pathophysiology of swallowing. The principal example is thermal (cold) stimulation of the oral cavity[40].

The work on thermal stimulation illustrates how further research is required to determine whether any of these therapies are of value (and under what circumstances). Lazzara et al[40] reported significant improvement in the triggering of swallowing after cold therapy. This study was criticised[41] on the grounds that the subjects were heterogeneous in terms of their stroke and nature of their swallowing problems. Furthermore, the duration and type of stimulation used were not clearly described. In a later paper, Rosebek et al[42] did not find any clear effect of thermal stimulation. More recently, oral electrical stimulation[43] and nifedipine[44] have been added to the number of therapies.

There have been few studies looking at the impact of specific interventions on aspiration pneumonia. An important factor is the origin of the infection. Murray *et al* found that accumulated oropharyngeal secretions predicted aspiration[45], which implies that pooling of saliva *per se* may be a major factor in developing pneumonia rather that feeding. Other studies have suggested that feeding tubes may not prevent aspiration[46] and that a major predictor of aspiration pneumonia is a previous episode[47]. In relation to acute stroke, it is possible that the aspiration of saliva occurs soon after the onset of symptoms, making it unlikely that stopping oral intake several hours later will have any impact on the development of pneumonia.

As with the prevention of aspiration pneumonia, it is not clear how an optimal level of hydration should be achieved in dysphagic patients following a stroke. Clearly, some fluid support is needed in those patients unable to take anything orally. However, due to the neuroendocrine response to acute stroke, some patients may have very high vasopressin levels[48]. It follows that these patients may need to be fluid restricted so that overhydration and hyponatraemia does not occur.

The major area in which a major impact on outcome following stroke may be possible is nutritional support. This is reviewed by Dennis[49] elsewhere in this issue, but, currently, there is only limited evidence for the use of PEG feeding or other nutritional support in patients with stroke.

Key points for clinical practice

- Screen all acute stroke patients for dysphagia using: disturbance of consciousness, wet voice, weak cough and cough on taking small amounts of water. Use pulse oximetry if available.
- If any doubt about presence of swallowing impairment, refer to a speech and language therapist
- Use videofluoroscopy only where the speech and language therapist needs information to guide choice of therapy
- Consider entering patients into the FOOD study[6,49] to determine fluid and nutritional support
- Monitor (and treat) for aspiration pneumonia

References

1   Smithard DG, O'Neill PA, England RE *et al*. The natural history of dysphagia following a stroke. *Dysphagia* 1997; **12**: 188–93
2   Smithard DG, O'Neill PA, Park C *et al*. Complications and outcome following acute stroke: does dysphagia matter? *Stroke* 1996: **27**: 1200–4

3   Kidd D, Lawson J, Nesbitt R, MacMahon J. The natural history and clinical consequences of aspiration in acute stroke. *Q J Med* 1995; **88**: 409–13

4   Barer DH. Dysphagia in acute stroke. *BMJ* 1987; **295**: 1137–8

5   Scottish Intercollegiate Guidelines Network (SIGN). *Management of Patients with Stroke: III: Identification and management of dysphagia*. Edinburgh: SIGN publications No 20, 1997

6   Dennis M. FOOD trial (feed or ordinary diet): a multicentre trial to evaluate various feeding policies in patients admitted to hospital with a recent stroke. *Trial Details Stroke* 1998; **29**: 2226–7

7   Hamdy S, Qasim A, Rothwell JC *et al*. The cortical topography of human swallowing musculature in health and disease. *Nat Med* 1996; **2**: 1217–24

8   Hamdy S, Qasim A, Rothwell JC *et al*. Explaining oropharyngeal dysphagia after unilateral hemispheric stroke. *Lancet* 1997; **350**: 686–92

9   Hamdy S, Aziz Q, Rothwell JC *et al*. Recovery of swallowing after dysphagic stroke relates to functional reorganisation in the intact motor cortex. *Gastroenterology* 1998; **115**: 1104–12

10 Daniels SK, Foundas AL. Lesion localization in acute stroke patients with risk of aspiration. *J Neuroimaging* 1999; **9**: 91–8

11 Gordon C, Langton-Hewer R, Wade DT. Dysphagia in acute stroke. *BMJ* 1987; **295**: 411–4

12 Wade DT, Hewer RL. Motor loss and swallowing difficulty after stroke: frequency, recovery, and prognosis. *Acta Neurol Scand* 1987; **76**: 50–4

13 Splaingard ML, Hutchins B, Sulton LD, Chaudhuri G. Aspiration in rehabilitation patients: videofluoroscopy versus bedside clinical assessment. *Arch Phys Med Rehabil* 1988; **69**: 637–40

14 Smithard DG, O'Neill PA, Park C *et al*. Can bedside assessment reliably exclude aspiration following stroke? *Age Ageing* 1998; **27**: 99–106

15 Zaida NH, Smith HA, King SC, Park C, O'Neill PA, Connelly MJ Oxygen saturation on swallowing as a potential marker of aspiration in acute stroke. *Age Ageing* 1995; **24**: 267–70

16 Collins MJ, Bakheit AMO. Does pulse oximetry reliably detect aspiration in dysphagic stroke patients. *Stroke* 1997; **28**: 1773–5

17 Kidd D, Lawson J, Nesbitt R, MacMahon J. Aspiration in acute stroke: a clinical study with videofluoroscopy. *Q J Med* 1993; **86**: 825–6

18 Gottilieb D, Kipnis M, Sister E, Vardi Y, Brill S. Validation of the 50 ml drinking test for evaluation of post stroke dysphagia. *Disabil Rebabil* 1996; **18**: 529–32

19 Hinds NP, Wiles CM. Assessment of swallowing and referral to speech and language therapists in acute stroke. *Q J Med* 1998; **91**: 829–3

20 Logemann JA, Veis S, Colagelo L. A screening procedure for oropharyngeal dysphagia. *Dysphagia* 1999; **14**: 44–51

21 Horner J, Massey EW, Riski JE, Lathrop DL, Chase KN. Aspiration following a stroke: clinical correlates and outcome. *Neurology* 1988; **38**: 1359–62

22 Horner J, Massey EW. Silent aspiration following stroke. *Neurology* 1988; **38**: 317–9

23 Horner J, Buoyer FG, Alberts MJ, Helms MJ. Dysphagia following brain-stem stroke. *Arch Neurol* 1991; **48**: 1170–3

24 Mann G, Hankey GJ, Cameron D. Swallowing function after stroke: prognosis and prognostic factors at 6 months. *Stroke* 1999; **30**: 744–8

25 Kalra L, Smith DH, Crome P. Stroke in patients aged over 75 years: outcome and predictors. *Postgrad Med J* 1993; **69**: 33–6

26 Elliot JL. Swallowing disorders in the elderly: a guide to diagnosis and treatment. *Geriatrics* 1988; **43**: 95–113

27 Schmidt J. Holas M, Halvorson K, Reding M. Videofluoroscopic evidence of aspiration predicts pneumonia and death but not dehydration following stroke. *Dysphagia* 1994; **9**: 7–11

28 Ekberg O, Hildefors H. Defective closure of the laryngeal vestibule: frequency of pulmonary complications. *Am J Radiol* 1985; **145**: 1159–64

29 Axelsson K, Asplund K, Norberg A, Alafuzoff I. Nutritional status in patients with acute stroke. *Acta Med Scand* 1988; **224**: 217–24

30 Axelsson K, Asplund K, Norberg A, Eriksson S. Eating problems and nutritional status during hospital stay of patients with severe stroke. *J Am Diet Assoc* 1989; **89**: 1092–6

31 Davalos A, Ricart W, Gonzalez-Huix F *et al*. Effect of malnutrition after acute stroke on clinical outcome. *Stroke* 1996; **27**: 1028–32

32 Park C, O'Neill PA. Management of neurological dysphagia. *Clin Rehabil* 1994; **8**: 166–74
33 Lucas C, Rodgers H. Variation in the management of dysphagia after stroke: does SLT make a difference. *Int J Lang Commun Disord* 1998: **33 (Suppl.)**: 284–9
34 Jacobsson C, Axelsson, Norberg A, Asplund K, Wenngren BI. Outcomes of individualised interventions in patients with severe eating difficulties. *Clin Nurs Res* 1997; **6**: 25–44
35 Sorin R, Somers S, Austin W, Bester W. The influence of videofluoroscopy on the management of the dysphagic patient. *Dysphagia* 1988; **2**: 127–35
36 Logemann JA. *Evaluation and Treatment of Swallowing Disorders*. San Diego: College-Hill, 1983
37 Field FH, Weiss CJ. Dysphagia with head injury. *Brain Inj* 1989; **3**: 19–26
38 Logemann JA. Approaches to the management of disordered swallowing. *Baillières Clin Gastroenterol* 1991; **5**: 269–80
39 Jordan K. Rehabilitation of patients with dysphagia. *Ear Nose Throat J* 1979; **58**: 86–7
40 Lazzara G de L, Lazarus C, Logemann JA. Impact of thermal stimulation on the triggering of the swallow reflex. *Dysphagia* 1986; **1**: 73–7
41 Warms T. Impact of thermal stimulation on the triggering of the swallow reflex. *Dysphagia* 1987; **2**: 55–8
42 Rosenbek JC, Robbins J, Fishback B, Levine RL. Effect of thermal application on dysphagia after stroke. *J Speech Hearing Res* 1991; **34**: 1257–68
43 Park CL, O'Neill PA, Martin DF. A pilot exploratory study of oral electrical stimulation on swallow function following stroke: an innovative technique. *Dysphagia* 1997; **12**: 161–6
44 Perez I, Smithard DG, Davies H, Kalra L. Pharmacological treatment of dysphagia in stroke. *Dysphagia* 1998; **13**: 12–6
45 Murray J, Langmore SE, Ginsberg S, Dostie A. The significance of accumulated oropharyngeal secretions and swallowing frequency in predicting aspiration. *Dysphagia* 1996; **11**: 99–103
46 Croghan JE, Burke EM, Caplan S, Denman S. Pilot study of 12-months outcomes of nursing home patients with aspiration on videofluoroscopy. *Dysphagia* 1994; **9**: 141–6
47 Hassett JM, Sunby C, Flint LM. No elimination of aspiration pneumonia in neurologically disabled patients with feeding gastrostomy. *Surg Gynec Obstet* 1988; **167**: 383–8
48 O'Neill PA, Davies I, Fullerton KJ, Bennett D. Fluid balance in elderly patients following acute stroke. *Age Ageing* 1992; **21**: 280–5
49 Dennis M. Nutrition after stroke. *Br Med Bull* 2000; **56**: 466–75

Nutrition after stroke

Martin Dennis

Department of Clinical Neurosciences, University of Edinburgh, Edinburgh, UK

Decisions about feeding are amongst the most difficult to face those managing stroke patients. About a fifth of patients with acute stroke are malnourished on admission to hospital. Moreover, patients' nutritional status often deteriorates thereafter because of increased metabolic demands which cannot be met due to feeding difficulties. Poor nutritional intake may result from: (i) reduced conscious level; (ii) an unsafe swallow (iii) arm or facial weakness; (iv) poor mobility; or (v) ill fitting dentures. Malnutrition is associated with poorer survival and functional outcomes, although these associations may not be causal. Patients often receive support with oral supplements or enteral tube feeding via nasogastric or percutaneous endoscopic gastrostomy. Although these probably improve nutritional parameters, it is unclear whether they improve patients' outcomes. Also the optimal timing, type and method of enteral feeding is uncertain. Large randomised trials are now in progress to identify the optimum feeding policies for stroke patients.

The influence of nutrition on the risk of stroke has been the subject of much research. In contrast, few studies of nutrition after stroke, especially that during the first few days and weeks, have been reported. This is surprising because feeding problems are amongst the most common and difficult management issues which confront the clinician caring for stroke patients.

This review aims to define what is known, what is not known and areas where more research is needed. It will not address the issue of dietary modification in secondary prevention nor provide a detailed account of swallowing problems and their assessment in stroke patients which have been covered elsewhere[1]. This review will focus on several clinically important questions including:

1 How can malnutrition be identified?

2 How common is malnutrition after a stroke?

3 Which patients are likely to have malnutrition?

4 Does malnutrition matter after a stroke?

5 Will nutritional support improve the patient's outcome?

Correspondence to:
Dr Martin Dennis,
Department of Clinical
Neurosciences, Western
General Hospital,
Crewe Road,
Edinburgh EH4 2XU, UK

6 How should stroke patients be fed?

7 When should tube feeding start after stroke?

8 Is feeding via a percutaneous endoscopic gastrostomy (PEG) better than that via a nasogastric (NG) tube?

How can malnutrition be identified?

In routine clinical practice there are practical difficulties in assessing stroke patients' nutritional status. A dietary and weight history may not be available because of patients' communication problems and an alternative source of this information may not be available if, as is common, the patient lives alone. Simple assessments of weight and height to estimate the body mass index (BMI) pose problems in immobile stroke patients. Specialised equipment, of limited availability, such as weighing beds or scales which accommodate wheelchairs, may be required and height may need to be estimated from the patient's demi-span or heel-knee length. More complex anthropometric measures, e.g. mid-arm circumference (MAC) and triceps skin-fold thickness (TFT) which allow the mid-arm muscle circumference (MAMC) to be calculated, require not only a tape measure and skin-fold callipers but training for the assessor to obtain reproducible measures. Anthropometric measures may also change because of paralysis of the arm after stroke. Laboratory parameters such as haemoglobin, serum protein, albumen and transferrin, are readily available but low levels occur in many conditions and do not necessarily reflect nutritional status. Indeed, in any acute illness, the serum albumen tends to fall due to increased catabolism and preferential production of acute phase proteins. More specialised measures such as vitamin estimations, antigen skin testing and bioelectric impedance (the latter to estimate body fat mass, body lean mass, body cell mass and total body water) are used in research, but are not widely available and are not suited to routine clinical practice. An awareness of the possibility of malnutrition is a key factor in identifying malnourished patients. A simple end of the bed assessment reliably identifies most stroke patients with low BMI and abnormal anthropometry[2]. Estimation of the BMI, serial weights to identify weight loss and monitoring of dietary intake could be used to screen patients on admission and monitor patients on stroke units although no specific assessment tool has been developed and tested for use in stroke patients[3]. Some assessment of patients' nutritional status should be routinely applied on admission to the stroke unit and periodically thereafter.

How common is malnutrition after a stroke?

Malnutrition is a common and often unrecognised problem in patients, especially the elderly, admitted to hospital. Those who remain in hospital for prolonged periods are also at risk[4]. Inevitably, the reported frequency of malnutrition after stroke has varied depending on patient selection, the definitions of malnutrition and the method and timing of assessments. Table 1 shows the various estimates of the frequency of malnutrition on admission to hospital after an acute stroke. Studies have varied in the number of nutritional parameters measured, their reference ranges and the number of abnormal results required to categorise patients as malnourished. Most have focused on undernutrition, but overnutrition with obesity is probably more common in Western countries and poses practical difficulties for patients[9]. Transfers, walking, continence and skin hygiene may all be compromised by obesity.

Several studies have shown that stroke patients' nutritional status may worsen during hospital admission[5-8,11]. However, these rely on grouped data where estimates of nutritional status later in the admission exclude those who have died or have already been discharged. Few studies have provided serial measurements in surviving patients, but those that have inevitably show that some patients improve, some deteriorate and some remain stable with respect to nutritional indices[5].

Which patients are likely to have malnutrition?

The factors which have been associated with malnutrition on admission to hospital are shown in Table 1, but few conclusions can be drawn.

Table 1 Estimates of the frequency of malnutrition in various studies

Study	n at baseline	Type of patients	n (%) with low albumen	n (%) classified as malnourished and criteria	Factors associated with malnutrition on admission
Axelsson[5]	100	Acute admissions	23 (23%)	16 (16%) > 2 low values	Increased age* Females* Prior peptic ulcer* Atrial fibrillation**
Unosson[6]	50	Acute admissions	31 (62%) < 36g/l	4 (8%) > 2 low values	n/a
Davalos[7]	104	Acute admissions	8 (8%)	17 (16%) either low albumen or TSF/MAMC	n/a
Gariballa[8]	201	All acute admissions	38 (19%) < 35g/l	n/a	n/a
Choi-Kwon[9]	88	Acute females only (highly selected)		30 (34%) > 2 low	Haemorrhagic stroke
Finestone[10]	49	Rehabilitation only	n/a	Mild 7 (14%) Moderate 9 (19%) Severe 8 (16%) > 1 low level	Dysphagia* Diabetes** Previous stroke**

British Medical Bulletin 2000;**56** (No. 2)

Drawing on the non-stroke literature, one would expect malnutrition to be more frequent in older patients, those living in institutions and poor social circumstances, those with prior cognitive impairment, physical disability or gastrointestinal disease. Stroke, like any acute illness, may lead to a negative energy balance and greater nutritional demands, but stroke patients may be less able to meet these increased demands[12]. Davalos et al[7] showed that patients with severe strokes have a greater stress response (based on cortisol levels) than those with milder strokes and that this was associated with a more marked deterioration in nutritional status. Complications such as infections which increase the patients' metabolic demands are associated with deteriorating nutritional status[5]. To compound the general problem of malnutrition, it has been estimated that up to 50% of hospitalised stroke patients are unable to swallow safely, although again the reported frequency depends on the selection of cases, the timing of assessments and the sensitivity of the method used to detect swallowing problems[11,13,14]. In most studies, deterioration in nutrition occurred more often in dysphagic patients[7,11] or in those who need help with feeding[6]. Even patients who are capable of swallowing liquids and food may have a poor appetite because of the effects of intercurrent illness or medication and they may eat more slowly or be less keen to eat because of facial weakness, lack of dentures or poor arm function[15].

Does malnutrition matter after stroke?

Poor nutrition, although not specifically in stroke patients, has been associated with reduced muscle strength, reduced resistance to infection and impaired wound healing[16,17]. Among patients with stroke, most of whom are elderly, muscle weakness, infections and pressure sores are common and account for significant mortality and morbidity[18]. It is plausible that malnutrition could increase the frequency of these problems and result in poorer outcomes. Davalos et al[7] showed that malnutrition after the first week of admission was associated with an increased risk of a poor outcome (dead or Barthel index ≤50) at 1 month, death, a greater frequency of infections and pressure sores, and longer length of stay. However, these associations were not statistically significant after adequate adjustment for stroke severity, using the Canadian Stroke Scale. More recently, Gariballa et al[8] showed that serum albumen, which may reflect nutritional status, predicted post-stroke survival, but did not adequately adjust for baseline stroke severity in their Cox proportional hazards' model. Although the Modified Rankin and Orpington Prognostic score at baseline was collected, the authors only included the former in their model, even though the latter is the better validated prognostic indicator. Based on these studies, there appears to be an association between malnutrition and poor outcome, but this is not necessarily independent of other prognostic factors and may not be causal.

Will nutritional support improve the patient's outcome?

Evidence of a causal relationship between malnutrition and poor outcome could come from intervention studies if improving nutrition resulted in better outcomes. There have been a large number of randomised trials testing the effects of providing protein calorie supplementation to diverse groups of patients. These studies have been individually too small to reliably demonstrate an effect on their own, but a recent systematic review of all of the available trials suggested that oral or enteral (*i.e.* via a feeding tube) nutritional supplementation definitely improves nutritional parameters and may reduce the odds of death (odds ratio = 0.66; 95% CI 0.48–0.91)[19]. However, this review included trials of differing methodological quality and when only more rigorous studies were included in the analysis the effect was statistically non significant (odds ratio = 0.81; 95% CI 0.44–1.50). None of these studies were specifically for stroke patients and few stroke patients were included. One small randomised trial (*n* = 42) has suggested that oral supplementation after stroke improves nutritional parameters[20] and a retrospective non-randomised study showed that early enteral nutrition after stroke reduced length of stay in hospital[21]. Thus, nutritional support probably improves nutritional parameters, but it is unclear whether this leads to improved clinical outcomes.

How should stroke patients be fed?

Even if there is little evidence to support nutritional supplementation, it is obvious that stroke patients require feeding. Ideally, patients would eat normally, but this is not possible for the important minority of patients who cannot swallow safely. Patients with swallowing difficulties are usually put 'nil by mouth' and given parenteral fluids believing (but with little scientific justification) that this will reduce the risk of aspiration pneumonia. Of course, these patients must still cope with their saliva. Patients' swallowing usually recovers over the first few days or weeks to an extent which allows most patients to safely take fluids and food, if necessary with a modified consistency[13,14,22,23]. Indeed, many patients can swallow safely if carefully positioned, given food and fluids of appropriate consistency and using a variety of compensatory strategies.

It is unclear how we should best support patients' nutritional status during the period when their oral intake is inadequate. How long is it reasonable to wait before starting feeding and what is the best route? Intravenous feeding can be used, but in practice is rarely justified in stroke patients who are able to absorb nutrients from their gut. Peripheral total parenteral nutrition (TPN) offers a less invasive option than that delivered via central venous line and may become more widely used where enteral routes are impractical. In most settings, the choice of support lies between enteral feeding via a nasogastric (NG) or percutaneous endoscopic gastrostomy (PEG) tube (Fig. 1) or one of the closely related alternatives, *e.g.* a radiologically-guided gastrostomy or a jejunostomy.

When should tube feeding start after stroke?

Whilst the patient cannot swallow adequate food, their nutritional status will inevitably deteriorate unless supported. If tube feeding was well tolerated and carried no hazard, then one would lose nothing by starting early. However, patients find tube feeding uncomfortable and it carries a risk of complications which have to be set against the benefits. By filling the patient's stomach, enteral feeding inevitably increases the risk of aspiration in patients who do not adequately protect their airway. In theory, early feeding might be associated with metabolic changes (*e.g.* hyperglycaemia) which could be detrimental to the ischaemic penumbra[24]. The balance of risk and benefit will vary depending on the nutritional status of the patient and whether they are taking any food orally. The risk associated with tube feeding, in turn, will depend on the method used, its duration and local factors (*e.g.* complication rates associated with PEG insertion). Some clinicians prefer to introduce tube feeding very soon after the stroke, others delay for days and sometimes weeks. There are no completed large randomised trials to guide our use of enteral feeding.

Is feeding via a PEG better than that via an NG tube?

Nasogastric (NG) tubes are often inserted to allow fluid and food to be given to patients. However, in patients who are unable to swallow, they are not always easy to insert and they are often pulled out by patients and have to be replaced, because they are uncomfortable. This adds to patients' distress, may necessitate a further X-ray to check position and interrupts any feeding regimen. NG tubes, especially the fine bore variety, may become displaced and cause aspiration. If left *in situ* for prolonged periods, ulceration of the nostril, oesophageal strictures and oesophagotracheal fistulae have been described. Because of these problems, some workers

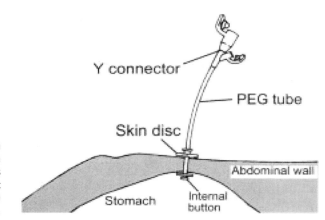

Y connector

PEG tube

Skin disc

Abdominal wall

Stomach   Internal
           button

Fig. 1 A diagram showing a percutaneous endoscopic gastrostomy (PEG) tube *in situ*.

advocate the increased and earlier use of PEG tubes. This technique, which can be performed with little or no sedation, provides an effective and quite acceptable method of enteral feeding (Fig. 1). However, any advantages of PEG over NG tubes, as far as improved delivery of nutrition is concerned, have to be carefully weighed against their relative complication rates. Unfortunately, despite the frequency of their use, there are few data concerning the complication rates associated with NG tubes in stroke patients. In contrast, literally hundreds of series have been published reporting the experience with PEG tubes, although relatively few specifically in stroke patients. A systematic review of a large number (but not all) of these studies[25] suggested that there was a 0.3% risk of death related to the procedure itself and a 10% risk of major complications (Table 2). However, these figures are likely to underestimate the risks in stroke patients because: (i) specialist centres which achieve better results are more likely to publish than those with less interest or higher complication rates; (ii) many studies are retrospective and rely on routine recording of complications; and (iii) stroke patients who tend to be elderly and frail may have higher complication rates.

Table 2 Reported frequency of major complications after percutaneous endoscopic gastrostomy (from Wollman[25])

Wound related	3.3%
Abscess	
Septicaemia	
Necrotising faciitis	
Aspiration pneumonia	2.1%
Peritonitis	0.5%
Other GI	2.4%
Perforation	
Gastro-colic fistula	
Haemorrhage	
Dislodged tube requiring repeat procedure	0.9%

Recently, several reports of the complication rates of PEG insertion amongst stroke patients have been published[26-30]. These included a total of 310 patients of whom about 8% died within a week or two of the procedure and 25% died during the hospital admission. The rates of various complications during variable follow-up periods were: aspiration pneumonia 19%, tube blockage/breakage or removal 11%, wound infection 8%, gastrointestinal haemorrhage 0.6% (one fatal), and fatal perforation 0.3%. Unfortunately, such studies are of limited value in guiding practice and indirect comparisons of complication rates between NG and PEG tubes are bound to be unreliable.

There have been only three small randomised comparisons of NG and PEG tube feeding. These suggested that the latter provided more effective nutritional support with less interruption of feeding[30-32]. One of these trials[30] was in severe stroke patients and showed that those fed by PEG had an implausibly large (70% relative) reduction in case fatality compared with those fed via NG tube. However, this trial only included 30 patients and little data were provided to allow an assessment of the effectiveness of randomisation in achieving balanced groups. It seems most likely that some imbalance in baseline factors accounted for much of the observed difference in outcome. Thus, the relative merits of the two types of tube are uncertain, at least in the first month or so after the stroke. There is little doubt that a PEG tube is a better option if feeding is to be prolonged. Also, in practice, there may be no alternative to a PEG tube if feeding is required and nasogastric feeding has been unsuccessful.

The need for more research

A survey of almost 3000 physicians who manage stroke in the UK demonstrated wide variation in the use of oral supplements and in the timing and method of feeding in dysphagic stroke patients[33]. Such variation reflects the lack of clear evidence to guide practice. There is clearly a need for large randomised trials to establish how best to feed patients after a stroke. Trials are needed to address several important questions including:

1 Should patients who can take adequate fluids orally routinely receive nutritional supplements to improve their outcome? If not are there particular groups of patients who should?

2 In patients who are unable to take adequate fluid and food orally immediately after the stroke, should we start tube feeding early or wait for a few days to allow their swallowing to improve?

3 If tube feeding is required, is feeding via a percutaneous endoscopic gastrostomy (PEG) superior to that via the traditional nasogastric tube (NG)?

The FOOD trial (Feed Or Ordinary Diet; www.dcn.ed.ac.uk/food) is an on-going multicentre international randomised trial which aims to address these and other important questions relating to nutrition after stroke.

Ethical considerations

Feeding is regarded by some as a basic component of care and by others as a medical intervention. Decisions about whether to feed, when to feed and how to feed stroke patients are among the most difficult to confront the professions involved in their care[34,35]. Many patients who are unable to eat normally are likely to have a poor functional outcome and perhaps a quality of life which some would judge to be worse than death. It is far from clear whether judgements regarding the quality of life in a dependent state made by the person before their stroke, or by their relatives or involved professionals are valid in making decisions about starting or continuing nutritional support. Unfortunately, most patients in whom this issue arises are unable to communicate their own wishes. Relatives may or may not be able to speak on their behalf. Nurses, doctors and therapists will all have an opinion, but these may not converge and may differ from those of the family. Moreover, the lack of reliable information about the benefits and risks of feeding techniques adds further uncertainty to decision making. Because of these difficulties, it is essential that issues surrounding nutritional support are discussed openly with all concerned, and that lines of communication are kept open so that the best decision can be made to minimize potential conflict.

References

1 O'Neill PA. Swallowing and prevention of complications. *Br Med Bull* 2000; **56**: 457–65

2 Mead GE, Donaldson L, North P, Dennis MS. An informal assessment of nutritional status in acute stroke for use in an international multicentre trial of feeding regimens. *Int J Clin Pract* 1998; **52**: 316–8

3 Nightingale JMD, Walsh N, Bullock ME, Wicks AC. Three simple methods of detecting malnutrition on medical wards. *J R Soc Med* 1996; **89**: 144–8

4 Sullivan DH, Sun S, Walls RC. Protein-energy undernutrition among elderly hospitalized patients: a prospective study. *JAMA* 1999; **281**: 2013–9

5 Axelsson K, Asplund K, Norberg A, Alafuzoff I. Nutritional status in patients with acute stroke. *Acta Med Scand* 1988; **224**: 217–24

6 Unosson M, Ek AC, Bjurulf P, von Schenck H, Larsson J. Feeding dependence and nutritional status after acute stroke. *Stroke* 1994; **25**: 366–71

7 Davalos A, Ricart W, Gonzalez-Huix F *et al*. Effect of malnutrition after acute stroke on clinical outcome. *Stroke* 1996; **27**: 1028–32

8 Gariballa SE, Parker SG, Taub N, Castleden CM. Influence of nutritional status on clinical outcome after stroke *Am J Clin Nutr* 1998; **68**: 275–81

9 Choi-Kwon S, Yang YH, Kim EK, Jeon MY, Kim JS. Nutritional status in acute stroke: undernutrition versus overnutrition in different stroke subtypes. *Acta Neurol Scand* 1998; **98**: 187–92

10   Finestone HM, Greene-Finestone LS, Wilson ES, Teasell RW. Malnutrition in stroke patients on the rehabilitation service and at follow up: prevalence and predictors. *Arch Phys Med Rehabil* 1995; **76**: 310–6

11   Smithard DG, O'Neill PA, Park C *et al*. Complications and outcome after acute stroke. Does dysphagia matter? *Stroke* 1996: **27**: 1200–4

12   Klipstein-Grobusch K, Reilly JJ, Potter J, Edwards CA, Roberts MA. Energy intake and expenditure in elderly patients admitted to hospital with acute illness. *Br J Nutr* 1995; **73**: 323–34

13   Gordon C, Langton Hewer R, Wade DT. Dysphagia in acute stroke. *BMJ* 1987; **295**: 411–14

14   Barer DH. The natural history and functional consequences of dysphagia after hemispheric stroke. *J Neurol Neurosurg Psychiatry* 1989; **52**: 236–41

15   Carr EK, Hawthorn PJ. Lip function and eating after a stroke: a nursing perspective. *J Adv Nurs* 1988; **13**: 447–51

16   Fiatarone MA, Evans WJ. The etiology and reversibility of muscle dysfunction in the aged. *J Gerontol* 1993; **48**: 77–83

17   Chandra RK. Graying of the immune system. Can nutrient supplements improve immunity in the elderly? *JAMA* 1997; **277**: 1398–9

18   Davenport RJ, Dennis MS, Wellwood I, Warlow CP. Complications following acute stroke. *Stroke* 1996; **27**: 415–20

19   Potter JN, Langhorne P, Roberts M. Routine protein energy supplementation in adults: systematic review. *BMJ* 1998; **317**: 495–501

20   Gariballa SE, Parker SG, Castleden CM. A randomised controlled trial of nutritional supplementation after stroke. *Age Ageing* 1998; **27** (**Suppl 1**): 66

21   Nyswonger GD, Helmchen RH. Early enteral nutrition and length of stay in stroke patients. *J Neurosci Nurs* 1992; **24**: 220–3

22   Smithard D, O'Neill P, England RE *et al*. The natural history of dysphagia following a stroke. *Dysphagia* 1997; **12**: 188–93

23   Mann G, Dip PG, Hankey GJ, Cameron D. Swallowing function after stroke. Prognosis and prognostic factors at 6 months. *Stroke* 1999; **30**: 744–8

24   Scott JF, Gray CS, O'Connell JE, Alberti KGMM. Glucose and insulin therapy in acute stroke; why delay further? *Q J Med* 1998; **91**: 511–5

25   Wollman B, D'Agostino HB, Walus-Wigle JR, Easter DW, Beale A. Radiologic, endoscopic and surgical gastrostomy: an institutional evaluation and a meta-analysis of the literature. *Radiology* 1995; **197**: 699–704

26   Wanklyn P, Cox N, Belfield P. Outcome in patients who require a gastrostomy after stroke *Age Ageing* 1995; **24**: 510–4

27   Wijdicks EFM, McMahon MM. Percutaneous endoscopic gastrostomy after acute stroke: complications and outcome. *Cerebrovasc Dis* 1999; **9**: 109–11

28   James A, Kapur K, Hawthorne AB. Long-term outcome of percutaneous endoscopic gastrostomy feeding in patients with dysphagic stroke. *Age Ageing* 1998; **27**: 671–6

29   Skelly R, Terry H, Millar E, Cohen D. Outcomes of percutaneous endoscopic gastrostomy feeding. *Age Ageing* 1999; **28**: 416

30   Norton B, Homer-Ward M, Donnelly MT, Long RG, Holmes GKT. A randomised prospective comparison of percutaneous endoscopic gastrostomy and nasogastric tube feeding after acute dysphagic stroke. *BMJ* 1996; **312**: 13–6

31   Park RH, Allison MC, Lang J *et al*. Randomised comparison of percutaneous endoscopic gastrostomy and nasogastric tube feeding in patients with persisting neurological dysphagia. *BMJ* 1992; **304**: 1406–9

32   Baeten C, Hoefnagels J. Feeding via nasogastric tube or percutaneous endoscopic gastrostomy. A comparison. *Scand J Gasterenterol* 1992; **27** (**Suppl 194**): 95–8

33   Ebrahim S, Redfern J. *Stroke Care – A matter of chance. A national survey of stroke services*. London: Stroke Association, 1999

34   Rabeneck L, McCullough LB, Wray NP. Ethically justified, clinically comprehensive guidelines for percutaneous endoscopic tube placement. *Lancet* 1997; **349**: 496–8

35   Macfie J. Ethics and nutritional support. *Wien Klin Wochenschr* 1997; **109**: 850–7

Management of spasticity in stroke

Bipin B Bhakta

Rheumatology and Rehabilitation Research Unit, University of Leeds, Leeds, UK

Spasticity treatment must be considered in relation to other impairments with functional goals defined prior to intervention. The effects of muscle co-contraction and involuntary limb movement associated with exaggerated cutaneous reflexes or effort as well as stretch reflex hyperexcitability need to be considered. Exacerbating factors such as pain must be identified. Physical therapy and conventional orthoses are the mainstays of spasticity management during acute rehabilitation. Botulinum toxin shows promise but needs further evaluation in the context of acute rehabilitation. Phenol chemodenervation can produce good results in spasticity refractory to standard treatments. Muscle strengthening exercises may be appropriate in chronic hemiparesis without adversely affecting tone. Electrical stimulation may be a useful adjunct to other spasticity treatments. Difficulty demonstrating functional benefit from antispasticity treatment may imply that interventions directed at single motor impairments whether weakness or spasticity are not likely to result in functional benefit, but it is their combination that is important.

Correspondence to:
Dr Bipin B Bhakta,
Rheumatology and
Rehabilitation Research
Unit, School of Medicine,
University of Leeds, 36
Clarendon Road,
Leeds LS2 9NZ, UK

Spasticity is abnormal muscle tone recognised clinically as resistance to passive muscle stretch which increases with velocity of stretch. It is more formally defined as: 'a motor disorder characterised by velocity dependent increase in tonic stretch reflexes with exaggerated tendon jerks, resulting from hyperexcitability of the stretch reflex'[1]. While these definitions are useful for diagnostic purposes, they are too restrictive in terms of understanding and managing the consequences of inappropriate muscle activity found after stroke. While paresis and loss of dexterity are the main causes of motor dysfunction, the impact of spasticity as defined by Lance remains controversial[2]. This controversy partly reflects lack of functional benefit found in some earlier studies of antispasticity treatments. For the purposes of understanding the role of antispasticity treatments on motor recovery following stroke, this article includes the effects of muscle co-contraction and involuntary limb movement associated with exaggerated cutaneous reflexes or effort (associated reactions), in addition to stretch reflex hyperexcitability.

Pathophysiology

Central to the generation of spasticity is overactivity of the alpha motor neuron (α-MN) pool, which also causes some of the other 'positive' manifestations described above. Lesions restricted to corticospinal tracts cause muscle weakness, loss of dexterity and a Babinski response, but not spasticity. Loss of descending input from cerebral cortex and basal ganglia, through medial and dorsal reticulospinal and vestibulospinal fibres, is thought to be important in causing impaired modulation of monosynaptic input from primary afferent (Ia) fibres (segmental myotatic reflex), and polysynaptic afferent input from cutaneous receptors and Golgi tendon organs contributing to α-MN hyperexcitability[1]. Spinal interneurons play a crucial part in this modulation, in particular through presynaptic and reciprocal Ia inhibition. Inappropriate muscle co-contraction may arise through reduced reciprocal Ia inhibition impeding voluntary limb movement[3]. In addition, nocioceptive and motor pathways have considerable influence on each other, emphasising the clinical importance of pain management in treating spasticity.

Consequences of spasticity

Stroke affecting the motor cortex or internal capsule commonly produces initial hypotonia and absent tendon jerks, followed several days or weeks later by spastic hypertonia in the antigravity muscles. The upper limb adopts an adducted posture at the shoulder and a flexed posture at the elbow and wrist, with the fingers flexed into the palm. In the lower limb there is hip and knee extension, with plantarflexion at the ankle.

In patients with no functionally useful voluntary limb movement, spasticity can maintain an abnormal resting limb posture leading to contracture formation. In the arm, severe flexion deformity of the fingers and elbow may interfere with hand hygiene and dressing, as well as affecting self image. In the leg, abnormal resting posture of the hips and knees may cause difficulty with wheelchair seating and transferring, as well as popliteal fossa and groin hygiene. In severe cases, the heel may be in contact with the buttock, with risk of pressure sores. Severe equinus deformity interferes with donning footwear and use of wheelchair foot plates. Spasticity, therefore, indirectly affects many aspects of self-care through the maintenance of abnormal limb posture. Articular and peri-articular pain caused by the abnormal resting position and immobility of the joints can exacerbate spasticity. Exaggerated reflex responses to cutaneous stimuli may cause painful flexor or extensor spasms, which can interfere with seating, transferring and cause sleep disturbance. In some patients, heterotopic calcification may cause pain and further encourage abnormal limb posture. The importance of pain relief in the management of spasticity should not be underestimated.

In patients with functionally useful voluntary limb movement, inappropriate co-activation of agonist and antagonist muscles can impede normal limb movement. In the arm, co-activation of the biceps and triceps may affect the placement function. Co-contraction of the forearm flexor and extensor muscles may prevent voluntary extension of the fingers and thus impede relaxation of grip. In the leg, involuntary knee flexion caused by inappropriate hamstring muscle activity with the effort of standing may interfere with weight bearing and walking. Dynamic equinus deformity of the ankle from calf muscle spasticity can impede toe clearance during the swing phase of gait causing the patient to fall as a result their toe 'catching' on the ground. The presence of clonus may have a direct effect on walking by affecting foot placement during standing. Inappropriate activity in the intrinsic muscles of the foot and long toe flexors may cause painful toe flexion and difficulty walking and running. Involuntary big toe hyperextension from extensor hallucis longus overactivity may interfere with donning footwear. Effortful activities (*e.g.* self-propelling a wheelchair, standing and walking) may generate inappropriate muscle activity causing involuntary movements in the paretic limbs (associated reactions). Although the role of associated reactions (AR) during motor recovery is debated, a direct impact is often implied when patients report involuntary limb movement (*e.g.* elbow flexion) interfering with standing or walking balance. In individuals where recovery is arrested during the synergistic stages, AR can become a long-term problem. Not all the consequences of spasticity are negative, for example hip and knee extensor spasticity may allow weight bearing, with the affected limb acting like a splint.

Management

Effective management of spasticity requires a multidisciplinary approach both for assessment and treatment and should not be viewed in isolation from the patient's other problems. Treatment should be directed at preventing abnormal limb or trunk posture and facilitate normal movement in the context of functional activities described above. Although the different approaches are described separately, for the management of an individual patient they should be integrated with one another as well as into the overall rehabilitation programme.

The management of spasticity can be broadly divided into: (i) identifying (usually painful) exacerbating factors (*e.g.* constipation, soft tissue rheumatism, pressure sores and deep venous thrombosis, post stroke pain syndrome) and their treatment; (ii) positioning the patient during sitting and lying to discourage the development of abnormal posture (therapeutic positioning of the patient aims to manipulate primitive reflexes, *e.g.* tonic neck reflexes and labyrinthine reflexes, released from higher motor control)[4]; and (iii) having access to treatments directed at established spasticity. Physical, pharmacological, electrical stimulation and surgical methods are used in spasticity treatment following stroke.

Physical treatment

Physiotherapy techniques aim to improve motor performance partly through manipulation of muscle tone. Several approaches are used during rehabilitation, although there is lack of evidence to show which is most effective[5]. The Bobath approach[6] advocates reduction of spasticity and primitive postural reflexes prior to facilitating voluntary activity in paretic muscles through attention to trunk posture and controlled muscle stretch of the limbs. Reduction in segmental reflex hyperexcitability through inhibition of distal segmental reflexes via Ib inhibitory interneurons is reported using this approach. The Brunnstrom approach[7] advocates techniques to promote activity in weak agonists by facilitating contraction of either corresponding muscles in the unaffected limb or proximal muscles on the paretic side. This technique focuses on individual muscle groups with the underlying concept that stimulation of the weak agonist muscle will result in Ia mediated reciprocal inhibition in the spastic antagonist muscle. Unfortunately, reduction in Ia reciprocal inhibition often accompanies spasticity and, therefore, this avenue of reflex suppression may not be available. In some patients where weakness predominates, resistive muscle strength training may improve motor performance without necessarily increasing limb spasticity[8]. Concurrent sensory stimulation using heat and cold can cause short-term reduction in spasticity[9] which can be useful adjunct to physical therapy treatment.

An important aspect of preventing and treating abnormal limb posture is maintaining full range of joint movement through regular mobilisation (at least 2 h during a 24 h period is suggested) and the appropriate use of orthoses and serial plaster casting to maintain muscle stretch. Orthotic prescription depends on the type of deformity that needs to be accommodated, the degree of voluntary limb movement and patient usability. Improvements in walking pattern have been demonstrated with ankle foot orthosis in patients with equinovarus deformity[10]. Thermoplastic splints are advocated for the arm while rigid or hinged polypropylene splints are needed to withstand forces in the leg produced during walking. Inflatable pressure splintage is used when rigid splints are not tolerated, particularly for severe finger flexion.

Lycra orthoses offers an alternative to thermoplastic and polypropylene splints for postural management of the upper limb[11].

Drug treatment

The rationale for the type of drug treatment used should reflect the functional problem and the pattern of muscle involvement. With the development of targeted antispasticity treatments, the role of systemic antispasticity agents (*e.g.* baclofen, dantrolene) in a disease which causes 'focal spasticity problems' is likely to diminish, particularly in the context of acute rehabilitation.

Oral baclofen, an effective antispasticity agent which is well tolerated if gradually increased to the maintenance dose (up to 100 mg/day), has an adverse effect on muscle strength (particularly in unaffected muscles), which may increase disability and, therefore, should be used cautiously in stroke patients and certainly should not be a first line antispasticity agent. It still has a role in patients with refractory generalised bilateral limb spasticity, particularly if pain is present. Attention to concurrent medication is important because non-tricyclic antidepressants (*e.g.* fluoxetine) may antagonise the effect of baclofen. If the role for oral baclofen is limited, is there a role for intrathecal administration of baclofen in stroke? Intrathecal baclofen infusion *via* pump is effective in refractory lower limb spasticity where several muscles groups in both legs are affected (*e.g.* spinal cord injury, multiple sclerosis). In stroke patients with unilateral spasticity, there is risk of weakening muscles on the 'normal' side and, therefore, intrathecal baclofen should not be used. Nevertheless, a small study including 3 stroke patients with severe chronic lower limb spasticity, reported tone reduction on the affected side with preservation of muscle strength on the 'normal' side following continuous intrathecal baclofen infusion[12].

A newer systemic drug, **tizanidine** (an α_2-adrenergic receptor agonist) is effective in reducing spasticity in patients with multiple sclerosis and spinal cord injury. Its effects are thought to be mediated via neurons in the locus ceruleous and inhibitory spinal interneurons. Like baclofen, tizanidine also appears to have an anti-nocioceptive effect. Use in multiple sclerosis and spinal cord injury suggests muscle weakness occurs less frequently than with baclofen. Evidence of effectiveness in stroke is limited because comparisons have only been made with diazepam[13] and, therefore, it is not recommended for routine use in stroke.

Dantrolene, while an effective antispasticity agent, causes muscle weakness as well as hepatotoxicity and has not been shown to be useful in stroke[14]. **Diazepam** adversely affects walking and increases the risk of cognitive dysfunction. These drugs should not be used for the routine management of spasticity in stroke. Although there has been recent interest in the antispasticity effects of **gabapentin**, there is no evidence to support its routine use for spasticity in stroke.

Disability attributable to inappropriate activity in a muscle or group of muscles would suggest an important role for targeted 'local' anti-spasticity treatment, given that oral treatments may cause generalised weakness. Percutaneous nerve and/or motor point blocks using phenol or alcohol, and intramuscular botulinum toxin type A are currently available targeted treatments.

Phenol nerve blocks have been used to successfully manage abnormal arm and leg posture in chronic hemiparesis (> 6 months post-stroke). In the leg, chemodenervation of the posterior tibial nerve can reduce equinovarus deformity[15], and in the sciatic nerve reduces inappropriate knee flexion. The effect may last from a few months to several years. Following phenol, painful dysaesthesia may occur through damage to the sensory fibres of mixed nerves (*e.g.* median), and vascular occlusion through damage to adjacent blood vessels. Phenol nerve blocks are no longer recommended for treatment of upper limb spasticity[16], although phenol motor point blocks reduce the risk of sensory disturbance. Alcohol (50%) has been used as an alternative to phenol, but it is less effective.

Botulinum toxin type A (BT-A) offers the possibility of local treatment of spasticity without affecting sensation. It is an established treatment for blepharospasm, hemifacial spasm and torticollis and has been used successfully (on an unlicensed basis) for spasticity treatment. BT-A, injected into the spastic muscle, produces chemodenervation by preventing release of acetylcholine at the neuromuscular junction[17]. BT-A acts peripherally to reduce muscle contraction caused by the hyperexcitable α-MN pool. The duration of muscle relaxation is usually 3 months, with loss of effect occurring through axonal sprouting proximal to the affected nerve terminal and the formation of new neuromuscular junctions. The preparations of BT-A currently available are Dysport® and BOTOX®. The potency, measured using a mouse bioassay, of these two preparations is different with 1 mouse unit of BOTOX® being equivalent to 3–5 mouse units of Dysport®[18].

The antispasticity effects of BT-A in stroke have been reported in short-term open studies, which often included patients with other diagnoses[19]. Impact on function has been more difficult to demonstrate, although improvement of limb posture following BT-A can translate into reduced disability and carer burden[20]. The largest reported placebo controlled study in 39 patients demonstrated a dose-dependent reduction in upper limb spasticity[21]. Investigation of BT-A treatment in the leg has been confined mainly to spastic equinus deformity. The largest placebo controlled study in 23 patients with hemiparesis, some of whom had traumatic brain injury, demonstrated reduction in calf spasticity and increased range of voluntary movement at the ankle after BT-A[22]. Walking speed was not significantly increased compared with placebo. To enhance the effect of BT-A, electrical stimulation of the treated muscles has been used[23] following animal experiments demonstrating increased uptake BT-A and reduced latency of muscle paresis following electrical stimulation. Current opinion advocates use of BT-A in conjunction with conventional physical therapy treatments and orthoses. BT-A may help to predict outcome from more permanent interventions such as phenol nerve blocks and surgery.

The advantages of BT-A over other antispasticity drug treatments is the ability to target specific muscle groups, lack of sensory disturbance, patient tolerability and ease of administration. The disadvantages of BT-A include short duration of action (which might be useful in acute stroke rehabilitation, but in patients with chronic spastic hemiparesis a longer term effect is often required). Distant unwanted muscle weakness may occur at a result of diffusion of toxin across fascial boundaries and systemic spread. Systemic effects such as generalised fatigue, flu-like symptoms, occur infrequently and are self-limiting. It is important to remember that antitoxin is of little value in iatrogenic botulism from overdosage or inappropriate placement of BT-A. Although the evidence to date relates to BT-A use in chronic hemiparesis, it may have a greater role in spasticity treatment during acute stroke rehabilitation. There is also the possibility of reducing contracture by early use of targeted antispasticity treatments[24]. Although animal experiments suggest that contracture may be prevented by BT-A, controlled studies investigating possible benefits of early intervention with BT-A are lacking.

Electrical treatment

Evidence for direct antispasticity effects of electrical stimulation is limited. Transcutaneous nerve stimulation applied over the dermatome corresponding to the nerve supply of the spastic muscle can produce short-lived reduction in spasticity. However, electrical stimulation directed at improving strength of paretic muscles[25] may augment the functional effects of BT-A treatment in the antagonist muscles. Electrical stimulation has also been used to compensate for muscle paresis causing equinus deformity. Electrical stimulation of the common peroneal nerve improved walking speed in patients with chronic hemiparesis whose walking was impaired because of equinus deformity with paresis and spasticity[26].

Surgical treatment

Surgical intervention can be broadly divided into procedures that interfere with the neuronal pathways and procedures that correct musculoskeletal deformity. Surgical ablation of peripheral nerves is usually reserved for patients in whom conservative antispasticity treatments have failed. Although this approach is inappropriate for mixed nerves, because of the risk of painful dysaesthesia, selective tibial neurotomy in patients with calf spasticity can improve the range of active ankle dorsiflexion[27]. Surgical sectioning of tendon and muscle combined with postoperative serial splintage can be used in patients with persistent deformity (*e.g.* Achilles tendon lengthening for equinus deformity at the ankle). In patients with potential for functional voluntary movement, fractional lengthening of forearm finger flexors, release of elbow flexors and tenodesis may facilitate arm placement and grip.

Key points for clinical practice

- While there is controversy regarding the role of spasticity on motor performance and the rationale for treating it, some of the later studies using targeted antispasticity treatment suggest aspects of motor performance may be improved[28]

- It remains difficult to demonstrate functional benefits from treatments directed at spasticity alone despite evidence of tone reduction. This may relate to the outcomes used, but perhaps reflects the fact that interventions directed at single motor impairments – whether weakness or spasticity – are not likely to result in significant functional benefit, but it is their combination that leads to benefit

- Not only must spasticity treatment be considered in relation to other impairments, but also functional goals defined prior to intervention

- Causes of pain must be identified and treated

- Physical therapy, attention to posture and seating, and conventional orthoses are the mainstays of spasticity management during acute rehabilitation

- Newer treatments – such as botulinum toxin-A and the use of Lycra splintage – show promise, but need further evaluation in the context of acute rehabilitation

- The role of muscle strengthening exercises in post acute rehabilitation may be appropriate for some patients without adversely affecting tone

- Electrical stimulation techniques, although used for movement loss related to muscle paresis may prove to be useful adjunct to other treatments (*e.g.* botulinum toxin-A) particularly for treating spastic equinus deformity

- Phenol nerve blocks can produce good results in leg spasticity refractory to standard treatments and can be useful in patients with chronic hemiparesis where botulinum toxin-A produces beneficial but short term effects

- Existing treatments in combination with the timely use of newer antispasticity drugs makes it likely that the number of patients with refractory spasticity requiring surgical intervention will diminish. Nevertheless, refractory spasticity will occur and, therefore, there is continued need for expertise in surgical interventions.

References

1 Brown P. Pathophysiology of spasticity. *J Neurol Neurosurg Psychiatry* 1994; **57**: 773–7

2 O'Dwyer NJ, Ada L, Neilson PD. Spasticity and muscle contracture following stroke. *Brain* 1996; **119**: 1737–49

3 Artieda J, Quesada P, Obeso JA. Reciprocal inhibition between forearm muscles in spastic hemiplegia. *Neurology* 1991; **4**: 286–9

4 Carr EK, Kenney FD. Positioning of the stroke patient: a review of the literature. *Int J Nurs Stud* 1992: **29**: 355–69

5 Basmajian JV, Gowland CA, Finlayson MA *et al*. Stroke treatment: comparison of integrated behavioural-physical therapy vs traditional physical therapy programs. *Arch Phys Med Rehabil* 1987; **68**: 267–72

6 Bobath B. (ed) *Adult Hemiplegia: Evaluation and Treatment*, 3rd edn, London: Heinemann, 1990

7 Brunnstrom S. (ed) *Movement Therapy in Hemiplegia*. New York: Harper and Row, 1970

8 Sharp SA, Brouwer BJ. Isokinetic training of the hemiparetic knee: effects on function and spasticity. *Arch Phys Med Rehabil* 1997; **78**: 1231–6

9 Price R, Lehmann JF, Boswell-Bessette S, Burleigh A, deLateur B. Influence of cryotherapy on spasticity at the human ankle. *Arch Phys Med Rehabil* 1993; **74**: 300–4

10 Hesse S, Werner C, Matthias K, Stephen K, Berteanu M. Non-velocity related effects of a rigid double-stopped ankle-foot orthosis on gait and lower limb muscle activity of hemiparetic subjects with equinovarus deformity. *Stroke* 1999; **30**: 1855–61

11 Gracies D-M, Fitzpatrick R, Wilson L, Burke D, Gandevia SC. Lycra garments designed for patients with upper limb spasticity: Mechanical effects in normal subjects. *Arch Phys Med Rehabil* 1997; **78**: 1066–71

12 Meythaler JM, Guin-Renfroe S, Hadley MN. Continuously infused intrathecal baclofen for spastic/dystonic hemiplegia. *Am J Phys Med Rehabil* 1999; **78**: 247–53

13 Bes A, Eyssette M, Pierrot-Deseilligny E, Rohmer T, Warter JM. A multicentre double blind trial of tizanidine as antispastic agent in spasticity associated with hemiplegia. *Curr Med Res Opin* 1988; **10**: 709–18

14 Katrak PH, Cole AM, Poulos CJ, McCauley JC. Objective assessment of spasticity, strength and function with early exhibition of dantrolene sodium after cerebrovascular accident: a randomised double blind study. *Arch Phys Med Rehabil* 1992; **73**: 4–9

15 Petrillo CR, Knoploch S. Phenol block of the tibial nerve for spasticity: a long term follow-up study. *Int Dis Stud* 1988; **10**: 97–100

16 Skeil DA, Barnes MP. The local treatment of spasticity. *Clin Rehabil* 1994; **8**: 240–6

17 Blasi J, Chapman ER, Link E *et al*. Botulinum neurotoxin A selectively cleaves the synaptic protein SNAP-25. *Nature* 1993; **365**: 160–3

18 First ER, Pearce LB, Borodic GE. Dose standardisation of botulinum toxin. *Lancet* 1994; **343**: 1035

19 Dunne JW, Heye N, Dunne SL. Treatment of chronic limb spasticity with botulinum toxin A. *J Neurol Neurosurg Psychiatry* 1995; **58**: 232–5

20 Bhakta BB, Cozens JA, Bamford JM, Chamberlain MA. Use of botulinum toxin in stroke patients with severe upper limb spasticity. *J Neurol Neurosurg Psychiatry* 1996; **61**: 30–5

21 Simpson DM, Alexander DN, O'Brien CF *et al*. Botulinum toxin type in the treatment of upper limb spasticity: a randomised double blind placebo controlled trial. *Neurology* 1996; **46**: 1306–10

22 Burbaud P, Wiart L, Bubos JL, Gaujard E, Debelleix X, Joseph PA. A randomised double blind placebo controlled trial of botulinum toxin in the treatment of spastic foot in hemiparetic patients. *J Neurol Neurosurg Psychiatry* 1996; **61**: 265–9

23 Hesse S, Reiter F, Konrad M, Jahnke MT. Botulinum toxin type A and short term electrical stimulation in the treatment of upper limb flexor spasticity after stroke: a randomised double blind placebo controlled trial. *Clin Rehabil* 1998; **12**: 381–8

24 Cosgrove AP, Graham HK. Botulinum toxin A prevents the development of contractures in the hereditary spastic mouse. *Dev Med Child Neurol* 1994; **36**: 379–85

25 Powell J, Pandyan AD, Granat M, Cameron M, Stott DJ. Electrical stimulation of wrist extensors in poststroke hemiplegia. *Stroke* 1999; **30**: 1384–9

26 Burridge JH, Taylor PN, Hagan SA, Wood DE, Swain ID. The effects of common peroneal stimulation on effort and speed of walking: a randomised controlled trial with chronic hemiplegic patients. *Clin Rehabil* 1997; **11**: 201–10

27 Feve A, Decq P, Filipetti P *et al*. Physiological effects of selective tibial neurotomy on lower limb spasticity. *J Neurol Neurosurg Psychiatry* 1997; **63**: 575–8

28 Hesse S, Krajnik J, Luecke D, Jahnke MT, Gregoric M, Mauritz KH. Ankle muscle activity before and after botulinum toxin therapy for lower limb extensor spasticity in chronic hemiparetic patients. *Stroke* 1996; **27**: 455–60

Predicting outcome in acute stroke

S P Stone*, S J Allder† and J R F Gladman‡

Academic Department of Geriatric Medicine, Royal Free and University College Medical School, London and Divisions of †Clinical Neurology and ‡Rehabilitation and Ageing, University of Nottingham, Nottingham, UK

The natural history of acute stroke is well defined. Predicting outcome in individuals, however, remains difficult, because prognostic studies examining associations between clinical signs or syndromes and outcome differ in patient selection, timing and choice of neurological assessments and outcome measures. Accuracy has been disappointing. Osler in 1892 stated that the *'course of the disease ... is dependent on the situation and extent of the lesion'*. Until recently, it has not been possible to examine the stroke prognosis, using Osler's approach, with any great accuracy. The advent of diffusion weighted magnetic resonance imaging (DWI), which is highly sensitive to the pathophysiological changes underlying stroke, offers this possibility as it measures the site and extent of irreversible infarction. This review summarises the results of syndrome or sign-based predictive studies and shows how DWI may explain different outcomes in patients with identical neurological presentations, according to the 'situation and extent of the lesion'.

Correspondence to:
Dr S P Stone, Academic
Department of Geriatric
Medicine, Royal Free
Campus, Royal Free and
University College
Medical School,
Rowland Hill Street,
London NW3 2PQ, UK

One of the most important tasks a doctor can perform for a patient is to give an accurate prognosis in terms of survival and the quality of that survival[1]. Since Rankin published his major study in 1957, doctors have sought a simple, reliable means of predicting outcome in stroke. Predicting outcome might be expected to be simple as we now have a wealth of information on the natural history of stroke from community-based studies in Bristol, Oxford and Copenhagen[1-7]. There is a relatively rapid phase of recovery in the first 3 weeks, during which time most deaths occur and, in most patients, the majority of recovery occurs in 3 months. Significant recovery occurs in 30% over the next 3 months and, although this is not statistically significant at the group level, it is clinically significant for individuals[3,8]. Both the Oxford and Copenhagen studies showed that at 6 months about 20% of people with a stroke are dead, 50% are independent and 30% are dependent in self-care[5,6]. As Osler pointed out[8], 'the course of the disease...depends on the situation and extent of the lesion' and the Oxford and Copenhagen studies provide epidemiological proof of this. The Oxford Community Stroke Project[5] reported 6 month outcome in ischaemic stroke according to a quasi neuro-anatomical classification (Table 1) of LACI (lacunar anterior circulation infarct), TACI (total), PACI (partial) and POCI (posterior circulation infarct) and the Copenhagen study which classified stroke as 'mild', 'moderate', 'severe' and 'very severe', reported that 80% of patients in these groups made their maximum functional recovery at 3, 7, 12 and 13 weeks, respectively[7].

Predictive models and single clinical variables

It would seem that all researchers need to do is examine a large number of patients with acute stroke, assess their outcomes at 6 months, use statistical techniques to identify significant predictor variables and then assign probabilities of outcome group membership to individual patients according to the presence of these variables. It has not proved as simple in practice and the literature offers a huge variety of predictive models. Some use single signs (e.g level of consciousness or incontinence)[1,10–13], others use combinations of signs (e.g visual neglect, level of consciousness, hemiplegia)[14,15]. Some use neurological scales or have investigated neuro-imaging (CT scan, NMR, SPECT, PET)[16–18]. However, the doctor wishing to advise patients with stroke on the basis of these studies may find them difficult to apply to their clinical practice for a number of reasons.

What a clinician requires of a good prognostic model is that it be based on a representative sample of patients, make clinical sense, be accurate and simple. However, studies often differ in their selection of patients, e.g community based[19], hospital based[12–15,20], stroke unit based[21] or restricted to patients under 75 years[19]. Timing of the neurological assessment that predicts outcome varies from 24 h[20], to 1 month[12]. Methods of neurological assessment may be part of standard clinical practice or may include new measures, which may or may not have been validated[22]. Timing of outcome assessment varies from 2 months, to 4 months, to 6 months, or at discharge and may vary within the study. Outcome measures vary between studies from 'place of discharge' to 'independence in self-care' to Barthel or other ADL score and the means used to classify people as 'independent' or 'dependent' may vary and may or may not have been standardised[22]. Outcome groups may be merged, e.g 'dead and dependent', even though they are clinically very different. There may be significant variation within any one outcome group, e.g 'dependent in personal ADL' covers the whole range from doubly incontinent and requiring PEG feeding to being able to do everything except get in and out of the bath unaided. Few studies[15,19] grade dependency as 'mild', 'moderate' or 'severe', and none have tried to predict specific activities of daily living, such as 'able to transfer with one', but it is these categories that may be clinically relevant to the difficulty of arranging a discharge home or elsewhere, and resource use thereafter. There is usually significant variation in patient management within individual studies as well as between studies. The Stroke Unit Triallists Collaboration's systematic review indicates that those managed on a stroke unit[2,3,23] or geriatric units[23] may well receive better management and have a better outcome than those managed on general medical wards[14,15,20]. Stroke is a disease primarily of old age[5], but pre-existing disability[23] and general cognition[2,14,23] are rarely taken into account. Presentation of results varies. The most useful, clinically, is recording the sensitivity, specificity, accuracy and likelihood ratio of any one predictor variable or equation. Studies giving statistical correlations between predictor variables and outcome are less immediately useful. Odds ratios are useful in identifying factors, such as fever or hypoglycaemia, that worsen prognosis and whose modification should, therefore, be the focus of a randomised controlled trial, but do not help with individual patient prediction. Some multi-variate models use complicated predictive equations[2,3,14,15]. Although not in itself a major criticism, this inconvenience makes it less likely that such models will be used. Finally, most models do not differentiate between patients with haemorrhage and those with an infarct, although there is evidence from the Copenhagen studies that outcome is no different once the level of severity of stroke is adjusted for.

Kwakkel et al[22] reviewed 78 prognostic studies and set up 10 criteria of internal, external and statistical validity. Only 13 (17%) studies met 8 or more of these criteria and many studies failed to meet some of the most basic, such as the use of reliable and valid outcome measures or predictor variables. Of the 13 studies, Kwakkel chose 8 that met all criteria for internal and statistical validity[2,12,15,18–20,24,25] and selected from those studies only the findings based on valid and reliable predictor variables. Urinary continence, loss of consciousness, disorientation, age, degree of paralysis were common predictors of outcome, with individual studies also identifying social support[25], visual neglect[15], tactile extinction[24] and visual field defects[2]. Scrutiny of these studies illustrates the difficulty of applying even these carefully selected findings to groups of stroke patients in general. One study only looked at outcome in those under 75 years[19]. Another study only recruited patients who were conscious and able to swallow medication at 48 h[20,24]. Some[2,15,25] used measures that are not yet part of standard clinical practice and one[18] depended on PET scanning, which may not be routinely available, particularly in the UK. Some presented results as correlation coefficients rather than giving sensitivity and specificity. Some merged death and dependency into one outcome[12,20,24] and most excluded death altogether[2,15,18,19,25].

Kwakkel et al[20] noted that few studies have been revalidated on a fresh sample of patients. Where this has happened, there may be good correlation between actual and predicted outcome but not so close as to be clinically useful in individual patients[21]. Indeed complex multivariate models had little advantage[1,11,13,26] over simple clinical predictors such as level of consciousness or incontinence. Even the most well validated predictors are not very accurate and there is little to support the use of predictive models in the clinical setting. They are more likely to be useful in stratifying clinical trials or in case mix analysis[15,20]. Simple predictors, such as level of consciousness[1,10–12,26], have a sensitivity for predicting death that varies from 40–78%, specificity that varies from 72–96% and overall accuracy of 60–80%. There is similar variation in the ability of level of consciousness to predict 'death or dependency'. Incontinence at 1 month predicts 'death or dependency' at 6 months[1,11,12,26], but sensitivity (57–92%), specificity (84–90%) and accuracy (75–89%) varies. More complex models, such as the Guy's Index or its modification, the 'G' score[20], predict 'death or dependency' with sensitivity of 34–86%, specificity of 63–99% and overall accuracy of 70–86%[20,26]. Most models are derived from clinical findings in the acute stage, but none seem able to account for the heterogeneity of stroke and accurately reflect 'the situation and extent of the lesion'.

Prediction and syndromes

Advice to patients and their relatives might, therefore, be better based on the epidemiological studies carried out in Oxford and Copenhagen, which have used a syndromic approach. Clinical syndromes combine individual signs, not in a mathematically generated fashion, as in a predictive model, but in a way that makes pathophysiological sense. They are used to diagnose stroke, and have, in the Oxford studies in particular, been used to study natural history. It would be reasonable to tell a patient with a LACI, for example, that their chances of survival are good and that two-thirds of patients with LACIs become independent in self-care and that a quarter are dependent to varying degrees (Table 1). The general discussion with them and their family would then include the fact that actual outcome remains uncertain. A similar 'syndromic'

Table 1 Natural history of stroke by subtype

Outcome at 6 months	LACI	TACI	PACI	POCI
Dead	7%	56%	10%	14%
Dependent	26%	39%	34%	18%
Independent	66%	4%	55%	68%

LACI, lacunar anterior circulation infarct; TACI, total circulation infarct; PACI, partial circulation infarct; and POCI posterior circulation infarct.

approach, not relying on acute stage signs, but on findings several weeks post-stroke, divides patients into three groups: those with only motor deficits, those with motor and sensory deficits and those with motor deficits, sensory deficits and hemianopia[27]. Studies using this simple scheme, which ignores higher cortical function, appears to identify different recovery patterns. Nearly 90% of 'motor only' patients became independently mobile (at a mean of 2.5 months post-stroke), 55% of 'motor and sensory' became mobile at a mean of 4.5 months, and 30% of 'motor, sensory and hemianopia' became mobile at 5.5 months. More work is required to examine the value of this classification in an unselected population at different times post-stroke.

Pathophysiologically based prediction

Until recently it has not been possible to examine the prognosis of stroke using Osler's approach, that the outcome depends upon the site and extent of the lesion, because at least 30% of patients have a normal CT. The future direction of prognostic studies may be dictated by developments in neuro-imaging (see Jäger in this issue). Diffusion and perfusion weighted imaging MRI (DWI and PWI) and MRI angiography allow the arterial territory of cerebral infarction to be accurately identified, whereas clinical examination (and hence the use of syndromic classification) is inaccurate. Furthermore, studies beginning in the first few hours after stroke may show significant pathophysiological differences in the state of the ischaemic insult present in patients with identical stroke syndromes. DWI lesions in patients who have undergone spontaneous recannalisation do not increase in size, whereas in patients with a persisting arterial occlusion and an ischaemic penumbra (DWI–PWI mismatch) further increases in the volume of infarction may occur. This might explain some of the variability in outcome even within groups of patients with infarction in the same arterial territory. We are not alone in believing that such MRI studies have the potential to help clinicians make the most accurate prediction of prognosis for individual patients. Pritchard and Grossmann commented that MRI techniques are 'unique among all imaging methods in their sensitivity to the pathophysiological changes underlying acute stroke' and are likely to become the investigations of choice in the acute management of stroke[28].

To give examples of the way in which the accurate localisation of the lesion obtained by these techniques might be used to predict outcome we present three cases. Figures 1–3 show the DWI images taken within 24 h of stroke, of 3 patients with identical TACI-type syndromes presenting with hemiparesis, the PWI and MRA images were normal in each case

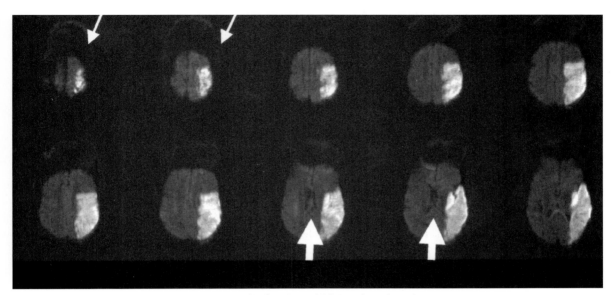

Fig. 1 The DWI lesion reveals extensive cortical infarction which involves the primary motor cortex.

implying spontaneous recanalization so there was no risk of developing further ischaemic damage. The white areas represent acute infarction. The contrast that can be seen between damaged and normal tissue is very easy to see, and this demonstrates how precisely these images can localise cerebral infarction. In case 1 (Fig. 1), the primary motor cortex was involved (thin arrows). Although the subcortical section of the pyramidal tracts was intact (thick arrows), the patient made little motor

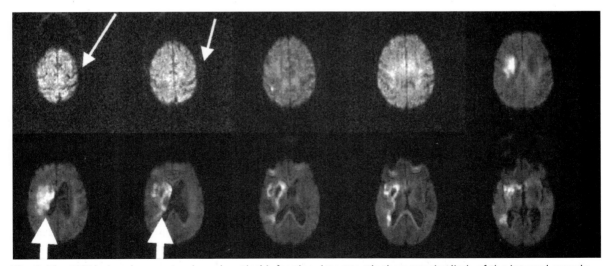

Fig. 2 The DWI lesion shows extensive subcortical infarction, importantly the posterior limb of the internal capsule, hence motor tract, is involved in the lesion.

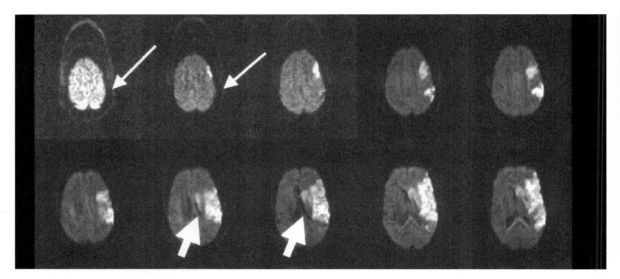

Fig. 3 The DWI lesion shows extensive cortical and subcortical infarction, however both the motor cortex and internal capsule are spared.

recovery (Barthel 20 out of 100). In case 2 (Fig. 2), the primary motor cortex was spared (thin arrows), but the subcortical corticospinal tract was damaged (thick arrows), and the patient made little motor recovery (Barthel 15). In case 3 (Fig. 3), with a similar volume infarct to case 1, the primary cortex and the subcortical region carrying the pyramidal tracts were spared (arrows) and the patient made considerable motor recovery (Barthel 80). This patient had some sub-cortical damage, but the rim of non-infarcted tissue indicated by the thick arrow, which is supplied by the anterior choroidal artery, is not infarcted. This type of region can only be identified by techniques with this degree of resolution. Conventional CT scanning can not distinguish between patients with persisting occlusion and spontaneous recanalization and the resolution of infarction of DWI is far beyond that of conventional CT scan imaging; this may explain the relatively small contribution made by CT to prediction of outcome[16]. Thus, although all three patients were clinically indistinguishable, only one of them (case 3) had an intact cortico-spinal tract and this was the patient who made a motor recovery. We suspect that further work using this technique will enable, for the first time, the stroke syndrome to be classified into coherent physiological categories, and that having done so, the logical and expected relationship between damage and outcome will be revealed. Further studies will determine whether this is so, and whether such imaging can reliably predict death, dependency, recovery of individual deficits (*e.g.* dysphasia and neglect), or even specific activities of daily living, such as walking or transfers.

Until these techniques become widely available, perhaps the information we give patients should be based on the large scale epidemiological studies and the most valid prognostic studies. This means defining the stroke syndrome and routinely measuring the single clinical variables identified as important by previous prognostic studies, such as consciousness, paralysis, continence and neglect. An experienced clinician can then tailor his or her prediction, and refine it as the patient's clinical course is revealed. Even experienced clinicians will be wise to admit that their predictions are fallible. Uncertainty should worry us as clinicians, because if we can not predict the outcome of a disease, then we almost certainly do not know enough about it. The recent developments in neuro-imaging may remedy this by providing adequate information about 'the situation and extent' of the cerebral lesion to enable prognostication to take place along the lines Osler first suggested.

Acknowledgement

SJA is supported by the Stroke Association

References

1 Wade DT, Hewer RL. Outlook after acute stroke: urinary incontinence and loss of consciousness compared in 532 patients. *Q J Med* 1985; **56**: 601–8

2 Wade DT, Hewer RL. Functional abilities after stroke: measurement, natural history and prognosis. *J Neurol Neurosurg Psychiatry* 1987; **50**: 177–82

3 Wade DT, Skilbeck CE, Hewer RL. Predicting Barthel ADL score at 6 months after acute stroke. *Arch Phys Med Rehabil* 1983; **64**: 24–7

4 Wade DT, Wood VA, Hewer RL. Recovery after stroke: the first three months. *J Neurol Neurosurg Psychiatry* 1985; **48**: 7–13

5 Bamford JM, Sandercock PAG, Dennis MS, Burn J, Warlow CP. Classification and natural history of identifiable sub-types of cerebral infarction. *Lancet* 1991; **337**: 1521–6

6 Jorgensen HS, Nakayama H, Raaschou HO *et al.* Outcome and time course of recovery in stroke Part 1: Outcome. Copenhagen Stroke Study. *Arch Phys Med Rehabil* 1995; **76**: 399–406

7 Jorgensen HS, Nakayama H, Raaschou HO *et al.* Outcome and time course of recovery in stroke Part 2: Time course of recovery. Copenhagen Stroke Study. *Arch Phys Med Rehabil* 1995; **76**: 406–12

8 Andrews K, Brockelhurst JC, Richards B, Laycock PJ. The rate of recovery from stroke and its measurement. *Int J Rehabil Res* 1981; **3**: 155–61

9 Osler W. *The Principles and Practice of Medicine*. New York: Appleton, 1892

10 Oxbury JM, Greenhall RCD, Grainger KMR. Predicting the outcome of stroke: acute stage after cerebral infarction. *BMJ* 1975; ii: 125–7

11 Gladman JRF, Harwood DMJ, Barer DH. Predicting the outcome of acute stroke: prospective evaluation of five multivariate models and comparison with simple methods. *J Neurol Neurosurg Psychiatry* 1992; **55**: 347–51

12 Barer DH. Continence after stroke: useful predictor or goal of therapy. *Age Ageing* 1989; **18**: 183–91

13   Barer DH, Mitchell JRA. Predicting the outcome of acute stroke: do multivariate models help? *Q J Med* 1989; **261**: 27–39

14   Fullerton KJ, Mackenzie F, Stout RW. Prognostic indices in stroke. *Q J Med* 1988; **250**: 146–72

15   Stone SP, Patel P, Greenwood RJ. Selection of patients for trials of treatment of visual neglect. *J Neurol Neurosurg Psychiatry* 1993; **56**: 463–6

16   Wardlaw JM, Lewis SC, Dennis MS *et al*. Is visible infarction on computed tomography associated with an adverse prognosis in acute ischaemic stroke? *Stroke* 1998; **29**: 1315–

17   Saunders DE, Clifton AG, Brown MM. Measurement of infarct size using MRI prediction prognosis in middle cerebral artery infarct. *Stroke* 1995; **26**: 2272–6

18   Heiss WD, Edmunds HG, Herholz K. Cerebral glucose metabolism as a predictor of rehabilitation after ischaemic stroke. *Stroke* 1993; **24**: 1784–8

19   Taub NA, Wolfe CDA, Richardson E *et al*. Predicting the disability of first time stroke sufferers at one year. *Stroke* 1994; **25**: 352–7

20   Kwakkel G, Wagenaar RC, Kollen BJ *et al*. Predicting disability in stroke – a critical review of the literature. *Age Ageing* 1996; **25**: 479–89

21   Gompertz P, Pound P, Ebrahim S. Predicting stroke outcome: Guy's prognostic score in practice. *J Neurol Neurosurg Psychiatry* 1994; **57**: 932–5

22   Kalra L, Crome P. The role of prognostic scores in targeting stroke rehabilitation in elderly patients. *J Am Geriatr Soc* 1993; **41**: 396–400

23   Glass TA, Matchar DB, Belyea M *et al*. Impact of social support on outcome in first stroke. *Stroke* 1993; **24**: 64–70

24   Barer DH. The influence of visual and tactile inattention on predictions for recovery from acute stroke. *Q J Med* 1990; **273**: 21–32

25   Lincoln NB, Jackson JM, Edmans JA *et al*. The accuracy of predictions about progress of patients on a stroke unit. *J Neurol Neurosurg Psychiatry* 1990; **53**: 972–5

26   Burn J, Sandercock P. Predicting the outcome of acute stroke. *J Neurol Neurosurg Psychiatry* 1993; **56**: 576

27   Sanchez-Blanco I, Ochoa-Sangrador C, Lopez-Munian L *et al*. Predictive model of functional independence in stroke patients admitted to a rehabilitation programme. *Clin Rehabil* 1999; In press

28   Prichard JW, Grossman RI. New reasons for early use of MRI in stroke. *Neurology* 1999; **52**: 1733–36

Improving long-term rehabilitation

John R F Gladman

Division of Rehabilitation and Ageing, University of Nottingham, Nottingham, UK

The long-term problems of stroke are both physical and mental. Rehabilitation (active promotion of recovery), maintenance (active prevention of deterioration), and care (support for those with disabilities) are intertwined elements of service provision aimed at reducing these problems. Over time, the prevention of deterioration becomes dominant.

Currently there is interest in 'intermediate care' – services aiming to provide choices other than inadequate care at home, inappropriate care in hospital, or expensive care in long-term institutions. There is also interest in stroke co-ordinators to manage community services. These developments have exposed problems of inequity (*e.g.* minority groups) and service provision (*e.g.* a shortage of trained staff). This had led to experiments in novel approaches such as generic workers and co-workers.

There is interest too in examining ways in which the social and built environment can be altered to increase the participation of disabled people in society.

Follow-up studies of stroke units show that half of all stroke patients are dead by 5 years[1–3] and only 10–20% are alive after 10 years[4]. These studies also show that the survival benefits of stroke units persist for these periods of time. Better still, improved survival does not seem to be at the expense of increased disability.

But long-term stroke survivors have long-term problems. About 10% of survivors will have severe disability (Barthel score < 10/20) and many of these will live in institutional care[5]. But even in those that make a good physical recovery, there is a poor quality of life[6,7]. Niemi and colleagues followed up 46 stroke patients under the age of 65 years over a 4 year period and found leisure activities and family relationships were severely affected[6]. Problems with long-term quality of life were particularly associated with depressive symptoms. Many non-specific symptoms are prominent in long-term stroke survivors, including tiredness, irritability, intolerance of bustle, increased need for sleep, forgetfulness, mental slowness, poor concentration, inability to do two things simultaneously, crying more readily and loss of initiative[6,7].

In its strict sense, rehabilitation is the active promotion of recovery. It is a labour intensive process and such activity is not generally applicable in the longer term. However, rehabilitation services in practice do more than

*Correspondence to:
Dr J R F Gladman,
Division of Rehabilitation
and Ageing, School of
Community Health
Sciences, B Floor Medical
School, University
Hospital, Nottingham
NG7 2UH, UK*

provide rehabilitation in its strict sense. For example, they provide care or support, whilst disability is being overcome, and they arrange for long-term care needs to be met. They also deal greatly with the prevention of deterioration, for example by attempting to prevent painful shoulders, pressure sores, malnutrition and contractures. They also provide curative treatment for complications, *e.g.* depression or urinary sepsis. They are also involved in medical secondary prevention of stroke, *e.g.* the use of antiplatelet drugs, and in the primary prevention of other vascular diseases in helping to stop smoking and modify life-style. In the early phase after a stroke, while a patient is in hospital, all these activities are provided by a rehabilitation service. Once the patient leaves hospital, the scope for recovery is more limited, and services aimed at promoting recovery tend to be used less. As time goes by and services withdraw, the long-term outcome of the patient depends upon the residual problems left after the stroke, and the ability of the patient and his/her support and care mechanism to resist decline.

There is evidence that 'late' rehabilitation interventions (in the strict sense of the word) can produce measurable benefits, at 9 months, 1 year or even several years after a stroke. In a randomised cross over study in Nottingham, Walker and Drummond[8] showed that focused dressing therapy about 9 months after a stroke could improve performance. Tangeman and colleagues in Oregon[9] showed that intensive intervention at one year could improve performance. This was a non-random study, but the size of the benefits appeared to be much greater than would have been expected without the intervention. Collen and colleagues' randomised study in Oxford[10] showed that gait speed could be improved even after up to 5 years post-stroke.

Whilst these studies attest to the efficacy of rehabilitation interventions, they do not offer a great solution to the long-term problems of stroke survivors. All three studies did not aim to treat the neuropsychiatric problems after stroke. In the Oxford study, the benefits of intervention were quickly lost. The intensity of treatment given in the Oregon study was greater than would be possible in the UK, and would be hard to justify on cost-effectiveness grounds.

There has been too great an attention on the narrow focus of the word rehabilitation, and too little attention to some of the other important functions performed by rehabilitation services. Little is known about the sorts of services that can be used after a spell in hospital to protect against poor long-term outcome, nor about models of care in the community or about the role of the social and built environment in maximising quality of life.

Service delivery – intermediate care

One of the most important adverse long-term outcomes of stroke is institutionalisation. In a study in Nottingham, we found that a quarter of survivors of acute stroke admitted to hospital went into institutional care on discharge, at a mean time of less than 3 months after the stroke[11]. This study was conducted in the late 1980s when the availability of private nursing homes was rising exponentially, and without any major development in community care. In the late 1990s, attention was been brought to bear on this problem by the Audit Commission's report *Coming of Age*[12]. It describes a vicious cycle, wherein the majority of the budget designated for community care actually pays for institutional care, thereby allowing no funding for community alternatives. Attention has focused on these community alternatives for two reasons. The first is that older people, whether disabled by stroke or other conditions, do not want to end their days in an institution. The other is that if they avoid institutionalisation, they may reduce long-term care costs. These community alternatives go under the title 'intermediate care'[13] and include the following.

Community hospitals

These are typically small hospitals, often supervised primarily by GPs, suitable for temporary care, either rehabilitation or convalescence. They often provide a range of services. They may provide a community safety net for unstable patients, who might otherwise go into institutional care. They have been closing around the UK on economic grounds, but their effectiveness in this role is unknown.

Community care centres

These are like community hospitals, but tend to have been created more recently, and do not aim to duplicate hospital services. They are often nurse-led. They may use health or social services facilities. Evaluation is limited.

Hospital at home

These may be schemes to avoid admission to hospital or an institution, or expedite discharge. They are essentially augmented domiciliary rehabilitation and care services, to be targeted at short-term needs. Evaluations to date suggest that they can reduce the use of hospital care, but it is not known if they influence the rate of long term institutionalisation.

There is currently much experiment in these sorts of services, and it seems likely that some version of them will, increasingly, be part of the pattern of service delivery in the future, as hospitals become more and more sophisticated high technology centres with shorter lengths of stay. Careful use of these services may break the vicious circle, and avoid diverting frail or vulnerable people unnecessarily into institutions, thereby improving their longer term outcome.

Service delivery – stroke co-ordinators

If such services are developed, they will augment the existing community rehabilitation and care services, which are patchy and vary from region to region. Patients in the community need a wide range of services, including the traditional rehabilitation services of physiotherapy, occupational therapy and speech therapy. But they also need chiropodists, dentists, dieticians, GPs, orthotists, social workers, nurses, and so on. In hospital, the stroke unit provides the organisational focus to allow these services to be brought together and focused upon the patients. In the community, the role of 'stroke co-ordinator' has been invented, with the objective of bringing the appropriate services to bear upon properly identified needs. Little is known about what sort of training stroke co-ordinators should have, nor the degree to which the services they co-ordinate should be specific for stroke. More importantly, little is known about whether stroke co-ordination in the community produces the benefits of organised stroke care in hospital. After all, organised in-patient stroke care saves lives and there is no reason why organised out-patient care might do likewise.

Little is written about what stroke co-ordinators do, but it is my observation that there is a great deal of experimentation. For example, the national shortage of trained therapists has prompted the development of generic workers – members of staff from one discipline who learn and are authorised to act in other professional roles. Community working has identified groups of patients from ethnic minorities who are often not well served by the hospital service. The lack of a range of trained professionals who speak the language of each of these minorities has meant that the idea of the 'bilingual co-worker' has needed to be invented. These are often bilingual people who receive a simple training allowing them to interface between a professionally trained person and a patient from an ethnic minority. As in much of this field, there is much experiment, but little research.

Just as one can expect that the primary/secondary care interface will be populated by intermediate care schemes, so longer term community stroke care will be populated by new breeds of health care professionals, managing increasingly complicated services.

Environment

Short-term rehabilitation interventions seem to produce measurable benefits, but these appear to be lost over time. Furthermore, the benefits that are seen are often in terms of improved ADL ability or gait speed. But, in the longer term, the objective is to reduce handicap, or increase participation (as new terminology has it). Another ambition is to reduce the number of psychological symptoms and complaints that longer term stroke survivors report. There seems to be a need to find ways to achieve rehabilitation gains that are resistant to decline and which are ultimately satisfying to the patient. This is where the social and built environment comes in.

Stroke patients report a sense of abandonment after discharge from hospital[14], and this indicates that the rehabilitation was incomplete because it failed to achieve re-integration into society. Yet integration to society may also be the key step to sustainability of function. For example, in some cases, patients are left house-bound because of the lack of ramps, or wheelchairs. In other cases they live too far away from bus-stops, or the bus service is infrequent, or the buses do not go where the patient needs to go. Public transport does not easily accommodate wheelchair users. If the environment were more carefully designed to meet the needs of all its potential users (the able-bodied and the disabled), then perhaps the effect on life-style of a particular disability would be less. In a modern population there are large numbers of people with disabilities, from stroke, arthritis, blindness, dementia, and so on. Many of the structural changes to the environment would help all of them, and most changes would make it easier for the 'able-bodied' too (*e.g.* access to buses for mothers carrying shopping and pushing buggies).

Aiming to re-integrate people back into society after an illness may require some radical thought. For example, perhaps rehabilitation should take place in ordinary community settings, *e.g.* shopping centres or leisure centres, rather than in hospitals or in patients' homes. It would then be a much smaller leap from therapeutic activity to ordinary activity. 'Patients' having rehabilitation could more easily become 'shoppers' or 'leisure centre clients' on discharge instead of becoming lonely, house-bound, excluded individuals. Clearly, if rehabilitation did take place in such settings, there would be much more emphasis on getting access to transport and in making these settings more suitable for users with disabilities, whereas at present the containment of these people in hospital settings does not.

All this sort of activity will have a financial cost. But on the other hand, if it sustains the more frail and vulnerable members of society outside of institutions, then there is the opportunity for savings. Unfortunately, the evaluation of the cost-efficacy of such environmental changes is not easy to do. It is a challenge for health and social scientists and policy makers alike.

Conclusions

Good long-term outcome for stroke patients requires organised acute and hospital management. It also requires careful attention to the more disabled survivors who are at risk of institutionalisation and, in the near future, this is likely to require the judicious use of intermediate care services. Community rehabilitation services themselves will need greater organisation, especially as the range of community services develops, and the benefits of so doing could be considerable. Re-integration into society is a particular goal of community rehabilitation in that it might ensure that rehabilitation achievements are sustained in the long-term.

References

1 Indredavik B, Slørdahl SA, Bakke F, Rokseth R, Håheim LL. Stroke unit treatment, long-term effects. *Stroke* 1997; **28**: 1861–6
2 Jorgensen HS, Nakayama H, Kammersgaard LP, Larsen K, Hubbe P, Olsen T. Marked reduction in mortality 5 years after Stroke Unit treatment [Abstract]. *Cerebrovasc Dis* 1999; **9 (Suppl 1)**: 123
3 Husbands SL, Lincoln NB, Drummond AER, Gladman J, Trescoli C. Five year results of a randomized controlled trial of a stroke rehabilitation unit [Abstract]. *Clin Rehabil* 2000; In press
4 Indredavik B, Slordahl SA, Bakke F, Haheim LL. Stroke unit treatment – 10 years follow up [Abstract]. *Cerebrovasc Dis* 1999; **9 (Suppl 1)**: 124
5 Gladman JFR, Sackley CM. The scope for rehabilitation in severely disabled stroke patients. *Disabil Rehabil* 1998; **10**: 391–4
6 Niemi M-J, Laaksonen R, Kotila M, Waltimo O. Quality of life 4 years after stroke. *Stroke* 1988; **19**: 1101–7
7 Hochstenbach J. *The Cognitive, Emotional and Behavioural Consequences of Stroke*. Thesis, University of Nijmegen, 1999
8 Walker MF, Drummond AER, Lincoln NB. Evaluation of dressing practice for stroke patients after discharge from hospital: a cross-over design study. *Clin Rehabil* 1996; **10**: 23–31
9 Tangeman PT, Banaitis DA, Williams AK. Rehabilitation of chronic stroke patients: changes in functional performance. *Arch Phys Med Rehabil* 1990; **71**: 876–80
10 Wade DT, Collen FM, Robb GF, Warlow CP. Physiotherapy intervention late after stroke and mobility. *BMJ* 1992; **304**: 609–13
11 Gladman JRF, Albazzaz M, Barer D. A survey of survivors of acute stroke discharged from hospital to private nursing homes in Nottingham. *Health Trends* 1991; **23**: 158–60
12 Audit Commission. *Coming of Age*. London: HMSO, 1997
13 Steiner A. *Intermediate Care. A conceptual framework and review of the literature*. London: Kings Fund, 1997
14 Anderson R. *The Aftermath of Stroke. The experience of patients and their families*. Cambridge: Cambridge University Press, 1992

AUTHOR QUERY 3 Husbands SL, Lincoln NB, Drummond AER, Gladman J, Trescoli C. Update?

Anticoagulants

Graham S Venables

Department of Neurology, Central Sheffield University Hospitals NHS Trust, Sheffield, UK

Anticoagulation is a treatment with significant and life threatening complications requiring that the balance of risk and benefit be individually assessed in each patient. The risks are greater in the elderly and those with hypertension, falls and gastrointestinal disease. The use of anticoagulants is now established in patients with symptomatic non-rheumatic atrial fibrillation, especially older patients with hypertension, cardiac failure or a large left atrium or left ventricular dysfunction. There is, however, no place for the routine use of anticoagulants in acute stroke or as part of secondary prevention in patients in sinus rhythm. There may be a place, though as yet the evidence would not support this, for the limited use of anticoagulants in special situations such as cortical venous thrombosis or carotid dissection.

Stroke, in 80% of cases, is the result of the consequences of arterial occlusion from fibrin, platelets, red cells, cholesterol or fragments of atheroma. Therefore, drugs known to reduce the effects of arterial occlusion elsewhere in the body have, historically, been used to reduce the consequences of occlusion within the arteries supplying the brain. The downside of this argument for both patient and clinician is that such agents also cause both extra and intra-cranial haemorrhage, the consequences of which are rarely trivial and often fatal. Their use, therefore, must be based on an assessment of not only their theoretical benefit but also knowledge of the balance of benefit and risk in real life clinical practice.

Primary prevention

Atrial fibrillation

*Correspondence to:
Dr Graham S Venables,
Department of
Neurology, Central
Sheffield University
Hospitals NHS Trust,
Glossop Road,
Sheffield S10 2JF, UK*

Approximately 20% of strokes are associated with non-valvular atrial fibrillation (AF), especially in the elderly. The annual rate of stroke varies from 0.5–11% depending partly on the age of the patient and on the other vascular risk factors. Hypertension, prior TIA/stroke and left ventricular systolic dysfunction are independent predictors of stroke. One-third of events occur in those with paroxysmal AF. These patients tend to be younger and have less underlying cardiac disease with a lower risk of stroke.

Five randomised trials[1-5] of anticoagulants for primary prevention of AF with oral vitamin K antagonists have been reported showing a mean risk reduction for those treated with anticoagulants compared with those on no treatment of 68% for stroke and 48% for stroke, systemic embolism, and death. Risk stratification for patients with non valvular AF is set out in Table 1[6].

There is clearly serious concern about the potential for haemorrhagic complications in any population, especially those at greatest risk, the elderly. Patients entering clinical trials tend to have closer monitoring of their anticoagulant control than other populations and in these trials target international normalised ratios (INR) ranged from 1.4–4.5. The greatest efficacy was reported with INR 1.4–2.8 and Stroke Prevention in Atrial Fibrillation III (SPAF III)[7] suggested that the optimal INR was 2.0. INR less than 3 was associated with a very low rate of intracranial bleeding complications (0.3%/year); however, one trial that included AF patients >75 years with a mean INR 2.6 had a rate of 1.8%/year intracranial haemorrhage which offset any reduction in ischaemic stroke[8]. A recent consensus conference recommended INR 2.0–3.0 with a lower target range for those over 75 years (1.6–2.5)[6].

Because of the wide variation in risk between different groups of patients, there is a corresponding variation in benefit from anticoagulants and, in general, it is appropriate for patients at high risk to be treated with anticoagulants and those at lower risk only to receive antiplatelet therapy.

If all eligible patients are to be treated with anticoagulants sufficient resources would need to be made available for the identification of at risk individuals and anticoagulant monitoring. A recent study would suggest that 4.7% of the population over 65 years might be in atrial fibrillation and many of these would benefit from anticoagulants[9]. Overall, in the UK, if such a screening and treatment policy were put

Table 1 Risk stratification for patients with non valvular atrial fibrillation

	High risk	Moderate risk	Low risk
AFI/ACCP	History of hypertension Diabetes Prior stroke/TIA Coronary artery disease Congestive cardiac failure	Age > 65 years no high risk features	Age < 65 years no high risk features
Stroke risk without treatment	6%/year	2%/year	1%/year
SPAF III	Systolic BP > 160 mmHg Left ventricular dysfunction Prior stroke/TIA Female > 75 years	History of hypertension	No risk factors
Stroke risk on ASA	8%/year	3.5%/year	1%/year

into effect then there might be a reduction of 3000–5000 (2.5%) in the total number of strokes. Poor anticoagulant control with significant bleeding complications would minimise any benefit.

Structural heart disease

There exists little by way of randomised evidence to guide the clinician on the use of anticoagulants in those with structural heart disease. Most patients with rheumatic heart disease or mechanical heart valves are anticoagulated by custom and have an overall risk of embolism of 2%/year. Mitral valve replacements have a greater risk of stroke than aortic valve replacements. There is slightly better evidence for the efficacy of anticoagulants in second generation valves. There are no guidelines based on randomised evidence as to the use of anticoagulants in patients with rheumatic valve disease, patent foramen ovale, atrial septal aneurysm, mitral valve prolapse, mitral annular calcification, aortic valve disease, cardiomyopathy, or left ventricular aneurysm.

Early secondary prevention

Elsewhere in this issue, the therapeutic effects of anticoagulation in acute stroke are discussed. This section deals with the effects of anticoagulation on early secondary prevention of stroke.

There are now in excess of 16 randomised-controlled trials of anti-coagulants in acute stroke involving over 20,000 patients. The methodology of these studies varies widely; some patients received low molecular weight heparins but the vast majority was treated with standard heparin. There was a variation in practice with regard to brain imaging prior to treatment and not all patients underwent CT. In some studies treatment was initiated early and in other was delayed up to 7 days after onset. The dose of heparin varied with some patients given low or medium dose subcutaneous heparin, others full strength intravenous heparin. Whilst various efficacy measures have been used, this section will concentrate on the effects of anticoagulants on stroke recurrence within 14 days.

A systematic review of 21 trials of the consequences of a policy of early anticoagulation[10] involving 23,427 patients would suggest that there is no benefit to the application of this policy to patients in the first week after stroke. Eight trials included 22,450 patients and showed that anticoagulant therapy was associated with 9 fewer recurrent ischaemic strokes per 1000 patients treated and an additional 9 intracranial haemorrhages per 1000 treated. Whilst 4/1000 pulmonary emboli might be avoided the benefit was offset by 9/1000 additional major extra-cranial bleedings. Any benefit in the use of heparin is offset by the number of patients who sustained disabling intra-cranial haemorrhage. There exist four trials, involving 493 people, of low molecular weight heparins. None has provided data on early secondary prevention of stroke.

Patients in atrial fibrillation fare no differently from those in sinus rhythm and no special case should be made for them in the acute phase of stroke[11].

There remains anecdotal evidence of benefit in the use of anticoagulants in special circumstances preventing deterioration in special circumstances, *e.g.* a thrombosing basilar artery, but the use of anticoagulants cannot be recommended on the basis of randomised evidence.

Late secondary prevention

Patients in sinus rhythm

Historically, there have been a number of small studies that have attempted to address the place of anticoagulants in secondary stroke prevention, after stroke or TIA in patients in sinus rhythm. These include nine trials with a total of 1214 patients. Many were done before the advent of CT and prior to the use of the INR in monitoring anticoagulants and it may be that these studies included some patients with primary intra-cranial haemorrhage. There was no reduction in the risk of death or dependency (odds ratio 0.83, 95% confidence limits 0.52–1.34) or the risk of recurrent stroke (odds ratio 0.79, 95% confidence limits 0.56–1.13). There was an excess of fatal intracranial haemorrhage (odds ratio 2.54, 95% CI 1.19–5.45) and major extra-cranial haemorrhage (odds ratio 4.87, 95% confidence limits 2.50–9.49), *i.e.* there were 11 additional fatal intracranial haemorrhages and 25 additional extracranial haemorrhages per year per 1000 patients given anticoagulant therapy. Whatever their deficiencies, a recent systematic review[12] showed intra-cranial haemorrhage amounted to a significant excess which may have offset any benefit in terms of pre-venting ischaemic stroke in patients in sinus rhythm.

One recent trial has disclosed results of comparing a policy of prevention with anticoagulants compared with a policy of stroke prevention with aspirin. This study of patients with recent (< 6 months) TIA, minor or major non-disabling stroke who were not in atrial fibrillation and in whom there was < 70% carotid stenosis showed that the policy of anticoagulant treatment was associated with significant hazard in terms of fatal and non-fatal intra-cranial haemorrhage[13]. For the primary outcome event (death from all causes, non-fatal stroke, non-fatal MI, non-fatal major bleeding complications) the hazard ratio for the use of anticoagulants was 2.3 (95% confidence limits 1.6–3.5). The hazard ratio for major ischaemic events was 1.03 (95% CI 0.06–1.75). Certain subgroups appeared to be at greater risk than others, *e.g.* patients > 65 years (HR 1.9, 95% CI 1.0–3.4), and with extensive subcortical white matter disease (leukoaraiosis) (HR 2.7, 95% CI 1.4–5.3). The incidence of intracranial bleeding was 3.7% and this increased by 1.37 for each 0.5 unit INR. Comparing this study with EAFT, there was a 19-fold excess risk of brain haemorrhage in patients with ischaemia of arterial origin compared with that due to atrial fibrillation.

This study has been criticised because of the target INR (3.0–4.0), however this was the target used in previous studies and that widely used in European clinical practice.

Two further studies have yet to report; however, in this group of patients the evidence would suggest that at the present time there is no benefit, and some hazard, to the policy of treatment with anticoagulants. Anti-platelet drugs remain the treatment of choice.

Structural cardiac disease

There exists almost no randomised data about the use of anticoagulants in patients with structural heart disease who have already had stroke. The ASPECT study suggested that for every 1000 patient years of anti-coagulation, there were 5 fewer strokes and 10 additional major bleedings as well as 28 fewer first re-infarctions[14]. It has been conventional practice that in acute MI, heparin should be reserved for those at special risk, *e.g.* those in heart failure, but there are no data to support this and patients are probably safer on antiplatelet drugs.

Non-rheumatic atrial fibrillation (NRAF)

There is level Ia evidence for the efficacy of anticoagulants in the prevention of first-ever stroke in patients with atrial fibrillation[15]. The EAFT was published in 1993 and included 1007 patients with NRAF; 669 patients were randomised to take open anticoagulants with a target INR 2.5–4.0 or double blind aspirin 300 mg daily or placebo. Mean follow-up was 2.3 years. The primary outcome event was vascular death, non-fatal stroke, non-fatal MI or systemic embolism. The annual event rate was reduced from 17% in the placebo treated group to 8% in the anticoagulant treated group (HR 0.53, 95% CI 0.36–0.79). The stroke risk reduced from 12% to 4% annually (HR 0.34, 95% CI 0.20–0.57) suggesting that 90 vascular events would be prevented per 1000 patients treated each year. There were no intracranial haemorrhages. The optimal INR was between 2–4 and any significant (extracranial) bleedings occurred above INR 5.0. Three other smaller trials that also in part addressed the same question showed results consistent with those found in the EAFT; these included the VA-SPINAF, SPAF-III and Studio Fibrillazione Atriale.

When these data are included with data from primary prevention studies, it remains clear that higher risk patients (*i.e.* older patients with additional risk factors such as hypertension, diabetes or heart failure) should be offered anticoagulants, whilst younger patients without other risk factors need only be offered treatment with anti-platelet drugs. The EAFT randomised patients up to 3 months after their event and data from acute trials referred to above would suggest that patients are not disadvantaged by waiting until their neurological deficit has stabilised before starting long-term treatment with anticoagulants. A more detailed discussion of the present position can be found in the recent Sir James MacKenzie Consensus Conference[16].

The prevention of stroke in patients with paroxysmal atrial fibrillation is more contentious. Patients with paroxysmal AF were included in some of the clinical trials and, whilst there is argument about the time at which they are most at risk, in general they should be treated as though they have established atrial fibrillation and considered, if at high risk, for anti-coagulation.

A special consideration needs to be given to the very elderly. It has already been stated that increasing age is a risk for stroke in the presence of AF and the elderly should be excluded from those being offered treatment. However, there are relatively few patients over the age of 80 years in clinical trials and the relative (and absolute) contra-indications to the use of anticoagulants should not be forgotten in this group of patients.

Clinical trials are only conducted over a finite period of time and, whilst the treatment effect obtained with anticoagulation appears durable over time, the mean period in the EAFT was only 2.3 years. In general, however, it is recommended that patients continue therapy until contraindications to the use of anticoagulants become apparent.

Patients in whom thyrotoxicosis is causing their atrial fibrillation are also at risk of stroke. No trials exist to assess the effectiveness of anti-coagulation; it is customary to offer them full anticoagulation until they are in sinus rhythm and their thyrotoxicosis is controlled.

Arterial dissection

Arterial dissection may predispose to artery-to-artery embolism and, on this basis, it has been traditional to offer patients anticoagulation. The risks of this policy are not only bleeding into the ischaemic brain, but also into the damaged arterial lining leading to further arterial occlusion. There exists no randomised data that would support the use of anticoagulants in this situation and present practice is dictated by uncontrolled natural history studies only. If treatment with anticoagulants is undertaken, then their use should be for a limited period only during which time arterial remodelling occurs.

Venous sinus thrombosis

Venous sinus thrombosis is less frequently diagnosed than arterial ischaemia, but with MR imaging becoming routine the diagnosis can be made easily using appropriate imaging sequences. Previously, custom was to treat patients with anticoagulants, based on retrospective non-randomised data. An early small randomised study in which 10 patients were treated with heparin and 10 with placebo suggested benefit to treatment with anticoagulants[17]. Patients treated with heparin had an improved clinical course after 3 days' treatment. This benefit was maintained during a 3 month follow-up period. The Cerebral Sinus Thrombosis Study[18], however, failed to confirm any statistically significant benefit in patients treated with low molecular weight heparins. Of the 60 patients who were enrolled after 12 weeks, there was a 7% benefit in favour of the heparin treated group (95% CI --26 to 12). The use of anticoagulants was, however, found to be safe even in patients in whom there had been intracranial haemorrhage. At present, therefore, randomised data would not justify the use of heparin on a routine basis in this group of patients.

Coagulation disorders

Coagulation disorders such as those associated with factor V Leiden, antithrombin III deficiency, protein C or protein S deficiency, activated protein C resistance and plasminogen abnormalities are associated with cerebral infarction of both arterial and venous origin. Their management in terms of prevention of thrombo-embolic events is controversial and lies outside the scope of this paper[19].

Key points for clinical practice

* Anticoagulation is a potentially dangerous procedure the use of which should be reserved for patients who will benefit most

- In daily clinical practice, this a the group of patients, often elderly with multiple vascular risk factors, who are in atrial fibrillation

- Patients require meticulous monitoring of their anticoagulant dose with appropriate patient education prior to starting and during treatment

- At present, in the UK, anticoagulant monitoring is often haphazard. It may be undertaken in anticoagulant clinics or in primary care and dosing is not infrequently left to the most junior member of the hospital team

- It is clear that, if the potential benefits of this type of treatment are to be maximised, dosing cannot be left to chance, but must be subject to rigorous quality control

References

1   Petersen P, Boysen G, Godtfredsen J et al. Placebo controlled, randomised trial of warfarin and aspirin for prevention of thromboembolic complications in chronic atrial fibrillation: the Copenhagen AFASAK Study. Lancet 1989; i: 175–9
2   Boston Area Anticoagulation Trial for Atrial Fibrillation Investigators. The effect of low dose warfarin on the risk of stroke in non-rheumatic atrial fibrillation. N Engl J Med 1990; 323: 1505–11
3   Connolly SJ, Laupacis A, Gent M et al. Canadian Atrial Fibrillation Anticoagulation (CAFA) Study. J Am Coll Cardiol 1991; 18: 349–55
4   Stroke Prevention in Atrial Fibrillation Investigators. The Stroke Prevention in Atrial Fibrillation Study. Circulation 1991; l84: 527–39
5   Veterans Affairs Stroke Prevention in Nonrheumatic Atrial Fibrillation Investigators. Warfarin in the prevention of stroke associated with non-rheumatic atrial fibrillation. N Engl J Med 1992; 327: 1406–12
6   Hart RG, Benavente O. Primary prevention of stroke in patients with atrial fibrillation. Proc R Coll Physicians Edinb 1999; 29 (Suppl 6): 20–6
7   Stroke Prevention in Atrial Fibrillation Investigators. Adjusted dose warfarin versus low intensity, fixed dose warfarin plus aspirin for high risk patients with atrial fibrillation; The Stroke Prevention in Atrial Fibrillation III randomised clinical trial. Lancet 1996; 348: 633–8
8   Stroke Prevention in Atrial Fibrillation Investigators. Warfarin versus aspirin for prevention of thromboembolism in atrial fibrillation. Stroke Prevention in Atrial Fibrillation II Study. Lancet 1994; 343: 687–91
9   Sudlow M, Thomsom R, Thwaites B, Rodgers H, Kenny RA. Prevalence of atrial fibrillation and eligibility for anticoagulants in the community. Lancet 1998; 352: 1167–71
10 Counsell C, Sandercock P. Efficacy and safety of anticoagulant therapy in patients with acute presumed ischaemic stroke: a systematic review of the randomised trials comparing anticoagulants with control. Oxford: Cochrane Collaboration, 1997
11 International Stroke Trial Collaborative Group. The International Stroke Trial (IST): a randomised trial of aspirin, subcutaneous heparin, both or neither among 19,435 patients with acute ischaemic stroke. Lancet 1997; 349: 1569–81
12 Liu M, Counsell C, Sandercock P. Anticoagulation versus no anticoagulation following non embolic stroke or transient ischaemic attack. Oxford: Cochrane Collaboration, 1997
13 The SPIRIT Trial Investigators. Secondary Prevention of Recurrent Ischaemia Trial. Ann Neurol 1997; 42: 857–65
14 ASPECT (Anticoagulants in secondary prevention of events in coronary thrombosis) Research Group. Effect of long term oral anticoagulant treatment and mortality and cardiovascular morbidity after myocardial infarction. Lancet 1994; 343: 499–503

15 Atrial Fibrillation Investigators. Risk factors for stroke and efficacy of antithrombotic therapy in atrial fibrillation. Analysis of pooled data from five randomised controlled trials. *Arch Intern Med* 1994; **154**: 449–57

16 Algra A, Koudstaal A, Koudstaal PJ. How do we prevent thromboembolism in atrial fibrillation? – Secondary prevention. *Proc R Coll Physicians Edinb* 1999; **29** (**Suppl 6**): 27–9

17 Einhaupl KM, Villringer A, Meister W *et al*. Heparin treatment in sinus venous thrombosis. *Lancet* 1991; **338**: 597–600

18 de Bruijn SF, Stam J. Randomised, placebo controlled trial of anticoagulant treatment with low molecular weight heparin for cerebral sinus thrombosis. *Stroke* 1999; **30**: 484–8

19 Greaves M. Coagulation abnormalities and cerebral infarction. *J Neurol Neurosurg Psychiatry* 1993; **56**: 433–9

Prevention of ischaemic stroke – antiplatelets

Dominick J H McCabe and **Martin M Brown**

Department of Clinical Neurology, Institute of Neurology, University College London, London, UK

Aspirin is the treatment of first choice for long-term secondary prevention of vascular events in patients with confirmed non-cardioembolic ischaemic stroke or TIA. However, there is no good evidence that it is of benefit in primary stroke prevention. If aspirin is contra-indicated, dipyridamole monotherapy is a relatively cheap, but slightly less effective, alternative. Aspirin and dipyridamole have an additive effect in secondary stroke prevention, but there is a high incidence of side effects and subsequent discontinuation of treatment with combination therapy. It is reasonable to consider clopidogrel for secondary prevention of vascular events in patients with ischaemic stroke who are intolerant of aspirin or dipyridamole, or who have a history of ischaemic heart disease. However, its cost is considerable. Over the next decade, oral antiplatelet agents directed against specific platelet receptors, or a combination of antiplatelet drugs inhibiting different aspects of platelet function, may improve secondary prevention of stroke.

Correspondence to:
Prof. Martin M Brown,
Institute of Neurology,
University College
London, National
Hospital for Neurology
and Neurosurgery,
Queen Square,
London WC1N 3BG, UK

Cerebral infarction is the underlying pathogenetic mechanism in approximately 80% of first strokes[1] and, in the Oxfordshire Community Stroke Project, the majority (78%) of patients with ischaemic stroke were alive one year later[2]. The risk of stroke recurrence was highest during this first year period at 13%, subsequently decreasing to approximately 4% per annum over the following 4 years[3]. Because patients with ischaemic stroke often have widespread vascular disease, they also have an increased risk of serious coronary events of about 3% per annum[4]. The majority of ischaemic strokes result from thromboembolism from a stenosing atheromatous plaque (9%), intra-cranial small vessel disease (27%) or embolism from the heart (19%)[5]. In the remainder, the origin of the infarction is not established by investigation, but it is likely that atherothrombosis is involved in the majority. Because platelets play a pivotal role in haemostasis and thromboembolism, antiplatelet agents have the potential to play a vital role in the prevention of vascular events in these patients. Aspirin is the most commonly prescribed antiplatelet agent, but, more recently, new approaches to antiplatelet therapy have been explored. This review focuses on the evidence regarding aspirin in the primary and secondary

British Medical Bulletin 2000; **56** (No. 2): 510–525

The beneficial effect of aspirin was similar and independent of the dose used in each of these four studies, and is consistent with the overall results of the meta-analysis performed by The Antiplatelet Trialists' Collaboration[16]. The Trialists analysed data from 145 trials of prolonged (1 month or more) antiplatelet therapy for any vascular indication available by March 1990[16]. Aspirin, at a dose of 75–1500 mg daily, was the most widely tested drug in these trials and treatment was continued for over 4 years in some cases[16]. It should be noted that the 'odds reductions' in outcome events associated with treatment, as calculated by the Antiplatelet Trialists, translate into slightly lower relative risk reductions quoted in other studies[16,21]. Antiplatelet therapy was associated with a proportional odds reduction in important vascular events (non-fatal stroke, non-fatal MI or vascular death) of 22% in patients presenting with a transient ischaemic attack (TIA) and 23% in those with completed stroke. Medium dose aspirin (75–325 mg daily) was equally protective against further vascular events compared to higher and more gastrotoxic doses (500–1500 mg daily)[16,17].

Algra and van Gijn performed an updated meta-analysis of 10 randomised trials of aspirin therapy *versus* control treatment in patients with a history of TIA or non-disabling stroke[21]. The relative reduction in the risk of subsequent vascular events was 13% with low dose (< 100 mg daily), 9% with medium dose (300 mg daily) and 14% with high dose aspirin treatment (> 900 mg daily) They concluded that doses of aspirin between 30–1500 mg daily were equally effective in secondary prevention after cerebral ischaemia, but cautioned that true differences in efficacy between the treatment regimens could not be excluded because of wide confidence intervals. These findings are consistent with those of a more recent report in which the authors conducted a metaregression analysis of 11 randomised, placebo-controlled trials of aspirin therapy in patients with a recent TIA, stroke or retinal artery occlusion[22]. Aspirin therapy, across a broad range of doses (50–1500 mg daily), significantly reduced the risk of stroke by about 15% compared to placebo (95% CI, 6–23%). There was no significant difference in efficacy between lower and higher doses of aspirin.

Until recently, aspirin was not routinely given in the acute phase of ischaemic stroke and the benefits of early secondary prevention were unknown. However, combining the results of two large trials (the Chinese Acute Stroke Trial (CAST)[23] and the International Stroke Trial (IST)[24] of aspirin therapy given within 48 h of acute ischaemic stroke (containing approximately 20,000 patients each) has confirmed that aspirin reduces both the early absolute risk of death or non–fatal recurrent stroke and the rate of death or dependency by about 1% (see elsewhere in this issue for a more detailed description of these two trials)[23,24].

Analysing the evidence from CAST[23] and IST[24], in addition to the other trials of delayed secondary prevention, one can conclude that all patients with suspected acute ischaemic stroke should have a CT of brain performed within 48 h of presentation to exclude intracerebral haemorrhage. Aspirin therapy should then be started and continued indefinitely unless some clear contra-indication to treatment develops, thus facilitating short-term and long-term secondary stroke prevention[16]. Because at least 160 mg (and perhaps 300 mg) of aspirin daily is required for the first few days[16] to 2 weeks[25] to maximally inhibit thromboxane biosynthesis, and due to the ease of availability of 300 mg tablets, patients should be treated with 300 mg initially, although reducing the dose to 50–150 mg daily may subsequently suffice.

Aspirin in subtypes of ischaemic stroke and high risk groups

There are limited data available on the efficacy of aspirin in the secondary prevention of specific subtypes of ischaemic stroke. Warfarin is significantly more effective than aspirin at preventing further stroke in patients who have had a recent cardioembolic TIA or minor ischaemic stroke associated with non-rheumatic atrial fibrillation[26]. In the European Atrial Fibrillation Trial (EAFT), the annual risk of recurrent stroke was reduced from 12% with placebo to 4% with warfarin (target INR 3.0, $P < 0.001$)[26]. However, aspirin (300 mg daily) did not significantly reduce the risk of recurrent stroke compared to placebo, although there was a trend towards a beneficial effect with treatment (10% *versus* 12% per annum, $P = 0.31$). The annual incidence of major bleeding complications was 0.9% and 2.8% in patients on aspirin and warfarin, respectively. Therefore, aspirin is a safe, though less effective, alternative when warfarin treatment is contra-indicated in this subgroup of patients.

The North American Symptomatic Carotid Endarterectomy Trial (NASCET)[27] and the European Carotid Surgery Trial (ECST)[28] compared the outcome of treatment with carotid endarterectomy to best medical care in patients who had a recent ischaemic stroke or TIA in association with > 70% carotid stenosis. 98% of endarterectomy patients and 94% of medical patients were taking aspirin in NASCET. Despite aspirin therapy, the risk of any ipsilateral stroke and the risk of major stroke or death in the medically treated patients during follow-up was 26% in NASCET and ECST, respectively. Therefore, aspirin fails to prevent a high rate of recurrent stroke in patients with recently symptomatic carotid stenosis, whereas endarterectomy markedly reduces the subsequent risk of stroke after the peri-operative period[27,28]. This may, in part, be related to the fact that an ulcerated atherosclerotic plaque causing vessel stenosis exposes platelets to increased shear stress[29] and aspirin is ineffective at preventing shear-induced platelet aggregation[30]. Recently, the Aspirin and Carotid Endarterectomy (ACE) Trial Collaborators have shown that patients undergoing carotid endarterectomy benefit more from lower than higher doses of aspirin in the peri-operative period[31]. The combined rate of stroke, MI or death at 3 months was significantly lower at 6.2% in patients receiving lower dose aspirin (81 mg or 325 mg) compared to 8.4% with higher doses of 650 mg or 1300 mg daily (*P* = 0.03).

There is no individual trial data comparing the effect of aspirin on other subtypes of ischaemic stroke. The meta-analysis performed by the Antiplatelet Trialists' Collaboration found no difference in the odds of subsequent vascular events with antiplatelet therapy between men and women, middle and older age groups, diabetic and non-diabetic patients, and hypertensive and normotensive patients[16].

Dipyridamole

Dipyridamole is believed to inhibit platelet aggregation by raising levels of cyclic adenosine monophosphate and cyclic guanosine monophosphate[20], and by inhibiting the uptake and metabolism of adenosine (a platelet-inhibiting vasodilator)[32]. Early trials investigating the relative effects of the combination of aspirin and dipyridamole versus aspirin alone were inconclusive, mainly due to their small sample size[33,34]. However, the European Stroke Prevention Study (ESPS) found that the combination of 225 mg dipyridamole and 990 mg aspirin daily reduced the relative risk of death or recurrent stroke by an impressive 33.5% compared to placebo in patients with a recent TIA or ischaemic stroke (*P* <0.001)[34]. However, this study had a number of methodological flaws and did not include an aspirin-only arm. A subsequent meta-analysis of the trials of combination antiplatelet therapy, including aspirin and dipyridamole, did not prove that these regimens were more beneficial than aspirin alone, but did not exclude this possibility either[16]. The Second European Stroke Prevention Study (ESPS–2), which was set up to address a number of issues raised by ESPS, showed that aspirin, dipyridamole, or a combination of aspirin and dipyridamole were superior to placebo in secondary stroke prevention[20]. The trial design and the results from the 'aspirin-alone' arm of the trial have been discussed earlier. In comparison to placebo, the overall reduction in stroke risk was 16% with dipyridamole alone, which was very similar to the 18% reduction associated with aspirin alone[20]. The combination of aspirin and dipyridamole led to a 37% reduction in stroke risk compared to placebo; this was significantly more beneficial than treatment with either agent alone (Fig. 1). The relative risk reductions for the combined endpoint of stroke or death were 15% with

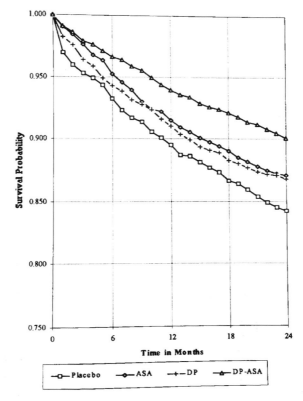

Fig. 1 Survival curves showing the probability of survival free of stroke over a 2 year period on treatment with placebo, aspirin (ASA), dipyridamole (DP) or combination therapy (DP-ASA) in ESPS–2 (from Diener et al[20]).

dipyridamole, and 24% with combination therapy. However, there was no significant reduction in the incidence of subsequent MI with any of the treatment regimens. In addition, treatment was very poorly tolerated initially, with 57% of placebo treated patients and over 60% of patients on aspirin, dipyridamole or combination therapy experiencing some adverse event. Treatment withdrawal occurred in 22% of patients in the placebo or aspirin-only groups, and in 29% of patients on dipyridamole (alone or in combination with aspirin). The most common adverse events leading to treatment withdrawal were headache (8%) and gastrointestinal disturbance (6–7%) in the dipyridamole groups. Bleeding from any site was approximately twice as common in the two aspirin groups (8.2%, 8.9%) compared to placebo (4.5%), but this was responsible for treatment withdrawal in only 1% of patients on aspirin (alone or in combination). However, there was no excess of bleeding in patients treated with dipyridamole alone (4.7%) compared to placebo.

A recent meta-analysis supports the view that a combination of aspirin and dipyridamole is superior to aspirin alone in preventing non-fatal stroke[35]. Combination therapy significantly reduced the odds of non-fatal recurrent stroke by 23% compared to aspirin alone, with no

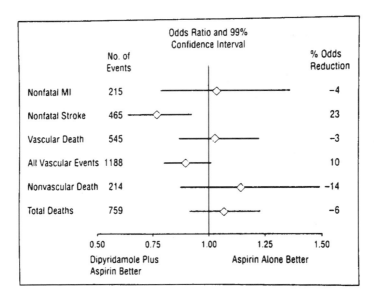

Fig. 2 Direct comparison of the proportional effects of treatment with dipyridamole plus aspirin *versus* aspirin alone on vascular events and non-vascular deaths. MI = myocardial infarction (from Wilterdink & Easton[35]).

significant effect on MI or other vascular events (Fig 2). Because ESPS–2 was the first study to show an unequivocal benefit of combination therapy with aspirin and dipyridamole over aspirin alone, and because of the unexplained and disparate effects of dipyridamole on the cerebrovascular and coronary circulation, further studies are warranted to confirm these findings. The efficacy and safety of the combination of aspirin and dipyridamole is currently being reassessed in an on-going study called the European and Australian Stroke Prevention in Reversible Ischaemia Trial (ESPRIT)[36].

Ticlopidine

Ticlopidine is a thienopyridine derivative that is believed to interfere with ADP-induced transformation of the glycoprotein IIb/IIIa receptor (GP IIb/IIIa) on platelet membranes, a complex that ultimately mediates platelet aggregation[10]. It has also been shown to inhibit aggregation induced by other agonists *ex vivo* in patients with cardiovascular disease[10]. The drug is inactive *in vitro* and must be activated by hepatic metabolism to exhibit its antiplatelet effects[7] which are maximal after 5–6 days of repeated oral therapy[37]. Ticlopidine has been shown to be more effective than placebo in reducing vascular events[38], and more effective than aspirin in secondary stroke prevention in patients with recent TIA or minor stroke[39].

In the Canadian American Ticlopidine Study, patients with recent thromboembolic stroke were randomised to receive either ticlopidine

250 mg twice daily or placebo[38]. Ticlopidine reduced the combined risk of stroke, myocardial infarction or vascular death by 23% compared to placebo ($P = 0.02$).

In the Ticlopidine Aspirin Stroke Study, ticlopidine (250 mg twice daily) was compared with aspirin (650 mg twice daily) in patients with a recent history of TIA, RIND, or minor stroke[39]. Ticlopidine reduced the 3 year risk of recurrent stroke by 21% compared to aspirin. However, there was no significant difference in the rate of vascular events in a subsequent direct comparison of the two drugs, combining all indications and outcome events, in a meta-analysis by the Antiplatelet Trialists' Collaboration[16]. Side effects were common in the ticlopidine group with diarrhoea occurring in 20% of patients, necessitating discontinuation of the drug in 6%[39]. Gastritis and gastrointestinal haemorrhage were more common in the aspirin group, but 'all site' haemorrhage was equally common in both treatment groups. More importantly, neutropenia occurred in 2.3% of patients on ticlopidine and was severe in 0.9%, necessitating regular haematological monitoring of patients. In most cases, neutropenia was first noted 1–3 months after commencing treatment, and resolved within 3 weeks of cessation of the drug[39]. Ticlopidine treatment was also associated with the development of hypercholesterolaemia (mean increase in total cholesterol level of 9 ± 20%), although the long-term implications of this finding are unknown. There have also been reports of thrombotic thrombocytopenic purpura in association with ticlopidine, with a mortality rate exceeding 20%[40]. Although recently licensed in the UK, ticlopidine is unlikely to be used widely for secondary stroke prevention due to the more favourable side effect profile associated with its chemically related compound, clopidogrel.

Clopidogrel

Clopidogrel is a new thienopyridine derivative, chemically related to ticlopidine, but with antithrombotic activity in animal models greater than ticlopidine[41]. A modest clinical benefit of clopidogrel over aspirin has been demonstrated in the CAPRIE trial[41]: 19,185 patients with recent ischaemic stroke, MI or symptomatic atherosclerotic peripheral arterial disease were randomised to receive clopidogrel (75 mg daily) or aspirin (325 mg daily). The relative risk reduction in the average annual incidence of ischaemic stroke, MI or vascular death was 8.7% with clopidogrel compared to aspirin (absolute risk reduction of 0.51%, $P = 0.04$; Fig. 3). The trend towards a reduction in the relative risk of subsequent events with clopidogrel compared to aspirin in the subgroup of patients presenting with stroke was not statistically significant (7.3%, $P = 0.26$), but the study was not adequately powered to detect treatment

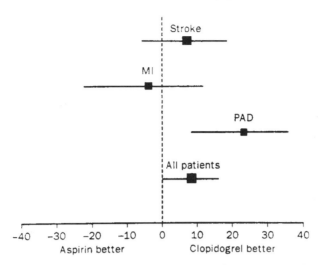

Fig. 3 Percentage relative risk reduction in the primary outcome of ischaemic stroke, myocardial infarction (MI), or vascular death in patients presenting with stroke, MI, or peripheral arterial disease (PAD) in the CAPRIE trial (from CAPRIE Steering Committee[41]).

effects in different subgroups. However, among the subgroup of patients presenting with ischaemic stroke or peripheral vascular disease who had a previous history of MI, clopidogrel significantly reduced the relative risk of subsequent vascular events by 22.7% compared to aspirin. In comparison to aspirin, severe rash (0.3%) and diarrhoea (4.5%) occurred more commonly with clopidogrel, but there was no excess of neutropenia (0.1%) or hypercholesterolaemia. Gastrointestinal haemorrhage was significantly less common with clopidogrel than aspirin (1.99% *versus* 2.66%, P <0.05), and there was a non-significant trend towards a lower rate of intracranial haemorrhage with clopidogrel (0.35% *versus* 0.49%, P = 0.23). Therefore, although the trend towards the efficacy of clopidogrel in the stroke subgroup was not significant, this trial was not designed to detect differences within patient subgroups, and the true potential of clopidogrel in patients with stroke may have been underestimated.

Glycoprotein IIb/IIIa antagonists

Regardless of the stimulus to activation, platelet aggregation is ultimately mediated by GP IIb/IIIa, and individual platelets possess 60,000–80,000 copies of GP IIb/IIIa on their surface membrane[42]. In resting platelets, this receptor has a low affinity for its major ligand, fibrinogen, and the surface receptor must undergo a conformational change to allow ligand binding. This change is the final common pathway in platelet aggregation[10]. GPIIb/IIIa blocking drugs bind to this receptor on both resting and non-resting platelets and itravenous preparations have been shown to be beneficial in acute coronary syndromes and trials of percutaneous transluminal coronary intervention[43]. There is insufficient evidence to recommend therapy with GPIIb/IIIa antagonists in patients with ischaemic stroke at the present time. However, the efficacy and safety of long-term secondary prevention with lotrafiban, an oral GPIIb/IIIa antagonist, is being studied[43], and subsequent to a recently published pilot study, a further trial of treatment with an intravenous GPIIb/IIIa antagonist (abciximab) in acute ischaemic stroke is being planned[44].

Key points for clinical practice – choice of antiplatelet agent

Aspirin is a moderately effective agent for secondary stroke prevention, but there is no evidence from prospective randomised trials that it is of benefit in primary stroke prevention. Because of its low cost and favourable incidence of bleeding complications, it is likely to remain the treatment of first choice for long-term secondary prevention in patients presenting with an ischaemic stroke or TIA. If there is a history of aspirin allergy, aspirin intolerance, peptic ulcer disease, or another contra-indication to its use, dipyridamole monotherapy is a relatively cheap, but slightly less effective, alternative. Based on the evidence from ESPS–2, aspirin and dipyridamole have an additive effect in the secondary prevention of stroke, or the combined outcome of stroke or death. Our current practice is to reserve this treatment regimen for patients who have a further event on aspirin monotherapy, because of the additional cost of dipyridamole and because the side effects associated with combination therapy may lead to discontinuation of both drugs. There is currently insufficient evidence to determine whether or not certain 'high risk' patients with multiple vascular risk factors (e.g. patients with diabetes or hypertension) should be commenced on combination therapy for secondary stroke prevention after their first TIA/stroke. However, we do recommend combination therapy as first line treatment in these individuals. The on-going European Stroke Prevention in Reversible Ischaemia Trial (ESPRIT) will hopefully shed further light on the indications for dipyridamole when it is completed. It is reasonable to consider clopidogrel for secondary prevention of vascular events in patients with ischaemic stroke who are intolerant of aspirin or dipyridamole, or in patients with a history of ischaemic heart disease, in whom dipyridamole has not been shown to be effective. One must remember that its cost is considerable when compared to aspirin. 200 patients with a risk profile similar to those included in CAPRIE would have to be treated with clopidogrel rather than aspirin to prevent one additional vascular event[41]. However, clopidogrel should be more cost-effective if used for secondary prevention in subgroups of patients at high risk of vascular disease. Treatment must be tailored to suit the individual patient, and other agents considered when indicated, *e.g.* warfarin, for secondary stroke prevention in patients with non-rheumatic atrial fibrillation. There is no evidence regarding optimal secondary prevention in patients who have a further TIA or stroke on aspirin monotherapy. However, we favour the use of aspirin (50–75 mg daily) and dipyridamole (200 mg modified-release b.d.) in these individuals, unless they have a history of ischaemic heart disease when we favour changing to clopidogrel (75 mg daily).

Over the next decade, oral antiplatelet agents directed against specific platelet receptors, *e.g.* GP IIb/IIIa, may improve secondary prevention of stroke. In addition, a combination of antiplatelet drugs inhibiting different aspects of platelet function, such as aspirin and clopidogrel, or aspirin and a GP IIb/IIIa antagonist, may prove to be the most effective treatment option. There is certainly much to be gained from more effective antiplatelet therapy.

Acknowledgement

DJHM is supported by a grant from the Brain Research Trust.

References

1 Warlow CP, Dennis MS, van Gijn J, Sandercock PAG, Bamford JM, Wardlaw J. What pathological type of stroke is it? In: Warlow CP, Dennis MS, van Gijn J, Hankey GJ, Sandercock PAG, Bamford JM, Wardlaw J, eds. *Stroke. A practical guide to management.* Oxford: Blackwell Science Ltd, 1996: 146–189

2 Dennis MS, Burn JPS, Sandercock PAG, Bamford JM, Wade DT, Warlow CP. Long-term survival after first-ever stroke: The Oxfordshire Community Stroke Project. *Stroke* 1993; **24**: 796–800

3 Burn J, Dennis M, Bamford J, Sandercock P, Wade D, Warlow C. Long-term risk of recurrent stroke after a first-ever stroke: The Oxfordshire Community Stroke Project. *Stroke* 1994; **25**: 333–7

4 Warlow CP. Epidemiology of stroke. *Lancet* 1998; **352 (Suppl III)**: 1–4.

5 Sacco RL, Ellenberg JH, Mohr JP *et al.* Infarcts of undetermined cause: The NINCDS Stroke Data Bank. *Ann Neurol* 1989; **25**: 382–390

6 Delanty N. Secondary prevention after cerebral ischaemia of presumed arterial origin: Is aspirin still the touchstone? *J Neurol Neurosurg Psychiatry* 1999; **67**: 832

7 Harker LA. Therapeutic inhibition of platelet function in stroke. *Cerebrovasc Dis* 1998; **8 (Suppl 5)**: 8–18

8 Peto R, Gray R, Collins R *et al.* Randomised trial of prophylactic daily aspirin in British male doctors. *BMJ* 1988; **296**: 313–316

9 Steering Committee of the Physicians' Health Study Research Group. Final report on the aspirin component of the ongoing Physicians' Health Study. *N Engl J Med* 1989; **321**: 129–135

10 Moran N, Fitzgerald GA. Mechanisms of action of antiplatelet drugs. In: Colman RW, Hirsh J, Marder VJ, Salzman EW. (eds) *Haemostasis and Thrombosis: Basic Principles and Clinical Practice*, 3rd edn. Philadelphia: JB Lippincott, 1994; 1623–37

11 Bronner LL, Kanter DS, Manson JE. Primary prevention of stroke. *N Engl J Med* 1995; **333**: 1392–400

12 Manson JE, Stampfer MJ, Colditz GA *et al*. A prospective study of aspirin use and primary prevention of cardiovascular disease in women. *JAMA* 1991; **266**: 521–7

13 Iso H, Hennekens CH, Stampfer MJ *et al*. Prospective study of aspirin use and risk of stroke in women. *Stroke* 1999; **30**: 1764–71

14 Hansson L, Zanchetti A, Carruthers SG *et al*, for the HOT Study Group. Effects of intensive blood-pressure lowering and low-dose aspirin in patients with hypertension: principal results of the Hypertension Optimal Treatment (HOT) randomised trial. *Lancet* 1998; **351**: 1755–62

15 Côté R, Battista RN, Abrahamowicz M, Langlois Y, Bourque F, Mackey A, and the Asymptomatic Cervical Bruit Study Group. Lack of effect of aspirin in asymptomatic patients with carotid bruits and substantial carotid narrowing. *Ann Intern Med* 1995; **123**: 649–55

16 Antiplatelet Trialists' Collaboration. Collaborative overview of randomised trials of antiplatelet therapy – I: Prevention of death, myocardial infarction, and stroke by prolonged antiplatelet therapy in various categories of patients. *BMJ* 1994; **308**: 81–106

17 UK–TIA study group. The United Kingdom transient ischaemic attack (UK–TIA) aspirin trial: final results. *J Neurol Neurosurg Psychiatry* 1991; **54**: 1044–54

18 The SALT Collaborative Group. Swedish Aspirin Low-dose Trial (SALT) of 75 mg aspirin as secondary prophylaxis after cerebrovascular ischaemic events. *Lancet* 1991; **338**: 1345–9

19 The Dutch TIA Trial Study Group. A comparison of two doses of aspirin (30 mg vs. 283 mg a day) in patients after a transient ischemic attack or minor ischemic stroke. *N Engl J Med* 1991; **325**: 1261–6

20 Diener HC, Cunha L, Forbes C, Sivenius J, Smets P, Lowenthal A. European Stroke Prevention Study 2: Dipyridamole and acetylsalicylic acid in the secondary prevention of stroke. *J Neurol Sci* 1996; **143**: 1–13

21 Algra A, van Gijn J. Aspirin at any dose above 30 mg offers only modest protection after cerebral ischaemia. *J Neurol Neurosurg Psychiatry* 1996; **60**: 197–9

22 Johnson ES, Lanes SF, Wentworth CE, Satterfield MH, Abebe BL, Dicker LW. A metaregression analysis of the dose-response effect of aspirin on stroke. *Arch Intern Med* 1999; **159**: 1248–53

23 Chinese Acute Stroke Trial Collaborative Group. CAST: randomised placebo-controlled trial of early aspirin use in 20,000 patients with acute ischaemic stroke. *Lancet* 1997; **349**: 1641–9

24 International Stroke Trial Collaborative Group. The International Stroke Trial (IST): a randomised trial of aspirin, subcutaneous heparin, both or neither among 19,435 patients with acute ischaemic stroke. *Lancet* 1997; **349**: 1569–81

25 Sandercock P. Antiplatelet therapy with aspirin in acute ischaemic stroke. *Thromb Haemost* 1997; **78**: 180–2

26 EAFT (European Atrial Fibrillation Trial) Study Group. Secondary prevention in non-rheumatic atrial fibrillation after transient ischaemic attack or minor stroke. *Lancet* 1993; **342**: 1255–62

27 North American Symptomatic Carotid Endarterectomy Trial Collaborators. Beneficial effect of carotid endarterectomy in symptomatic patients with high-grade carotid stenosis. *N Engl J Med* 1991; **325**: 445–53

28 European Carotid Surgery Trialists' Collaborative Group. Randomised trial of endarterectomy for recently symptomatic carotid stenosis: final results of the MRC European Carotid Surgery Trial (ECST). *Lancet* 1998; **351**: 1379–87

29 Kroll MH, Hellums JD, McIntire LV, Schafer AI, Moake JL. Platelets and shear stress. *Blood* 1996; **5**: 1525–41

30 Uchiyama S, Yamazaki M, Maruyama S *et al*. Shear-induced platelet aggregation in cerebral ischaemia. *Stroke* 1994; **25**: 1547–51

31 Taylor DW, Barnett HJ, Haynes RB *et al*. Low-dose and high-dose acetylsalicylic acid for patients undergoing carotid endarterectomy: a randomised controlled trial. ASA and Carotid Endarterectomy (ACE) Trial Collaborators. *Lancet* 1999; **353**: 2179–84

32 Fitzgerald GA. Dipyridamole. *N Engl J Med* 1987; **316**: 1247–57

33 Diener H-C. Antiplatelet drugs in secondary prevention of stroke. *Int J Clin Pract* 1998; **52**: 91–7

34 ESPS Group. European Stroke Prevention Study. *Stroke* 1990; **21**: 1122–30

35 Wilterdink JL, Easton JD. Dipyridamole plus aspirin in cerebrovascular disease. *Arch Neurol* 1999; **56**: 1087–92

36 ESPRIT Investigators. Anticoagulants versus aspirin and the combination of aspirin and dipyridamole versus aspirin only in patients with transient ischaemic attacks or non-disabling ischaemic stroke: ESPRIT (European and Australian Stroke Prevention in Reversible Ischaemia Trial). Major ongoing stroke trials. *Stroke* 1999; **30**: 1301

37 Schrör K. The basic pharmacology of ticlopidine and clopidogel. *Platelets* 1993; **4**: 252–61

38 Gent M, Blakely JA, Easton JD *et al* and the CATS Group. The Canadian American Ticlopidine Study (CATS) in thromboembolic stroke. *Lancet* 1989; **i**: 1215–20

39 Hass WK, Easton JD, Adams HP *et al* for the Ticlopidine Aspirin Stroke Study Group. A randomised trial comparing ticlopidine hydrochloride with aspirin for the prevention of stroke in high risk patients. *N Engl J Med* 1989; **321**: 501–7

40 Steinhubl SR, Tan WA, Foody JM, Topol EJ. Incidence and clinical course of thrombotic thrombocytopenic purpura due to ticlopidine following coronary stenting. EPISTENT Investigators. Evaluation of platelet IIb/IIIa inhibitor for stenting. *JAMA* 1999; **281**: 806–10

41 CAPRIE Steering Committee. A randomised, blinded, trial of clopidogrel versus aspirin in patients at risk of ischaemic events (CAPRIE). *Lancet* 1996; **348**: 1329–39

42 Wagner CL, Mascelli MA, Neblock DS, Weisman HF, Coller BS, Jordan RE. Analysis of GPIIb/IIIa receptor number by quantification of 7E3 binding to human platelets. *Blood* 1996; **88**: 907–14

43 Topol EJ, Byzova TV, Plow EF. Platelet GPIIb-IIIa blockers. *Lancet* 1999; **353**: 227–31

44 Abciximab in Ischaemic Stroke Investigators Stroke Investigators. Abciximab in acute ischemic stroke, A randomised, double-blind, placebo-controlled, dose-escalation study. *Stroke* 2000; **31**: 601–609.

Who should have carotid surgery or angioplasty?

P M Rothwell

Department of Clinical Neurology, University of Oxford, Oxford, UK

Carotid endarterectomy reduces the overall risk of stroke in patients with [ECST]70–99% recently symptomatic stenosis, and to a lesser extent, at least in the short-term, in patients with severe asymptomatic stenosis. Whether angioplasty and stenting is a reasonable alternative will be decided by the results of on-going RCTs of angioplasty versus endarterectomy. The current policy of operating on all patients with a recently symptomatic severe carotid stenosis will, on average, do more good than harm. However, the number of patients needed to treat to prevent one stroke is still relatively high. The effectiveness of endarterectomy could be improved by selecting patients more rigorously. Subgroup analysis and risk factor modelling are likely to be of some value, but further testing is required before final models can be recommended for routine use in clinical practice. However, it is also likely that predictive models will eventually also take into account information on cerebral microemboli, cerebral perfusion, and genetic characteristics. The development and validation of integrated predictive models, combining these different modalities, will require large prospective clinical studies.

Correspondence:
Dr P M Rothwell,
Department of Clinical
Neurology, Radcliffe
Infirmary, Woodstock
Road, Oxford
OX2 6HE, UK

Most strokes are due to cerebral infarction, and the majority of these occur in the territory of the carotid arteries. Significant atherosclerotic narrowing of the origin of the internal carotid artery ipsilateral to the infarct is found in 20–30% of cases, compared with 5–10% of the general population in the same age range[1]. It was suggested at the beginning of the century that carotid atheroma may cause stroke, and this was eventually proven by the observation that endarterectomy of severe atherothrombotic stenosis markedly reduces the risk of subsequent ipsilateral carotid territory ischaemic stroke[2,3]. This chapter will review the results of the randomised controlled trials (RCTs) of carotid endarterectomy and percutaneous transluminal angioplasty (PTA) for recently symptomatic and asymptomatic carotid stenosis, and consider ways in which those patients with most to gain from these procedures might be selected.

Randomised controlled trials of endarterectomy for symptomatic carotid stenosis

About 150,000 carotid endarterectomies are performed each year in the US[4], and rates continue to rise in Europe. There have been five RCTs of endarterectomy for symptomatic carotid stenosis[5-9]. The first two were small, did not produce statistically significant results, and probably no longer reflect current surgical practice[5,6]. The larger VA trial (VA #309) reported a non-significant trend in favour of surgery[7], but was stopped early when the two largest trials, the European Carotid Surgery Trial (ECST) and the North American Symptomatic Carotid Endarterectomy Trial (NASCET), reported their preliminary results in 1991[2,3]. Because patients at high risk of stroke on medical treatment are likely to have the most to gain from surgery, the analyses of these trials were stratified by the degree of stenosis of the symptomatic carotid artery, which is a powerful predictor of stroke risk on medical treatment. However, different methods of measurement of the degree of stenosis on pre-randomisation angiograms were used; the NACSET method underestimating stenosis compared to the ECST method. Stenoses reported to be 70–99% in the NASCET trial were equivalent to 80–99% by the ECST method, and stenoses reported to be 70–99% by the ECST trialists were 50–99% by the NASCET method[10]. The ECST showed that surgery reduced the risk of stroke in patients with [ECST]70–99% stenosis[2]. The NASCET trial reported similar results in patients with [NASCET]70–99% ([ECST]80–99% stenosis)[3]. The ECST also reported that surgery was harmful in patients with mild stenosis ([ECST]0–29%), in whom the risk of stroke on medical treatment was too low to offset the operative risks[2]. Both trials continued to randomise patients with moderate stenosis, and reported their final results in 1998. The ECST showed that there was no benefit from surgery in patients with either [ECST]30–49% stenosis or [ECST]50–69% stenosis[8]. Indeed, when the results were stratified by decile of stenosis rather than the predefined stenosis groups, endarterectomy was only significantly beneficial in patients with [ECST]80–99% stenosis ([NASCET]70–99% stenosis). Only a very small trend in favour of surgery was seen in patients with [ECST]70–79% stenosis ([NASCET]50–69% stenosis). The absolute reduction in risk of major stroke or death at three years in patients with [ECST]80–99% stenosis ([NASCET]70–99% stenosis) was 11.6% ($P < 0.001$). This is consistent with the 10.1% ($P < 0.01$) reduction in major stroke or death at 2 years reported in NASCET in patients with [NASCET]70–99% stenosis[9]. However, NASCET also reported a 6.9% ($P = 0.03$) absolute reduction in risk of disabling stroke or death in patients with [NASCET]50–69% stenosis ([ECST]70–80% stenosis), although no benefit was seen in patients with less severe stenosis[9]. ECST did not show benefit within the [ECST]70–80% stenosis group, but the confidence interval of the estimate of treatment effect was wide. Taking the results of both trials together, it is reasonable to conclude that they have demonstrated some overall benefit from endarterectomy in patients with a recently symptomatic [ECST]70–99% stenosis ([NASCET]50–99% stenosis). It is necessary to operate on 8–10 patients to prevent one stroke over the next 3 years.

Randomised controlled trials of endarterectomy for asymptomatic carotid stenosis

There have been seven RCTs of endarterectomy for asymptomatic carotid stenosis[11], one of which is on-going[12]. The initial studies were small and did not produce statistically significant results.[11] The VA study (VA #167) demonstrated a significant reduction in the risk of the combined outcome of stroke and TIA in the endarterectomy group in patients with [NASCET]50–99% stenosis, but did not have the power to demonstrate a reduction in the risk of stroke alone[13]. In 1995, the Asymptomatic Carotid Artery Study (ACAS)[14] demonstrated a clearly significant reduction in the risk of ipsilateral ischaemic stroke in surgical patients with [NASCET]60–99% asymptomatic stenosis (assessed by Doppler ultrasound); a reduction in the 5 year actuarial risk of ipsilateral ischaemic stroke or operative death from 11% to 5.1% ($P < 0.001$). In other words, 17 operations are required to prevent 1 stroke over the next 5 years or 85 operations per year to prevent 1 stroke per year. This benefit is not regarded by many neurologists as sufficient to justify routine surgery for asymptomatic stenosis. The Asymptomatic Carotid Surgery Trial (ACST) is a large European RCT which is still recruiting and has now randomised in excess of 2000 patients[12]. It is expected to publish results sometime after 2002, and will more than double the existing randomised data.

Thus, there is some evidence of benefit from endarterectomy in patients with asymptomatic stenosis. However, the low short-term risk of ipsilateral ischaemic stroke on medical treatment distal to an asymptomatic stenosis (approximately 2% per annum) means that the overall short-term reduction in the absolute risk of stroke following endarterectomy will always be small[15]. However, short-term data may not be adequate. A younger patient with a severe asymptomatic stenosis may well survive for 10–20 years. The mean follow-up in the completed RCTs of endarterectomy for asymptomatic stenosis was little over 2 years. There are no detailed data on the long-term risk of stroke distal to different degrees of asymptomatic stenosis, but a preliminary analysis of a large collaborative natural history study has recently suggested that the

10 year stroke risk may be as high as that distal to symptomatic stenosis[16]. More detailed work is required to confirm or refute this observation. If true, it would have important implications for ongoing RCTs of endarterectomy and PTA, and for the use of endarterectomy in primary prevention of stroke. It is important to bear in mind that the risks of stroke and death due to endarterectomy for asymptomatic stenosis are significantly lower than for symptomatic stenosis[17].

Randomised controlled trials of carotid endarterectomy versus PTA

The operative risks of stroke and death within 30 days of carotid endarterectomy are not insignificant: 6.8% (95% CI = 5.6–8.0) in ECST and 6.7% (5.3–8.4) in NASCET[8,9]. These risks are higher than those reported in many surgical case-series[18], but these may be undermined by publication bias, and the trial risks are likely to be the most reliable guides to the real risks of the operation in good surgical practice. Angioplasty, with or without stenting, has been suggested as a potentially safer and less costly alternative to endarterectomy in patients with carotid stenosis. The 30 day risks of stroke and death due to PTA, and the rates of early and late restenosis have yet to be defined precisely. The Carotid and Vertebral Artery Transluminal Angioplasty Study (CAVATAS) has now provided useful data on which to base the further evaluation of angioplasty.[19] The main core of CAVATAS was a randomised comparison of angioplasty and endarterectomy. A total of 560 patients were recruited (504 randomised between angioplasty and endarterectomy). The 30 day risks of stroke and death were 10% in both treatment groups and there was no clear benefit for either treatment on initial follow-up. The 30 day risks in both groups had wide confidence intervals and were not statistically significantly different from the risks reported in ECST and NASCET. Follow-up continues in CAVATAS in order to determine the restenosis rate. A further small (17 patients) single centre RCT of angioplasty and stenting versus endarterectomy was stopped in 1998 due to an unacceptably high complication rate in the angioplasty group (5 out of 7 patients had strokes following angioplasty)[20]. Clearly, therefore, there is still uncertainty about the role of angioplasty[21], and further RCTs are necessary. A second and larger CAVATAS trial, in which angioplasty will be combined with routine stenting, will shortly begin recruitment. A similar large RCT of angioplasty and stenting *versus* endarterectomy is about to get underway in the US (CREST). At the present time, carotid angioplasty and stenting should only be performed within well-designed RCTs.

How can we identify the patients who are most likely to benefit from endarterectomy or PTA?

The overall results of RCTs of endarterectomy and PTA are useful, but they only go so far in helping patients and clinicians to make decisions in the clinic. For example, as described above, it has been shown that endarterectomy is beneficial in patients with a recently symptomatic ECST70–99% stenosis. However, although endarterectomy does indeed reduce the overall risk of ischaemic stroke by about 50% in relative terms over the next 3 years, only about 20% of such patients actually suffer a major stroke on medical treatment alone. Strictly speaking, therefore, the operation is of no value in the other 80% of patients who, despite having a severe symptomatic stenosis, are destined to remain stroke-free without surgery. Indeed, as a group, these patients will be harmed by surgery because of the significant operative risk of morbidity and mortality. Figure 1 illustrates the possible outcomes in patients undergoing endarterectomy for severe symptomatic carotid stenosis. The overall effect of surgery is shown as the point estimate and 95% confidence interval in the traditional meta-analysis format. The actual outcomes in individual patients are depicted by open dots (no stroke) or closed dots (stroke). The majority of patients (groups b and c) did not benefit from surgery, but were not harmed by the operation. Either they did not have an operative stroke, but would not have had a stroke

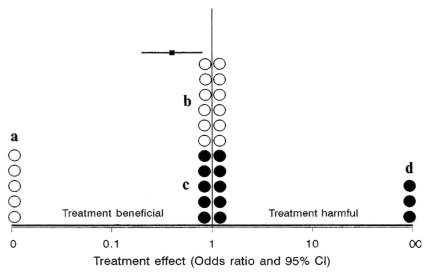

Fig. 1 The possible outcomes in patients undergoing endarterectomy for severe symptomatic carotid stenosis. The point estimate for the overall effect of surgery and the 95% confidence interval are shown in the traditional meta-analysis format. The actual outcomes in individual patients are depicted by the circles. See text for explanation.

anyway had they received medical treatment alone (group b) or they had an operative stroke, but would also have had a stroke if they had received medical treatment only (group c). A few patients (group d) were harmed by surgery, *i.e.* they had an operative stroke, but would not have had a stroke if they had not been operated. Only a relatively small proportion of patients (group a) actually benefited from surgery. These patients would have had a stroke had they only received medical treatment, but they did not have a stroke following endarterectomy. Clearly, if possible, it would be highly desirable to be able to identify in advance, and operate on, those individual patients who were most likely to fall into group a, and avoid surgery in all other patients. In this way, it would be possible, in theory at least, to prevent more strokes than would be prevented by operating on all patients, but only operate on a fraction of the patients. In practice, this ideal may not be achievable, but it is possible to go some way towards that goal by using as much prognostic information as is available to try to identify those individuals who are most likely to fall into group a, *i.e.* patients with a high risk of stroke on medical treatment alone, but a relatively low operative risk. Three techniques which might help us to do this are discussed below.

Subgroup analysis of data from RCTs

Subgroup analysis in clinical trials allows the effects of a treatment to be determined in patients with a particular characteristic. This allows clinicians to assess whether a particular patient with or without that characteristic might be more or less likely to benefit from treatment than suggested by the overall trial result. There are, of course, dangers with subgroup analysis[22]. Results are subject to the play of chance, and there have been many examples of misleading subgroup analyses which have led to particular groups of patients being denied treatments, which were subsequently shown to be effective when further trial data became available. Mistakes are particularly likely when multiple subgroup analyses are performed without correction of statistical significance for multiple comparisons. However, given a sufficient sample size and a statistically rigorous approach, subgroup analysis can be of some value. It should be borne in mind that stratification of trial results by severity of carotid stenosis is itself a subgroup analysis. In the final reports of the ECST and NASCET trials, other subgroups were examined in combination with severity of stenosis. In ECST, the benefit derived from endarterectomy in patients with ECST80–99% stenosis was reported to be greater in men than in women, with clear benefit in women only evident in patients with ECST90–99% stenosis[8]. In NASCET patients with moderate stenosis, endarterectomy was reported to be most beneficial in men, in patients with stroke as the qualifying event, and in patients with hemispheric (as opposed to ocular) symptoms[9]. Unfortunately, neither trial was powered to determine these relationships with certainty and the results cannot be relied upon. However, the individual patient data from the ECST, NASCET and VA trials have been combined in a single database in order to allow subgroup analyses with sufficient statistical power to influence clinical practice (The Carotid Endarterectomy Trialists' Collaboration). The collaboration includes detailed data on over 6000 randomised patients (95% of all patients randomised in RCTs of endarterectomy for symptomatic stenosis). It is proposed to determine the inter-relation between the effect of endarterectomy, the severity of carotid stenosis and each of the following characteristics: age, sex, diabetes, lacunar *versus* cortical presenting events, ocular *versus* cerebral presenting events, TIA *versus* stroke, contralateral carotid occlusion, ipsilateral plaque surface morphology, and post-stenotic collapse of the distal internal carotid artery.

Risk modelling using data from RCTs

Formal risk modelling or multivariate prognostic modelling has two main advantages over subgroup analysis. Firstly, it allows clinicians to take the effect of several different baseline characteristics into account, whereas traditional subgroup analysis is limited to one or two characteristics at a time. Individual patients may have several important risk factors each of which interact in a way which cannot be described using univariate subgroup analysis. In order to identify and operate only on those patients at high risk of stroke on medical treatment and a relatively low operative risk, a clinician must take all these characteristics into account[23]. Secondly, as discussed above, single variable subgroup analyses are subject to the play of chance and the problems of multiple *post hoc* comparisons, whereas stratification of trial results using an independently derived prognostic score is a single analysis based on the reasonable hypothesis that treatment effect is likely to vary with the risk of a poor outcome in the different treatment groups.

Previous prognostic models for the risk of stroke on medical treatment in patients with TIA or minor stroke have either been based on relatively small cohorts of patients, or not included the degree of stenosis of the symptomatic carotid artery[24]. No prognostic model has been validated in an independent group of patients and used routinely in clinical practice. However, several clinical and angiographic characteristics, in addition to the severity of carotid stenosis, have been shown to identify patients at high risk of stroke on medical treatment alone. For example, patients with recent cerebral ischaemic events are at higher risk of stroke than patients

Table 1 The hazard ratios (95% confidence intervals), statistical significance, derived risk points and points allocated in the predictive score for each of the independent predictors of outcome in the following models
Medical model: a Cox's proportional hazards model for ipsilateral carotid territory major ischaemic stroke (*i.e.* fatal or lasting longer than 7 days) on medical treatment derived from the 857 patients with 0–69% stenosis who were randomised to no-surgery in the ECST
Surgical model: a multiple logistic regression model for any major stroke (*i.e.* fatal or lasting longer than 7 days) or death from other causes within 30 days of carotid endarterectomy derived from 1203 patients with 0–69% stenosis who were randomised to surgery in the ECST

Prognostic variable	Hazard ratio	(95% CI)	P	Risk points[a]	Predictive score
Medical model					
Cerebral *versus* ocular events	2.45	(1.09–3.71)	0.02	1	1
Plaque surface irregularity	2.09	(1.21–3.62)	0.008	1	1
Any events within the last 2 months	1.82	(1.02–3.18)	0.04	1	1
Carotid stenosis (per 10% stenosis)	1.30	(1.10–1.40)	0.001	0–2	0–2
Surgical model					
Female sex	2.05	(1.29–3.24)	0.002	1	−0.5[c]
Peripheral vascular disease	2.48	(1.51–4.13)	0.0004	1	−0.5[c]
Systolic BP > 180 mmHg	2.21	(1.29–3.79)	0.004	1	−0.5[c]

The full lists of variables (and definitions) from which these models were derived are reported elsewhere.[28]
[a]Risk points were derived by rounding the hazard ratio to the nearest whole number and subtracting one.
[b]For application to the 70–99% stenosis group, points were allocated as follows: 70–79% (0); 80–89% (1); 90–99% (2).
[c]In the risk factor model which is applied to the 70–99% stenosis group, surgical risk points are subtracted (*i.e.* become negative) and their weighting is reduced by 50% as detailed in the methods.

with ocular events[25], patients with an irregular carotid plaque are at higher risk than patients with smooth plaques[26], and there are several risk factors for the operative risk of stoke and death due to endarterectomy[27].

A preliminary analysis of the ECST, using prognostic models to predict the risk of ipsilateral carotid territory ischaemic stroke on medical treatment and the risk of stroke and death within 30 days of carotid endarterectomy, suggests that benefit from surgery is confined to a subgroup of about 20% of patients with ECST70–99% stenosis[28]. Using data on the 2060 ECST patients with 0–69% carotid stenosis, two prognostic models were developed; one for the risk of ipsilateral carotid territory major ischaemic stroke (fatal of lasting longer than 7 days) on medical treatment and one for the risk of major stroke and death within 30 days of endarterectomy (Table 1). Using these models, a score was developed to identify patients with a high risk of stroke on medical treatment, but a relatively low operative risk. The utility of the score was tested on the ECST patients with 70–99% carotid stenosis. When the 990 patients with 70–99% stenosis were stratified using the scoring system, based on seven independent prognostic factors, endarterectomy was beneficial in only 162 (16%) patients with risk scores of 4 or more (Fig. 2). The odds of carotid territory ipsilateral major ischaemic stroke or

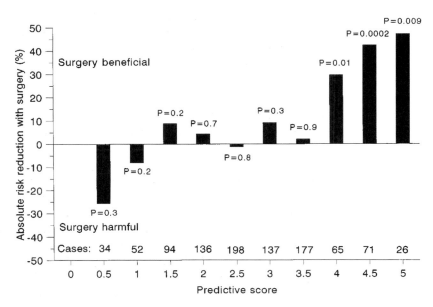

Fig. 2 The reduction in the 5 year actuarial absolute risk of ipsilateral carotid territory major ischaemic stroke or surgical major stroke or death in the surgery group compared with the medical group in patients with each predictive score. Statistical significance is tested at each score using the log rank test and the number of cases on which the estimate is based is given for each score.

operative major stroke or death were decreased considerably by surgery in this group (OR = 0.12, 95% CI = 0.05–0.29), but not in the other 828 (84%) patients (OR = 1.00, 95% CI = 0.65–1.54): the resulting 5 year actuarial absolute risk reductions were 33% (log rank = 20.5, P <0.00001) and 1% (log rank = 0.8, P = 0.7), respectively. Contrary to the overall results of ECST and NASCET, these data suggest that many patients with recently symptomatic ECST70–99% carotid stenosis do not benefit from carotid endarterectomy. Further work is required to refine and validate the predictive score on external datasets, but these preliminary results suggest that risk factor modelling might well be useful in identifying patients in whom endarterectomy is particularly beneficial. It may also be possible to use the same approach to identify a subgroup of patients with moderate stenosis in whom surgery is clearly beneficial. This will be pursued by the Carotid Endarterectomy Trialists' Collaboration. A similar approach is required for the RCTs for endarterectomy for asymptomatic stenosis.

Ancillary investigations

There have been several developments in stroke research which were unavailable at the time the when current and previous RCTs of endarterectomy and PTA were designed. However, these developments may be of value in identifying the individual patients who are most likely to benefit from these interventions. Three of the most promising areas are discussed below.

Detection of cerebral microemboli

It is possible to detect microemboli, made up of platelet emboli or plaque material, in the middle cerebral artery distal to a carotid stenosis using transcranial Doppler ultrasound (TCD; see also Markus elsewhere in this issue). TCD detection of microemboli has been shown to be reproducible and to have pathological validity[29,30]. Microemboli decrease with time after the last symptomatic ischaemic event[31], emboli are detected most frequently distal to carotid plaques which are subsequently found to have surface thrombus at endarterectomy[32], and the frequency of emboli is reduced considerably by surgery[30]. These findings suggest that emboli counting might be useful in identifying patients at particularly high early risk of ischaemic stroke. One recent pilot study has produced encouraging results[33], but large prospective cohort studies are clearly required in order to determine whether this technique will be clinically useful.

Cerebral perfusion studies

Cerebral infarction may also result from the reduction in cerebral perfusion pressure which occurs distal to a tight carotid stenosis or occlusion. A proportion of patients who have a recently symptomatic severe carotid stenosis or occlusion have significant hypoperfusion of the ipsilateral cerebral hemisphere and a loss of the ability to increase perfusion in response to raised levels of carbon dioxide[34,35]. This can be demonstrated using TCD, SPECT, ^{133}Xe radionuclide CT, functional MRI, and PET. It has also been shown, using magnetic resonance spectroscopy, that such patients have metabolic changes in the affected hemisphere which are consistent with chronic ischaemia in the absence of any evidence of cerebral infarction[36]. Both the perfusion deficit and the metabolic changes are reversed following carotid endarterectomy and extracranial-intracranial bypass grafting[37,38]. It is possible that cerebral hypoperfusion and ischaemic metabolic changes distal to severe carotid stenosis might also be useful in identifying patients at particularly high risk of stroke. Two small studies have recently suggested that hypoperfusion is associated with a high risk of stroke distal to a unilateral carotid occlusion[39,40], but no such link has yet been demonstrated in patients with carotid stenosis. It is possible to get indirect measures of cerebral perfusion distal to a carotid stenosis from traditional arterial imaging, and the presence or absence of angiographically defined collateral vessels and the degree of collapse of the post-stenotic internal carotid artery have recently been shown to predict the risk of stroke on medical treatment[41,42].

Genetic studies

Genetic characteristics might be useful in predicting the susceptibility to ischaemic stroke in individuals. Family history is an important independent risk factor for ischaemic stroke in man[43]. Twin studies have yielded proband concordance rates of about 20% for monozygotic twins and about 4% for dizygotic twins[44]. Work in animal models of stroke has shown that much of the genetic variation in susceptibility to stroke is independent of risk factors for vascular disease *per se*[45], and some potentially important unrelated polymorphisms have been identified[46,47]. Prediction of ischaemic stroke in individual patients with established cerebrovascular disease is likely to be improved by combining clinical and genetic risk factors. Thus far, studies have been too small and have, therefore, produced conflicting results[45]. Moreover, the vast majority have been case-control studies. What is required are large prospective cohort studies, detailed enough to take into account the pathological hetero-geneity of stroke, but large enough to define small relative risks with precision. There are already several interesting potential genetic risk factors, and it is highly likely that many other candidates of interest (as well as single nucleotide polymorphisms) will be identified over the next few years.

Key points for clinical practice

- Carotid endarterectomy reduces the overall risk of stroke in patients with [ECST]70–99% recently symptomatic stenosis. It is necessary to operate on 8–10 patients to prevent 1 stroke over the next 3 years

- Carotid endarterectomy reduces the overall risk of stroke in patients with severe asymptomatic stenosis. It is necessary to operate on about 17 patients to prevent 1 stroke over the next 5 years

- Carotid angioplasty and stenting may be a reasonable alternative to endarterectomy, but more data are required before it can be used routinely. Angioplasty should not currently be used outwith well-organised RCTs

- Carotid endarterectomy should be targeted at individual patients with a high risk of stroke on medical treatment alone and a reasonably low operative risk. The results of subgroup analyses and risk modelling using existing data from RCTs will help clinicians to do this

- Optimal prediction of the risk of stroke in individual patients is likely to require a combination of different types of data, probably including clinical data, imaging data, data on the frequency of cerebral microemboli, data on cerebral perfusion, and data on particular genetic characteristics

References

1 Ricci S, Flamini FO, Celani MG *et al*. Prevalence of internal carotid artery stenosis in subjects older than 49 years: a population study. *Cerebrovasc Dis* 1991; **1**: 16–9

2 European Carotid Surgery Trialists' Collaborative Group. MRC European Carotid Surgery Trial: interim results for symptomatic patients with severe (70–99%) or with mild (0–29%) carotid stenosis. *Lancet* 1991; **337**: 1235–43

3 North American Symptomatic Carotid Endarterectomy Trial Collaborators. Beneficial effect of carotid endarterectomy in symptomatic patients with high-grade carotid stenosis. *N Engl J Med* 1991; **325**: 445–53

4 Tu JV, Hannan EL, Anderson GM *et al*. The fall and rise of carotid endarterectomy in the United States and Canada. *N Engl J Med* 1998; **339**: 1441–7.

5 Fields WS, Maslenikov V, Meyer JS, Hass WK, Remington RD, MacDonald M. Joint study of extracranial arterial occlusion. V Progress report on prognosis following surgery or non-surgical treatment for transient cerebral ischaemic attacks and cervical carotid artery lesions. *JAMA* 1970; **211**: 1993–2003

6 Shaw DA, Venables GS, Cartilidge NEF, Bates D, Dickinson PH. Carotid endarterectomy in patients with transient cerebral ischaemia. *J Neurol Sci* 1984; **64**: 45–53

7 Mayberg MR, Wilson E, Yatsu F *et al*. Carotid endarterectomy and prevention of cerebral ischaemia in symptomatic carotid stenosis. *JAMA* 1991; **266**: 3289–94

8 European Carotid Surgery Trialists' Collaborative Group. Randomised trial of endarterectomy for recently symptomatic carotid stenosis: final results of the MRC European Carotid Surgery Trial (ECST). *Lancet* 1998; **351**: 1379–87

9 North American Symptomatic Carotid Endarterectomy Trialists' Collaborative Group. The final results of the NASCET trial. *N Engl J Med* 1998; **339**: 1415–25

10 Rothwell PM, Gibson RJ, Slattery J, Sellar RJ, Warlow CP. Equivalence of measurements of carotid stenosis: A comparison of three methods on 1001 angiograms. *Stroke* 1994; **25**: 2435–9

11 Benavente O, Moher D, Pham BA. Carotid endarterectomy for asymptomatic carotid stenosis: a meta-analysis. *BMJ* 1998; **317**: 1477–80

12 Halliday AW for the Steering Committee and for the Collaborators. The asymptomatic carotid surgery trial (ACST) rationale and design. *Eur J Vasc Surg* 1994; **8**: 703–10

13 Hobson RW, Weiss DG, Fields WS *et al*. Efficacy of carotid endarterectomy for asymptomatic carotid stenosis. *N Engl J Med* 1993; **328**: 221–7

14 Asymptomatic Carotid Atherosclerosis Study Group. Carotid endarterectomy for patients with asymptomatic internal carotid artery stenosis. *JAMA* 1995; **273**: 1421–8

15 Rothwell PM, Slattery J, Warlow CP on behalf of the ECST Collaborators. Risk of stroke in the distribution of an asymptomatic carotid artery. *Lancet* 1995; **345**: 209–12

16 Rothwell PM, Gutnikov S. The Asymptomatic Carotid Stenosis Study (ACSS): Differences in the time course of risk of ischaemic stroke distal to symptomatic and asymptomatic carotid stenoses. *Cerebrovasc Dis* 1999; **9 (Suppl 1)**: 66

17 Rothwell PM, Slattery J, Warlow CP. A systematic comparison of the risks of stroke and death due to carotid endarterectomy for symptomatic and asymptomatic stenosis. *Stroke* 1996; **27**: 266–9

18 Rothwell PM, Slattery J, Warlow CP. A systematic review of the risks of stroke and death due to endarterectomy for symptomatic carotid stenosis. *Stroke* 1996; **27**: 260–5

19 Brown MM for the CAVATAS Investigators. Results of the Carotid and Vertebral Artery Transluminal Angioplasty Study (CAVATAS). *Cerebrovasc Dis* 1998; **8 (Suppl 4)**: 21

20 Naylor AR, London NJM, Bell PRF. Carotid endarterectomy versus carotid angioplasty. *Lancet* 1997; **349**: 203–4

21 Beebe HG, Archie JP, Baker WH *et al*. Concern about the safety of carotid angioplasty. *Stroke* 1996; **27**: 197–8

22 Oxman AD, Guyatt GH. A consumer's guide to subgroup analysis. *Ann Intern Med* 1992; **116**: 78–84

23 Rothwell PM. Can overall results of clinical trials be applied to all patients? *Lancet* 1995; **345**: 1616–9

24 Kernan WN, Feinstein AR, Brass LM. A methodological appraisal of research on prognosis after transient ischaemic attacks. *Stroke* 1991; **22**: 1108–16

25 Hankey GJ, Slattery JM, Warlow CP. Transient ischaemic attacks: which patients are at high (and low) risks of serious vascular events? *J Neurol Neurosurg Psychiatry* 1992; **55**: 640–52

26 Eliasziw M, Streifler JY, Fox AJ *et al*. Significance of plaque ulceration in symptomatic patients with high-grade carotid stenosis. *Stroke* 1994; **25**: 304–8

27 Rothwell PM, Slattery J, Warlow CP. A systematic review of clinical and angiographic predictors of stroke and death due to carotid endarterectomy. *BMJ* 1997; **315**: 1571–77

28 Rothwell PM, Warlow CP on behalf of the ECST Collaborators. Prediction of benefit from carotid endarterectomy in individual patients: a risk-modelling study. *Lancet* 1999; **353**: 2105–10

29 Markus H, Loh A, Brown MM. Computerized detection of cerebral emboli and discrimination from artifact using Doppler ultrasound. *Stroke* 1993; **24**: 1667–72

30 Siebler M, Sitzer M, Rose G, Bendfeldt D, Steinmetz H. Silent cerebral embolism caused by neurologically symptomatic high-grade carotid stenosis. *Brain* 1993; **116**: 1005–15

31 Forteza AM, Babikian VL, Hyde C, Winter M, Pochay V. Effect of time and cerebrovascular symptoms on the prevalence of microembolic signals in patients with cervical carotid stenosis. *Stroke* 1996; **27**: 687–90

32 Sitzer M, Muller W, Seibler M *et al*. Plaque ulceration and lumen thrombus are the main sources of cerebral microemboli in high-grade internal carotid artery stenosis. *Stroke* 1995; **26**: 1231–3

33 Malloy JE, Markus HS. Asymptomatic embolism predicts stroke and TIA risk in carotid artery stenosis. *Stroke* 1999: **30**: 1440–3

34 Burt RW, Witt RM, Cirkit DF, Reddy RV. Carotid artery disease: evaluation with acetazolamide-enhanced with Tc-99m HMPAO SPECT. *Radiology* 1992; **182**: 461–4

35 Powers WJ. Cerebral haemodynamics in ischemic cerebrovascular disease. *Ann Neurol* 1991; **29**: 231–40

36 Van der Grond J, Balm R, Kappelle J, Eikelboom BC, Mali WPTM. Cerebral metabolism of patients with stenosis or occlusion of the internal carotid artery. A ¹H-MR spectroscopic imaging study. *Stroke* 1995; **26**: 822–8

37 Schroeder TB, Sillesen H, Engell HC. Haemodynamic effect of carotid endarterectomy. *Stroke* 1987; **18**: 204–9

38 Powers WJ, Grubb RL, Raichle ME. Clinical results of extracranial-intracranial bypass surgery in patients with hemodynamic cerebrovascular disease. *J Neurosurg* 1989; **70**: 61–7

39 Grubb RL, Derdeyn CP, Fritsch SM *et al*. Importance of hemodynamic factors in the prognosis of symptomatic carotid occlusion. *JAMA* 1998; **280**: 1055–60

40 Vernieri F, Pasqualetti P, Passarelli F, Rossini PM, Silvestrini M. Outcome of carotid artery occlusion is predicted by cerebrovascular reactivity. *Stroke* 1999; **30**: 593–8

41 Henderson R, Eliasziw M, Fox A, Rothwell PM, Barnett HJM. Importance of angiographically-defined collateral circulation in patients with severe carotid stenosis. *Stroke* 2000; **31**: 128–32

42 Rothwell PM, Warlow CP. Low risk of ischaemic stroke in patients with collapse of the internal carotid artery distal to severe carotid stenosis: cerebral protection due to low post-stenotic flow? *Stroke* 2000; **31**: 622–30

43 Welin I, Svardsudd K, Wilhelmsen L *et al*. Analysis of risk factors for stroke in a cohort of men born in 1913. *N Engl J Med* 1984; **311**: 501

44 Brass LM, Issacsohn JL, Merikangas KR, Robinette CD. A study of twins and stroke. *Stroke* 1992; **23**: 221–3

45 Boerwinkle E, Doris PA, Fornage M. Fields of need: the genetics of stroke. *Circulation* 1999; **99**: 331–3

46 Huang Z, Huang PL, Panahian M *et al*. Effects of cerebral ischaemia in mice deficient in neuronal nitric oxide synthase. *Science* 1994; **265**: 1883–5

47 Laskowitz DT, Sheng H *et al*. Apo E-deficient mice have increased susceptibility to focal cerebral ischaemia. *J Cereb Blood Flow Metab* 1997; **17**: 753–8

Making carotid surgery safer

A Ross Naylor

Department of Vascular and Endovascular Surgery, Leicester Royal Infirmary, Leicester, UK

Carotid surgery has been shown to be beneficial in level one randomised trials. However, evidence suggests that current outcomes do not match those published in 1991. In order to make carotid endarterectomy safer in the future, it is essential to optimise patient selection and risk factor management and to maintain an obsessional approach to surgical technique. A planned strategy of monitoring and quality control assessment can also contribute towards a sustained reduction in the peri-operative risk.

What is the current status of carotid endarterectomy?

Table 1 summarises the results from the European Carotid Surgery Trial (ECST), the North American Symptomatic Carotid Endarterectomy Trial (NASCET) and the Asymptomatic Carotid Atherosclerosis Study (ACAS)[1-3]. The reason for the apparent discrepancy between the ECST and NASCET data is the differing methods of quantifying carotid stenosis. In practice, a 50% NASCET stenosis corresponds to a 70% ECST stenosis.

There has been an increase in the number of carotid endarterectomies (CEAs) performed world-wide and, inevitably, an increasing proportion are undertaken in non-trial centres. For example, in the US, >93% of CEAs are currently performed in non-NASCET centres[4] and this has implications regarding the generalisability of the international trial results (see later).

Correspondence to:
Mr A Ross Naylor,
Department of Vascular
and Endovascular
Surgery, Leicester
Royal Infirmary,
Leicester LE1 5WW, UK

Table 1 Summary of results from ECST, NASCET and ACAS[1-3]

Stenosis	Trial	Stroke incidence (%)		Absolute risk reduction	Relative risk reduction
		Surgery	Medical		
0–30%	ECST	11.8%	6.2%	–5.6% at 3 years	None
31–69%	ECST	16.0%	15.0%	–1.0% at 5 years	None
70–99%	ECST	12.3%	21.9%	9.6% at 3 years	44% at 3 years
0–49%	NASCET	14.9%	18.7%	3.8% at 5 years	20%
50–69%	NASCET	15.7%	22.2%	6.4% at 3 years	34% at 3 years
70–99%	NASCET	9.0%	26.0%	17% at 2 years	65% at 2 years
60–99%	ACAS	5.1%	11.0%	5.9 % at 5 years	53% at 5 years

The long-term benefit of CEA is inextricably linked to the initial surgical risk, *e.g.* a unit with a 2% risk at 30 days will prevent 167 strokes/1000 CEAs long-term and only 6 operations need be performed to prevent one stroke. Conversely, a unit with a 7% complication rate will only prevent 117 strokes/1000 CEAs and 9 operations are required to prevent one stroke.[5]

Is there a current problem?

Although the randomised trials demonstrated a beneficial role for CEA, there are concerns about the generalisability of the results in everyday practice. Each international trial used highly selected surgeons, but current results may not match those that were published in 1991. At the same time that NASCET was being performed, Hsai audited outcome in all Medicare beneficiaries undergoing CEA. The operative mortality was almost 5 times that reported in the NASCET study. When the audit was repeated in 1996, the death rate had fallen to 1.6%[6], but was still more than twice that reported by NASCET in 1991. A further study has shown that the mortality rate following CEA is significantly lower in current NASCET centres, as opposed to non-NASCET centres, and that operative mortality is indirectly proportional to surgeon experience and annual operative volume[7]. There is also evidence from the surgical arm of the Carotid and Vertebral Artery Transluminal Angioplasty Study[8] that the 30 day risk of death by stroke was significantly higher than that reported by the ECST in 1991.

The net result of these larger, community-based studies has been to focus concern on the generalisability of the role of carotid surgery in the current era. Unless steps are taken to ensure that outcomes are at least equivalent to the international trials, the operation could fall into disrepute. Moreover, with the increasing moves towards refining the indications for CEA, surgeons could find that they are operating on a smaller proportion of symptomatic patients who are otherwise at very much higher risk of stroke, both in the natural history and possibly peri-operatively.

Can carotid surgery be made safer?

The simple answer to this is yes, but requires close attention to patient selection, optimisation of risk factors and modification of surgical technique. This chapter will not, however, discuss risk factor management any further.

Patient selection

In an ideal world, a multi-disciplinary team comprising neurologists, stroke physicians and surgeons should collaborate to ensure that appropriate patients are referred for carotid surgery. In the real world, this will largely be dictated by rapid access to neurologists who have an interest in stroke and the number of dedicated stroke physicians.

There is no proven role for CEA in patients with vertebrobasilar or non-hemispheric symptoms. At present, we advocate elective CEA in patients with a 70–80% stenosis (ECST criteria) who have had carotid territory symptoms within the preceding 6 months. The ECST and NASCET have both shown that patients with more severe degrees of stenosis continue to derive benefit from carotid surgery for 12 months following their most recent event[1,2]. Thus, we would now offer endarterectomy to patients with a symptomatic 80–99% stenosis for up to 12 months after their last event. The indications for surgery in asymptomatic patients remain controversial, despite the ACAS findings[3]. At present, CEA for asymptomatic disease comprises 15% of our operative workload and is almost exclusively applied to patients with severe bilateral disease or contralateral occlusion.

In practice, once a decision to operate has been made, the procedure should be performed as soon as possible because of the high risk of stroke in the first few weeks after onset of symptoms. In the past, there has been a policy of delaying endarterectomy for 6 weeks in patients with a completed stroke. This evolved because of fears of haemorrhagic trans-formation of an ischaemic infarct. However, there is increasing evidence that the improvements in peri-operative patient care and monitoring have made it safe to operate on these patients within 1 month of their stroke, provided they have made a good early recovery[9]. Our unit currently advocates urgent CEA in patients with crescendo TIAs and those very rare patients with stroke in evolution. In practice, urgent CEA comprise < 5% of our overall practice. We do not advocate emergency CEA following acute stroke unless this occurred in the immediate period following end-arterectomy.

It is hoped that combining the ECST and NASCET databases will enable clinicians to identify particularly high risk patient subgroups and also, perhaps, exclude lower risk patients from unnecessary surgery. It is also imperative that a uniform method of quantifying stenosis is agreed and future research must be directed at evaluating the role of plaque morph-ology and stroke risk.

Surgical technique

It seems intuitively obvious that by ensuring good training of young surgeons in the art of carotid surgery, early and late outcomes will improve. However, there may be a natural reluctance on the part of vascular surgeons to delegate CEA to their trainees because of a perception that the rate of complications will inevitably increase. However, there is increasing evidence that trainees can receive a comprehensive training in carotid surgery without compromising outcome[10]. Adherence to this training doctrine is essential if the current increase in operative workload continues. In order to ensure effective training, there must be a large enough case mix within individual centres as outcomes may be directly related to an individual surgeon's experience and annual operative volume[4,7]. In reality, it is difficult to define the exact number of cases required, but it would seem reasonable for a surgeon to perform a minimum of 25 CEAs per annum. It may be, therefore, that there will be increasing calls to centralise carotid surgery in larger regional centres. This will increase the experience within units and will inevitably facilitate better training, research and multi-disciplinary team input. In addition, it makes provision for peri-operative monitoring more cost-effective.

Operative technique

All surgeons must maintain obsessional attention to technical detail. A thorough knowledge of anatomy is essential to minimise cranial nerve injury. Surgeons should avoid undue dissection around the common carotid artery, carotid bifurcation and distal internal carotid artery. There are two reasons for this: the first is to minimise the risks of thromboembolism, while the second is to avoid the functional elongation of the carotid artery that occurs when the bifurcation is fully mobilised. Finally, surgeons should remain aware that inadvertent technical error is the principal cause of operation-related stroke[11] and avoid the tendency to ascribe blame to the shunt, patch, monitoring method, or even the patient, should adverse outcomes arise.

Much of the debate relating to improving the safety of CEA has been restricted to the role of patching and shunting. Each have their detractors and supporters and, for the most part, surgeon preference is largely dictated by how they were taught. An overview of the available randomised trials of routine patching versus routine primary closure has shown that patching confers a 3-fold reduction in the 30 day risk of stroke and carotid thrombosis[12]. There is no evidence that the type of patch (vein or prosthetic) influences outcome. Few randomised trials have evaluated whether a policy of routine shunting is preferable to either selective shunting or no shunting. At present, an overview of the published results shows no difference in outcome between routine and selective shunting, although methodological problems have confounded the interpretation of many of these studies[13]. However, there is increasing consensus that a policy of routine or selective shunting is preferable to a policy of routine no-shunting.

Monitoring and quality control assessment

Ever since the first CEA was performed, surgeons have been aware of the paradox that the very operation that is undertaken to prevent stroke in the long-term can itself precipitate a stroke in the early postoperative period. Accordingly, surgeons have developed a number of monitoring methods to improve outcome. However, despite the plethora of published literature, it is surprisingly difficult for an impartial reader to draw a firm conclusion as to whether such a policy alters outcome.

The principle underlying the role of monitoring is that prevention should be easier than treatment of an acute stroke following surgery. Relatively few studies have prospectively audited the exact cause of peri-operative events, but evidence suggest that the majority are intra-operative (i.e. apparent upon recovery from anaesthesia)[14]. Thrombo-embolism predominates over haemodynamic causes[11], even in high risk individuals with little or no reserve[15].

There are many reasons why a policy of monitoring and quality control assessment has failed to alter outcome in the past. The most obvious include a failure to ask the correct questions and the flawed assumption that one single monitoring modality is infallible and superior to all others[16]. For example, most monitoring techniques have been designed to identify haemodynamic failure during carotid clamping and thereafter to develop criteria for selective shunting. However, clamp ischaemia is a relatively rare cause of intra-operative stroke[14] and little attention has been directed towards identifying and preventing thromboembolism[11]. Thus, is it reasonable to blame the EEG for having failed to prevent a stroke secondary to embolisation of thrombus following restoration of flow if no attempt was made to identify and remove this beforehand?

There are a number of methods for monitoring cerebral perfusion intra-operatively (stump pressure measurement, cerebral blood flow measurement, transcranial Doppler (TCD) ultrasound, EEG, evoked potentials, near infra-red spectroscopy, awake testing and jugular venous oxygen saturation). The only method capable of detecting embolisation is TCD. Intra-operative quality control methods include angiography, duplex ultrasound assessment, continuous Doppler wave assessment and angioscopy. To date, no randomised trial has compared a programme of monitoring with no monitoring on overall outcome. However, a number of studies have shown that quality control methods will identify some form of technical error in about 25% of patients[17–19] and that introduction of some form of monitoring and quality control assessment may be associated with a reduction in peri-operative stroke risk[20,21].

Evolution of the Leicester monitoring protocol

The Leicester protocol evolved as a result of a systematic, prospective audit of 800 CEAs between 1992 and 1999. Prior to 1992, the 30 day risk of death or stroke in our unit was 6% and this was within national and international guidelines. In a pilot study of 100 patients, Gaunt compared intra-operative TCD, completion B-mode imaging, completion angioscopy and continuous wave Doppler assessment of the endarterectomy zone and noted that minor or major technical error was present in 12% of patients. No additional information was provided by B-mode imaging or continuous wave Doppler over TCD and angioscopy[22].

TCD immediately warns the surgeon of spontaneous embolisation during the dissection phase of the procedure thus enabling modification of operative technique. In our centre, the routine use of TCD has been associated with a 50% reduction in the incidence of intra-operative embolisation[23]. TCD also ensures that middle cerebral artery blood flow velocity (MCAV) remains in excess of 15 cm/s, a threshold previously shown to correlate with loss of cerebral electrical activity[24]. If necessary, this threshold can be achieved by pharmacological elevation of blood pressure. Transcranial Doppler monitoring also immediately identifies shunt malfunction. It is often naively assumed by surgeons that having inserted a shunt, no further problem can occur. However, evidence suggests that up to 3% of shunts malfunction[25]. In practice, one of the commonest reasons for poor shunt flow is impaction of the distal shunt lumen against a distal carotid kink or loop. Transcranial Doppler is also the only method capable of diagnosing on-table carotid thrombosis. This extremely rare condition can be diagnosed by a decline in MCAV to levels observed during carotid clamping in association with increasing rates of embolisation. In our last 800 CEAs, we have encountered two cases of on-table carotid thrombosis and on both occasions, the condition was immediately diagnosed by TCD thereby enabling the surgeon to re-explore the artery and remove the thrombus. In the absence of transcranial Doppler, the surgeon would only have become aware of a major problem when attempts were made to awaken the patient.

The benefit of completion angioscopy is that it can be performed prior to restoration of flow. Its main role is the detection of luminal thrombus and intimal flaps. The disadvantage of angiography and duplex assessment is that flow must be restored before any examination can be performed and thus any luminal thrombus may have embolised by then.

The original pilot study and a similar study performed two years later confirmed that a policy of intra-operative TCD and completion angioscopy was associated with virtual abolition of intra-operative stroke, but no change in the 3% rate of postoperative thrombotic stroke[22,26]. On two occasions, TCD monitoring was continued into the early post-operative period and we observed that the onset of thrombotic stroke was preceded by 1–2 h phase of increasing embolisation[22]. In a much larger series, Levi demonstrated that 60% of patients with sustained postoperative embolisation progressed on to a thrombotic stroke[27]. The association between increasing embolisation and postoperative carotid thrombosis has now been documented on three continents[22,25,27–29].

In an attempt to prevent postoperative thrombosis, we administered intravenous dextran therapy to all patients following restoration of flow. Although this was associated with abolition of thrombosis, there was an increased incidence of neck haematomas, cardiac failure and one death through dextran-mediated multi-organ failure[30]. We subsequently hypothesised that TCD could be used to monitor patients in the early postoperative period and, thereafter, identify those with increasing rates of embolisation in order to guide selective dextran therapy. In a pilot study of 100 patients, Lennard administered dextran to 5% of patients, embolisation ceased in every case and no patient suffered a stroke[30].

Since October 1995, we have implemented an integrated programme of monitoring comprising intra-operative TCD, completion angioscopy and 3 h of postoperative TCD monitoring in 500 patients[31]. Intra-operative TCD specifically altered management decisions in 1.8% of patients, including the diagnosis of one case of on-table carotid thrombosis. Intimal flaps were repaired in 3% and fragments of luminal thrombus were removed in 4% following angioscopy. The source of these luminal thrombi was bleeding from the vasa vasorum on to the highly thrombogenic endarterectomised surface. In practice, they can be surprisingly adherent and resistant to blind irrigation with heparinised saline.

TCD monitoring in the early postoperative period indicates that about 50% of patients will have one or more emboli detected, but only 5% will develop sustained embolisation within the first 3 h. Our current protocol is to administer an incremental dose of dextran to patients with more than 25 emboli detected in any 10 min period of monitoring, or who have large emboli which distort the MCA waveform. Dextran is administered as a 20 ml bolus followed by an infusion initially starting at 20 ml/h. If the rate of embolisation does not diminish, the dose is increased incrementally to a maximum of 40 ml/h. Once the rate of embolisation has started to decrease, the dextran is continued for a further 12 h. Since implementing this protocol, we have not had to re-explore any patient for postoperative carotid thrombosis, but 36% of patients receiving dextran have required increases in the dosage suggesting that administration of a single dose of dextran will not control the rate of embolisation in all patients[31].

Implementation of the current protocol has been associated with a 60% sustained decline in the peri-operative complication rate as compared to before 1992. The intra-operative stroke rate has fallen to 0.2% and no patient in the current series has progressed onto a thrombotic stroke. Overall, the death/disabling stroke rate in the 500 patients was 1.6% and the death/any stroke rate was 2.2%, despite the fact that > 50% of the procedures were performed by trainees under supervision[31]. Of particular note was the fact that >50% of the complications followed either intracranial haemorrhage or cardiac pathology. The incidence of ipsilateral embolic stroke was 0.8%.

Conclusions

Carotid surgery has been shown to be beneficial in level one randomised trials. However, evidence suggests that current outcomes do not match those published in 1991. In order to make CEA safer in the future, it is essential to optimise patient selection and risk factor management and to maintain an obsessional approach to surgical technique. It is our firm opinion that a planned strategy of monitoring and quality control assessment can also contribute towards a sustained reduction in the peri-operative risk. Finally, surgeons must never accept that peri-operative stroke is an inevitable and unavoidable complication of carotid surgery. Every surgeon is responsible for his/her own results and these must be quoted, rather than the results from the international trials, to justify practice. It is imperative that all surgeons continuously audit their own results, preferably independently, and continually strive to review all aspects of their practice.

References

1 European Carotid Surgery Trialists' Collaborative Group. Randomised trial of endarterectomy for recently symptomatic carotid stenosis: Final results of the MRC European Carotid Surgery Trial (ECST). *Lancet* 1998; **351**: 1379–87
2 Barnett HJM, Taylor DW, Eliasziw M *et al*. Benefit of carotid endarterectomy in patients with symptomatic moderate or severe stenosis. *N Engl J Med* 1998; **339**: 1415–25
3 Executive Committee for the Asymptomatic Carotid Atherosclerosis Study. Endarterectomy for asymptomatic carotid artery stenosis. *JAMA* 1995; **273**: 1421–8

4   Wennberg DE, Lucas FL, Birkmeyer JD, Bredenberg CE, Fisher ES. Variation in carotid endarterectomy mortality in the Medicare population: Trial Hospitals, volume and patient characteristics. *JAMA* 1998; **279**: 1278–81

5   Naylor AR, Rothwell PM. Should cost-effectiveness influence patient selection for carotid surgery? In: Naylor AR, Mackey WC. (eds) *Carotid Artery Surgery: A Problem Based Approach*. W.B, Saunders 2000 (pp 66–72)

6   Hsai DC, Krushat WM, Moscoe LM. Epidemiology of carotid endarterectomy among Medicare beneficiaries: 1985–1996 update. *Stroke* 1998; **29**: 346–50

7   Karp HR, Flanders D, Shipp CC, Taylor B, Martin D. Carotid endarterectomy among Medicare beneficiaries: a statewide evaluation of appropriateness and outcome. *Stroke* 1998; **29**: 46–52

8   CAVATAS Investigators. Results of the Carotid and Vertebral Artery Transluminal Angioplasty Study (CAVATAS). *Proceedings of the Annual Vascular Society Meeting of Great Britain and Ireland* (Hull, November 1998)

9   Eckstein HH, Schumacher H, Lanbach H *et al* Early carotid endarterectomy after non-disabling ischaemic stroke: Adequate therapeutical option in selected patients. *Eur J Vasc Endovasc Surg* 1998; **15**: 423–8

10 Naylor AR, Thompson MM, Varty K, Sayers RD, London NJM, Bell PRF. Provision of training in carotid surgery does not compromise patient safety. *Br J Surg* 1998; **85**: 939–42

11 Riles TS, Imparato AM, Jacobowitz GR *et al*. The cause of peri-operative stroke after carotid endarterectomy. *J Vasc Surg* 1994; **19**: 206–14

12 Counsell C, Salinas R, Naylor AR, Warlow CP. A systematic review of the randomised trials of carotid patch angioplasty in carotid endarterectomy. *Eur J Vasc Endovasc Surg* 1997: **13**: 345–54

13 Counsell C, Salinas R, Warlow CP, Naylor AR. The role of carotid artery shunting during carotid endarterectomy: a systematic review of the randomised trials of routine and selective shunting and the different methods of intra-operative monitoring. In: Warlow CP, van Gijn J, Sandercock P. (eds) *Stroke Module of the Cochrane database of Systematic Reviews, 1996* (issue 2). London: BMJ Publishing, 1996

14 Krul JM, van Gijn J, Ackerstaff RG, Eikelboom BC, Theodorides T, Vermeulen FE. Site and pathogenesis of infarcts associated with carotid endarterectomy. *Stroke* 1989; **20**: 324–8

15 Naylor AR, Merrick MV, Ruckley CV. Risk factors for intra-operative neurological deficit during carotid endarterectomy. *Eur J Vasc Surg* 1991; **5**: 33–9

16 Naylor AR. Prevention of operation related stroke: are we asking the right questions? *Cardiovasc Surg* 1999; **7**: 155–7

17 Blaisdell FW, Lim R, Hall AD. Technical result of carotid endarterectomy: arteriographic assessment. *Am J Surg* 1967; **114**: 239-45

18 Flanigan DP, Douglas DJ, Machi J *et al*. Intraoperative ultrasonic imaging of the carotid artery during carotid endarterectomy. *Surgery* 1986; **100**: 893–8

19 Schwartz RA, Peterson GJ, Noland KA *et al*. Intraoperative duplex scanning after carotid artery reconstruction: a valuable tool. *J Vasc Surg* 1988; **7**: 620–8

20 Scott SM, Sethi GK, Bridgeman AH. Perioperative stroke during carotid endarterectomy: the value of intraoperative angiography. *J Cardiovasc Surg* 1982; **23**: 353–8

21 Roon AJ, Hoogerwerf D. Intraoperative angiography and carotid surgery. *J Vasc Surg* 1992; **16**: 239–43

22 Gaunt ME, Smith JL, Martin PJ, Ratliff DA, Bell PRF, Naylor AR. A comparison of quality control methods applied to carotid endarterectomy. *Eur J Vasc Endovasc Surg* 1996; **11**: 4–11

23 Smith JL, Goodall S, Evans D, London NJM, Bell PRF, Naylor AR. Experience with transcranial Doppler reduces the incidence of embolisation during carotid endarterectomy. *Br J Surg* 1998; **85**: 56–9

24 Halsey JH, McDowell HA, Gelmon S, Morawetz RB. Blood flow velocity in the middle cerebral artery and regional cerebral blood flow during carotid endarterectomy. *Stroke* 1989; **20**: 53–8

25 Ghali R, Palazzo EG, Rodriguez DI *et al*. Transcranial Doppler intra-operative monitoring during carotid endarterectomy: experience with regional or general anaesthesia, with and without shunting. *Ann Vasc Surg* 1997; **11**: 9–13

26 Lennard N, Smith JL, Gaunt ME *et al*. A policy of quality control assessment reduces the risk of intra-operative stroke during carotid endarterectomy *Eur J Vasc Endovasc Surg* 1999; **17**: 234–40

27 Levi CR, O'Malley HM, Fell G *et al*. Transcranial Doppler detected cerebral embolism following carotid endarterectomy: high microembolic signal loads predict post-operative cerebral ischaemia. *Brain* 1997; **120**: 621–9

28 Spencer MP. Transcranial Doppler monitoring and causes of stroke from carotid endarterectomy. *Stroke* 1997; **28**: 685–91

29 Cantelmo NL, Babikian VL, Samaraweera RN, Gordon JK, Pochay VE, Winter MR. Cerebral microembolism and ischaemia changes associated with carotid endarterectomy. *J Vasc Surg* 1998; **27**: 1024–30

30 Lennard N, Smith JL, Abbott R *et al*. Prevention of post-operative thrombotic stroke after carotid endarterectomy: the role of transcranial Doppler ultrasound. *J Vasc Surg* 1997; **26**: 579–84

31 Naylor AR, Hayes PD, Allroggen H *et al*. Reducing the risk of carotid surgery: a seven year audit of the role of monitoring and quality control assessment. *Stroke* 2000; In press

Carotid angioplasty and stenting

P A Gaines

Sheffield Vascular Institute, Northern General Hospital, Sheffield, UK

The endovascular management of carotid artery disease is a rapidly developing area currently under evaluation in Europe and the US. The technique is a simple progression of those skills used in peripheral vessels and involves the percutaneous placement of a metallic stent. Current data indicate that it may well offer a similar safety profile and efficacy at stroke prevention as conventional endarterectomy, but as yet there has only been one randomised controlled trial (CAVATAS). Future developments include the identification of a cohort of patients best treated with this technology, the evaluation of cerebral protection systems, and optimisation of pharmacological support.

Correspondence to :
Dr P A Gaines, Sheffield
Vascular Institute,
Northern General
Hospital,
Sheffield S5 7AU, UK

Carotid endarterectomy combined with best medical treatment is a well validated technique to manage symptomatic high grade carotid disease. Two large randomised trials comparing carotid endarterectomy and best medical therapy against best medical therapy alone have been published and have shown additional benefit from surgery in symptomatic patients with high grade stenoses[1,2]. There are, however, significant problems with the technique, in particular the complications and costs associated with surgery of the neck. Thirty-day outcome following surgery in the European Carotid Surgery Trial (ECST) study was associated with a death and major stroke rate of 7.5%. Similarly, the North American Symptomatic Carotid Endarterectomy Trial (NASCET) had a corresponding rate of 5.8%. The NASCET study also highlighted a 7.6% rate of cranial nerve injury, wound complications in 8.9%, myocardial infarction in 0.9%, congestive heart failure in 0.6%, and other cardiovascular problems in 1.2% of patients. For some patients, serious cranial nerve injury is as incapacitating as stroke. Away from randomised trials performed by experienced surgeons in large units, the safety, and therefore the benefit, of surgery is less secure. When the American Heart Association performed an assessment of carotid endarterectomy in the community, the risks were substantially higher (death and major stroke 4.8–9%) than those reported in the American randomised trial[3]. Similarly, Rothwell performed a systematic review of carotid endarterectomy studies published since 1980 and demonstrated a risk of stroke and/or death of 5.64% with 95% confidence intervals of 4.4–6.9%[4].

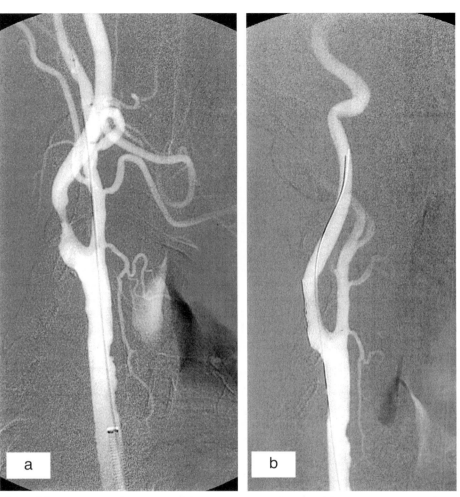

Fig. 1 (**a**) A symptomatic stenosis of the internal carotid artery. (**b**) The appearances after the endovascular placement of a stent (SMART stent, Cordis UK).

What then has the endovascular management of carotid disease got to offer (Fig. 1)? The value of carotid endarterectomy relies on the balance between the eventual stroke prophylaxis and the major events surrounding surgery. Clearly, any new therapeutic intervention that is not associated with the risks of general anaesthesia or neck incision and involved a short hospital stay would be worth pursuing, so long as it had a good risk benefit ratio and was financially prudent. Carotid angioplasty and stenting is performed from the groin under local anaesthesia. Significant costs are associated with the stent (currently approximately £700 in the UK) and in the future, with use of cerebral protection systems, costs will increase further. Balloon angioplasty and stent

significantly more cranial nerve palsies (0% *versus* 8.7%) and haematomas requiring intervention (1.2 *versus* 6.7%) in the surgical group.

The procedure is prophylactic with the intention of preventing stroke. At follow-up out to 3 years, there is no difference between the two techniques in preventing either ipsilateral stroke or disabling stroke and death.

There has been some criticism of the trial. The 30 day complication rate is high. To an extent this may reflect the outcome of patients treated outside the strict requirements of a surgical randomised trial when assessed by an independent neurologist. The endovascular complication rate may reflect the learning curves of the centres participating in new treatment, something that needs to be addressed by future trials. CAVATAS was not powered to show a difference in the 30 day complication rate and the confidence intervals surrounding this outcome are too broad to draw absolutely firm conclusions. The trial was also conducted during a period of change involving the technique of endovascular therapy. Future studies will probably involve cerebral protection, primary stent placement with low profile systems, optimised adjuvant pharmacology (particularly antiplatelet therapy) and better attention to post-procedure blood pressure management. Attention has been drawn to the randomisation process. This was performed using the 'grey area' principal similar to the ECST trial. Whilst a degree of prior selection was performed this is entirely in keeping with this type of trial involving new therapy.

Conclusions

Data are available to suggest that the endovascular management of carotid disease is a technique worthy of attention. Practitioners need to identify exactly where its role lies. Patients at high risk of stroke need to be better defined to reduce the number needed to treat to prevent stroke, and identify those who would most benefit from endovascular intervention. The new technologies need to be adequately assessed and already larger randomised trials are being proposed to address some of these issues. In the US, the NIH are funding a large multicentre randomised trial comparing surgery *versus* carotid stenting (CREST) and, in the UK, CAVATAS II is being developed.

References

1   North American Symptomatic Carotid Endarterectomy Trial Collaborators. Beneficial effect of carotid endarterectomy in symptomatic patients with high-grade carotid stenoses. *N Engl J Med* 1991; **325**: 445–53
2   European Carotid Surgery Trialists' Collaborative Group. MRC European Carotid Surgery Trial: interim results for symptomatic patients with severe (70–99%) or with mild (0–29%) carotid stenosis. *Lancet* 1991; **337**: 1235–41

3 Moore WS, Barnett HJM, Beebe HG *et al*. Guidelines for Carotid Endarterectomy. A multidisciplinary consensus statement from the *ad hoc* committee, American Heart Association. *Stroke* 1995; **26**: 188–201

4 Rothwell PM, Slattery J, Warlow CP. A systematic review of the risks of stroke and death due to endarterectomy for symptomatic carotid stenosis. *Stroke.* 1996; **27**: 260–5

5 Theron JG, Payelle GG, Coskun O, Guimaraens L. Carotid Artery stenosis: treatment with protection balloon angioplasty and stent placement. *Radiology* 1996; **201**: 627–36

6 Gaines PA. The endovascular management of symptomatic atherosclerotic carotid disease. *Eur J Vasc Endovasc Surg* 1998; **16**: 94–7

7 Crawley F, Brown MM. *Percutaneous transluminal angioplasty and stenting for carotid artery stenosis* (Cochrane Review). Oxford: The Cochrane Library, 1999

8 Gil-Peralta A, Mayol A, Marcos JRG *et al*. Percutaneous transluminal angioplasty of the symptomatic atherosclerotic carotid arteries. Results, complications and follow-up. *Stroke* 1996; **27**: 2271–3

9 Yadav JS, Roubin GS, Iyer S *et al*. Elective stenting of the extracranial carotid arteries. *Circulation* 1997; **95**: 376–81

10 Eckert B, Zanella FE, Thie A, Steinmetz J, Zeumer H. Angioplasty of the internal carotid artery: results, complications and follow-up in 61 cases. *Cerebrovasc Dis* 1996; **6**: 97–105

11 Gaines P, Cleveland T, Beard JD, Venables G. Endovascular carotid intervention – a single centre audit. *J Vasc Interv Radiol Suppl* 1999; **10**: 213

12 Brown MM for the CAVATAS investigators. Results of the Carotid and Vertebral Artery Transluminal Angioplasty Study (CAVATAS). *Cerebrovasc Dis* 1998; **8** (**Suppl 4**): 21

Cost-effectiveness of stroke prevention

Shah Ebrahim

MRC Health Services Research Collaboration, Department of Social Medicine, University of Bristol, Bristol, UK

Stroke is a preventable disease and there are several interventions that might have an important role in reducing the burden of disease. Economic appraisal of these different interventions is essential as resources are scarce and it is logical to attempt to obtain the greatest reduction in disease for the lowest cost. Anticoagulation for non-rheumatic atrial fibrillation is highly effective, but is expensive and cost-effectiveness analyses show that use of aspirin alone would prevent almost as many strokes at much lower cost. Antiplatelet drugs are both effective and inexpensive and their use in secondary prevention would potentially save the NHS about £900 per life year gained. Carotid endarterectomy and the associated screening costs are poor value for money but recent attempts to use predictive models to determine which patients will benefit from surgery may improve its cost-effectiveness. Current evidence is dominated by pharmacological interventions and much less good evidence is available for life-style modifications such as dietary change and physical exercise. Modification of major cardiovascular risk factors (blood cholesterol, high blood pressure and smoking) is very cost-effective but needs to be better targeted if potential health gain is to be realised.

The cost of stroke

Stroke kills over 70,000 people a year in the UK[1] and costs the NHS between 4–5% of its total budget – approximately £2 billion a year in 1999[2]. The bulk of this spending is on direct costs of acute and rehabilitation hospital care, but the estimate does not include indirect costs that fall on families and patients themselves or the so-called 'intangible' costs associated with suffering. The direct cost of an individual stroke patient is estimated to be between £4,600 (1988) in Scotland[2] and £5,900 (1983) in Sweden[3].

In considering direct costs, it is important in any chronic disease to examine costs over time and to include long-term care costs which may be almost as large as acute hospital costs[4]. In most costing studies, average costs per stroke have been reported, but many factors may cause costs to vary. For example, in Sweden the costs of stroke in women are almost double those for men, independent of age[3], and are probably

Correspondence to:
Prof. Shah Ebrahim, MRC HSRC, Department of Social Medicine, University of Bristol, Canynge Hall, Whiteladies Road, Bristol BS8 2PR, UK

explained by the unpaid care provided by women for men with stroke which is not reciprocated. Indirect costs, particularly those of unpaid carers, may make a major difference to the overall picture, but are rarely included in studies. With costs of this magnitude, even small reductions achieved by preventing stroke would be of considerable value.

Stroke is preventable

Epidemiological evidence shows that stroke is preventable. Variation between and within countries, trends over time, and variation between individuals who smoke, who take little exercise, and who have high blood pressure all suggest that stroke risk can be reduced[5]. Evidence from clinical trials of antihypertensive treatment confirms the preventability of stroke associated with high blood pressure, but in many areas, such as smoking cessation or promotion of physical activity, it is not possible to perform clinical trials.

The need for economic appraisal

While evidence of efficacy is very helpful in shaping clinical and public health policy, it is insufficient. The issue of cost is fundamental in deciding what to do and what not to do. Economic appraisal tends to have a bad reputation amongst doctors because it is invariably seen as part of rationing of health care. In fact, economic appraisal is concerned with achieving greater equity and openness in how decisions on resource use are made. Economic appraisal of health care aims to ensure that as much benefit as possible is obtained from available resources.

While there is much to criticise in the methods used by health economists, the alternatives are much less appealing. In the past, those who shouted loudest (teaching hospital consultants) and most dramatically (shroud-waving life and death specialities) got the bigger slice of the available cake. Political factors and special pleading by professionals and patient groups will inevitably continue to have an effect on decisions on how health care resources are used. Health economics provides a means of exposing how such decisions are made and provides the framework for a more rational approach.

Principles of economic appraisal

Health economics has basic principles: resources are limited (scarcity); demand tends to increase owing to ageing of populations, technological advances, and increasing aspirations of people (inflation); using resources on unproven or inefficient treatments is unethical (utilitarian ethics); linking costs to outcomes (cost-effectiveness); choices have to be made between alternative strategies (priority setting); choices between alternative options should maximise the benefits obtained for society (cost-benefit). All economic evaluations involve many assumptions, which must be made explicitly and their impact on the final analyses must be assessed (sensitivity analysis)[6]. In addition, economic appraisal often involves discounting of costs, and sometimes, of benefits as well. Discounting is a simple idea – £100 now is worth more than £100 in 10 year's time. Discounting future costs by a set amount – usually 5% – is a standard practice. With preventive interventions where costs come early but benefits come late, benefits may need to be discounted as well. If this is done, many preventive interventions look very poor value for money.

Cost-minimisation evaluation

The simplest method of evaluation does not even consider outcomes but simply compares costs between different options, making the assumption that either option is equally effective, and is a cost-minimisation evaluation. It would be rational to chose the cheapest option if both were equally effective.

Cost-effectiveness studies

Cost-effectiveness studies attempt to relate costs to some measure of outcome. This may be some clinical outcome (*e.g.* reduction in blood pressure or survival). If one intervention results in a greater increase in survival but at higher cost, a cost-effectiveness analysis may help to resolve the best policy.

Cost-utility studies

Cost-utility studies use a common measure of outcome, frequently the quality adjusted life year (QALY), as the yardstick of benefit and compare

Table 1 Cost per QALY of various interventions (1990 prices)

Intervention	Cost per QALY (£)
Smoking cessation advice from a GP	270
Antihypertensive treatment for stroke prevention (ages 45–64 years)	940
Hip replacement	1,180
Coronary artery bypass grafting (severe angina)	2,090
Kidney transplant	4,710
Home dialysis	17,260
Neurosurgery for malignant intracranial tumours	107,780

costs per QALY (Table 1). As can be seen, there is a very wide range of costs per QALY that the NHS considers reasonable to pay. Obviously, one of the difficulties of the cost-utility approach is that it does not make much sense to re-allocate resources solely to smoking cessation advice, when people suffer from and expect treatment for a wide range of conditions, many of which are not smoking related.

Cost-benefit

In cost-benefit analysis, the outcomes are measured in the same money units as the inputs. This means that lives saved or strokes avoided must be converted into their equivalent cash values. This raises many practical and ethical problems – what is a life worth? Where outcomes can be dealt with in this way, options which result in more overall benefits than costs would logically be chosen. A cost-benefit analysis of comprehensive primary prevention for stroke in Japan compared with the current *ad hoc* and inefficient arrangements found a cost:benefit ratio of 1:10, which supported the comprehensive care option[7].

Cost-effectiveness of stroke prevention

There are many interventions that have a role in the prevention of stroke (Table 2). In a short article, it is not possible to cover them all in detail, but rather some areas will be used to illustrate the approach of economic appraisal.

Anticoagulation for non-rheumatic atrial fibrillation

Long-term anticoagulation is probably more effective than aspirin in preventing stroke in patients with atrial fibrillation, but it costs considerably more and is risky, potentially causing serious bleeding. What is the best option to chose? In Sweden, a cost-effectiveness analysis was conducted[8] with a summary of the findings shown in Table 3.

Table 2 Interventions for stroke prevention

Anticoagulation for atrial fibrillation
Antiplatelet drugs for secondary prevention and for atrial fibrillation
Carotid endarterectomy
Carotid angioplasty
Lowering blood cholesterol
Treatment of high blood pressure
Smoking cessation
Multiple risk factor intervention

Table 3 Cost-effectiveness analysis comparing anticoagulation with aspirin in preventing stroke in patients with atrial fibrillation (data from Gustafsson et al[8]). Low and high risk refers to risk of bleeding on anticoagulation

	Anticoagulation only	Anticoagulation or aspirin	Aspirin only
No. eligible for treatment	22,000	75,000	75,000
Annual cost (£) of treatment	500	154	10
Net reduction in stroke, low risk	630	1,300	910
Net reduction in stroke, high risk	260	930	910
Cost (£) per stroke prevented, low risk	17,500	8,900	800
Cost (£) per stroke prevented, high risk	42,300	12,400	800

The most effective treatment is anticoagulation for those who can tolerate it and aspirin for the remainder. This prevents 1300 strokes a year, if complications of anticoagulation are kept low and, even if complications are high (intracranial bleeding rate of 2% per year), still prevents more strokes than simply giving everyone aspirin. Therefore, this would be the clinically preferred option if costs are ignored. However, when cost-effectiveness is considered, a different picture emerges. Aspirin treatment is so cheap (50 times cheaper than anticoagulation) that despite the greater efficacy of anticoagulation, it represents a poor value-for-money choice. If bleeding complications are high, cost-effectiveness of anticoagulation becomes even worse. The investigators in this study concluded that prophylactic treatment with anticoagulants in patients with chronic atrial fibrillation saves both strokes and money if bleeding complications are kept low. However, they ignored the greater savings of money obtained from the aspirin only policy.

A recent review of cost-utility analyses in stroke concluded that anticoagulation was the preferred treatment with a cost per QALY of the order of US$8000 in moderate risk patients[9]. However, most investigators have found that, while anticoagulation is more effective than aspirin, it is more expensive to use in practice and not as safe. The estimates of cost per QALY are very sensitive to assumptions made. For example, they can vary from −£400/QALY (*i.e.* a saving of £400) to £13,000/QALY depending on the amount of monitoring of anticoagulation[10], and from US$370,000/QALY for a 65-year-old patient with lone atrial fibrillation to US$8,000 for a similar patient with one additional risk factor[11].

Antiplatelet drugs

The evidence of efficacy of aspirin in secondary prevention is compelling[12]. The Second European Stroke Prevention Study[13] claims to have demonstrated independent and additive effects for aspirin 50 mg/day and dipyridamole 400 mg/day. The study had a 2 x 2 factorial design randomising 6602 patients post-stroke or TIA between aspirin, dipyridamole and placebo (so a quarter received each of the four possible combinations of active treatment and placebo). The primary analysis in such a design is aspirin against placebo (regardless of whether patients were given dipyridamole or not) and dipyridamole against placebo (regardless of whether aspirin was given or not). Factorial 2 x 2 design trials give, in effect, two trials for the price of one. The aspirin effect (reconstructing the secondary end-point of combined stroke, MI and sudden death from the published data for comparability) was an 18% relative risk reduction, whilst the dipyridamole effect was a 17% reduction. The effect of the combination (compared with the 'double' placebo group – those who did not receive either active drug) was a 33% reduction.

Does this demonstrate conclusively an additional effect for dipyridamole? Unfortunately not. Forty-three previous trials had evaluated aspirin plus dipyridamole combinations, with a total of 1750 events in 14,000 patients[12]. The relative odds reduction for these trials was 28%, identical to that for aspirin alone. Adding the new data increases the pooled relative odds reduction to 32% (95% CI 25–38%), still consistent with an identical effect to that of aspirin alone. Similarly, for the meta-analysis of the direct comparison studies, where previously 5300 patients had been randomised, no overall difference between regimens was found. Adding the new data gives a relative odds reduction for the risk of combined vascular events of 13% (95% CI –2% to 26%) in favour of the combination, again consistent with the hypothesis that the combination is no more effective than aspirin alone. On the other hand, the odds reduction in non-fatal stroke alone is significantly reduced by 23% for the combination compared to aspirin alone, with no significant effect on myocardial infarction or other vascular events (see Fig. 2 in McCabe & Brown, this issue). The apparently dramatic results in this single trial could be the results of two factors: a subgroup analysis giving undue prominence to extreme findings, and the dose of aspirin used was very small[5].

A further trial compared a new agent, clopidogrel, with 325 mg/day of aspirin in 19,185 patients at high vascular risk (including 6431 with ischaemic stroke)[14]. A small but significant relative risk reduction of 8.7% (95% CI 0.3–17%) for stroke, MI or vascular death in favour of clopidogrel over aspirin was found. The size of this trial illustrates what is required to demonstrate which of two active drugs is better. Clopidogrel is less toxic than ticlopidine, and is an alternative (along with dipyridamole) for patients intolerant of aspirin.

A recent review gave gross (i.e. no allowance made for possible cost savings) estimates of £30 per life year gained for aspirin and £1600 per life year gained for aspirin and dipyridamole combined[15]. When net costs (i.e. with allowance for reductions in hospital use, etc) were compared, aspirin achieved savings of £900 per life year gained, whereas aspirin and dipyridamole cost £740 per life year gained.

Carotid surgery

Carotid endarterectomy is effective in carefully selected patients with high degrees of stenosis. The European Carotid Surgery Trial[16] studied patients with TIA, minor ischaemic stroke or retinal infarct within the previous 6 months, and ipsilateral carotid artery stenosis. Participants were randomised to carotid endarterectomy plus best medical management or medical management alone, and according to the degree of carotid stenosis estimated from an angiogram. For patients with stenosis of 0–29%, there were no benefits. For patients with ipsilateral stenoses of 30–69% the rate of death or major stroke was 7.9% within 30 days of surgery. Over 8 years of follow-up, stroke-free survival was worse for the surgical group up to 3.4 years if carotid stenosis was 30–49%, and up to 2.3 years for stenosis of 50–69%. After that survival curves converged. Clearly for this group too, surgery is not indicated.

The group with symptomatic carotid stenoses of 70–99% (n = 778) did show a benefit from surgery. The benefit was concentrated in patients with stenosis greater than 80%, although this varied slightly with the age and sex of the patient[17]. Surgical mortality and morbidity was 7.5% (3.7% fatal or disabling stroke). Over the next 3 years, the risk of ipsilateral ischaemic stroke was 12.8% (8.4% disabling) in the control group and 2.8% (1.1% disabling) for the surgical group (odds ratio 0.16, upper 95% confidence limit 0.42). Risk of stroke in the control group was greatest in the first year after randomisation, and a net benefit of surgery was evident after about 6–9 months. The benefit for surgically treated patients persisted for 3 years, after which the ongoing risk in the two groups became the same[17]. In this patient group, and with these surgeons, 20 endarterectomies will cause one stroke and prevent two (over 3 years).

These results were confirmed in a similar North American trial of 659 patients with severe symptomatic stenosis (with stenosis severity defined slightly differently)[18]. Surgical mortality and stroke rate was 5.8%. After 2 years follow up, relative risk for surgical compared with control patients were was 0.35 for ipsilateral stroke, 0.46 for any stroke, and 0.49 for any stroke or death. In both trials, there was a gradient of increasing benefit with increasing severity of stenosis.

The question of relative risk and benefits is even more vexed for asymptomatic patients found to have carotid stenosis. There appears to be a small benefit for surgical over medical treatment, but the risk of stroke is low in these patients, and absolute net benefit is small[19].

Table 4 Factors determining cost effectiveness of carotid endarterectomy

Screening strategy used
Severity of carotid stenosis
Symptoms
Operative risk
Volume of operations
Time since operation
Quality of medical management
Individual prediction of benefit

Consequently, the cost-effectiveness of operation in asymptomatic people is low, with marginal lifetime (*i.e.* 30 years) cost-effectiveness of US$120,000 per quality adjusted life year[20]. These estimates compare with cost-effectiveness in symptomatic patients of between US$4000 to US$53,000 depending on the assumptions made[21].

If the screening strategy, an essential component of the overall service, is included in economic evaluations, the picture is even less clear with costs per QALY (1998) ranging from US$27,000 to US$138,000, and one analysis demonstrated that the no screening option was preferred on grounds of being cheaper and more effective[9] (Table 4).

A promising way to improve cost-effectiveness is to use a predictive model to determine which patients are very unlikely to benefit from surgery[22]. The current models increase the prediction obtained by just using degree of carotid stenosis but require validation in other datasets. This preliminary work suggests that the number needed to treat to avoid one stroke could be reduced from 14 patients to 3 patients with proportionate improvements in cost-effectiveness.

Carotid angioplasty

The efficacy of carotid angioplasty compared with carotid endarterectomy is uncertain. A recent study of the two procedures in a non-randomised comparison showed that costs were actually higher for the angioplasty group (US$30,000 per admission) compared with each carotid endarterectomy procedure (US$22,000). Moreover, strokes and deaths were more than twice as common in the angioplasty group[23]. On the other hand, in the Carotid and Vertebral Artery and Transluminal Angioplasty Study (CAVATAS) outcomes were identical in the two groups (see Gaines, this issue) and the costs in the angioplasty group were approximately half that of surgery (Brown MM, personal communication). At present, it seems that carotid angioplasty requires further development work to make the procedure safer and more efficient.

Lowering blood cholesterol

While some studies have suggested that stroke is not related to blood cholesterol[24], when risk of ischaemic stroke is considered, there is little doubt that blood cholesterol is an independent risk factor for ischaemic stroke[5]. Efforts to reduce blood cholesterol by use of statins in high cardiovascular risk patients (mostly following myocardial infarction) have also produced reductions in risk of stroke[25].

However, no trials of secondary prevention in people who have suffered TIA or stroke have been reported. It would seem reasonable to ascertain whether a patient with TIA or stroke has any clinical symptoms or signs of ischaemic heart disease, peripheral vascular disease, or diabetes and if so, to use guidelines for use of statins[26].

The cost-effectiveness of cholesterol lowering drugs has been widely investigated recently with the advent of statins – which, although very effective, are also very expensive. Current (1998) estimates of cost-effectiveness are of the order of £8000 per life year gained, but this figure is dependent on a number of assumptions[15]. The most important of these is the baseline level of cardiovascular risk in the patients treated as shown in Figure 1. The figure shows the discounted and undiscounted costs at different baseline rates.

The cost of statins is the other major determinant of cost-effectiveness. Reductions in price are to be expected, and the newer statins are considerably cheaper than those tested in trials of clinical outcomes. Pricing policy is suspect and the drugs can be produced at a fraction of the cost, as is occurring in India[27].

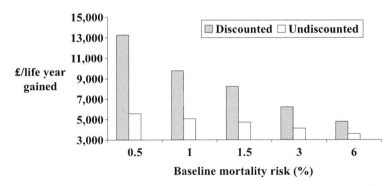

Fig. 1 Cost per life year gained of statins at different baseline levels of total mortality.

Treatment of high blood pressure

High risk and population approaches

Small downward shifts in the distribution of blood pressures would have a disproportionate effect on overall cardiovascular mortality and morbidity compared with treating those people at the top end of the blood pressure distribution[28,29]. Currently, there is debate about the role of salt reduction as a population intervention to reduce levels of blood pressure[30]. Most effort is currently spent on identifying and treating those people with raised blood pressures, usually using an arbitrary cut-off of 160/100, although more recent recommendations have suggest lower levels[31].

Systematic reviews of the hypertension treatment trials has demonstrated clear benefits in both stroke and coronary heart disease prevention[32,33]. These trials lasted, on average, 5 years and reduced diastolic blood pressure by 5–6 mmHg. Strokes in the trials therefore occurred, on average, after only 2–3 years of blood pressure reduction. There were 484 strokes in placebo groups, and 289 in active treatment groups, a relative risk on treatment of 0.58 (95% CI 0.50–0.67). The relative risk expected from the observational studies for such a blood pressure decrease was very similar, suggesting that virtually all the expected benefit of reducing blood pressure seems to be gained within 2–3 years of treatment[32,33]. The systematic reviews have also shown that treating older, rather than younger people produces greater absolute benefits[34].

Cost-effectiveness analyses of antihypertensive treatments usually cite the 'headline' figure of £940/QALY[35] (Table 5). However, these analyses are subject to large variations depending on the assumptions made. Two major factors dominate: the type of patient treated and the drug regimens used[36]. If young women with mild hypertension are treated with expensive drugs, it might be expected that cost-effectiveness would be low. However, the estimates are affected greatly by whether or not health benefits are discounted. If health benefits occurring in the future are discounted, this makes prevention a very bad option for younger people as the prevented events are so far in the future, their discounted value is almost negligible.

The high cost/QALY for diuretics in younger men is a direct result of the very small probability of benefiting and the high likelihood of adverse side

Table 5 Cost per QALY (£) – the effects of discounting on cost-effectiveness of antihypertensive drugs, pre-treatment diastolic blood pressure 100 mmHg

	Age (years)	Diuretic discounted	Diuretic undiscounted	ACE inhibitor discounted	ACE inhibitor undiscounted
Male					
	40	68,000	800	15,000	2,900
	50	4,000	800	10,000	3,100
	60	5,000	1,400	11,000	1,300
Female					
	40	*	800	21,000	2,800
	50	*	700	15,000	3,100
	60	*	500	15,000	4,300

*Treatment is of negative benefit. Re-drawn from Drummond and Coyle[36].

effects. The adverse side effects have a major effect on the estimates as they are felt immediately and reduce quality of life but the benefits are gained by only a few people and are far in the future.

Smoking cessation

Although GP advice to stop smoking has only a small effect, it is an inexpensive intervention and has no known side effects. Therefore, it scores well in cost-effectiveness analyses, and is usually at the top of the list (Table 1). No trials of the effects of advice on stopping smoking after stroke have been conducted, but simulations of very modest quit rates in stroke and myocardial infarction patients suggest that health care savings of US$3.2 billion could be made[37]. Cost-effectiveness of smoking cessation advice after myocardial infarction is estimated to be US$220/life year gained, assuming an intervention cost of US$100 per patient[38].

The cost-effectiveness of nicotine replacement therapy is claimed to be self-evident[39] on the grounds that nicotine replacement has been shown to double quit rates over placebo[40]. Estimates of cost per life year gained (discounting health benefits at 5%) of nicotine patches as an adjunct to physician advice have been made and are of the order of US$1000–1600 and US$1600–2300 for men and women, respectively[41].

Multiple risk factor interventions

Trials of multiple risk factor interventions in primary care or the workplace show that current approaches (usually nurse or doctor given advice to modify diet, take more exercise and stop smoking) are rewarded by only small changes in life-style risk factors and statistically insignificant reductions in mortality[42]. There is no clear evidence of benefit from these programmes and given the obvious cost-effectiveness of alternative interventions, multiple risk factor interventions should not be promoted.

Conclusion

The cost-effectiveness of a range of options for stroke prevention have been examined. Table 6 summarises the published estimates. It can be seen that, although all the interventions are well within the range of other commonly used interventions, there are some interventions that stand out as representing excellent value for money. It is also important to realise that the bulk of cost-effectiveness research concerns drugs rather than non-pharmacological interventions, such as dietary change

Table 6 Summary of cost-effectiveness of a range of preventive interventions for stroke

Intervention	Cost per QALY (£)
Aspirin for secondary prevention	30*
Aspirin for atrial fibrillation	40
Bendrofluazide, patient aged 69 years	50*
Smoking cessation, GP advice	270
Anticoagulation for atrial fibrillation	450–5,000
Nicotine replacement therapy + advice	600–1,500
Antihypertensives, medium cost regimen, patient aged 56 years	1,500*
Aspirin + dipyridamole for secondary prevention	1,600*
Carotid endarterectomy	4,000–53,000
Cholesterol lowering with simvastatin	8,000*
Carotid endarterectomy + screening	16,000–86,000

*Cost per life year gained.

and physical exercise. Greater efforts are needed to ensure that the options compared are not pharmacologically biased[43]. Achieving accurate identification and optimal coverage of the population at risk, and ensuring professional and patient adherence to treatment are essential if potential health gain is to be realised.

References

1 Office for National Statistics. *Mortality statistics 1996, general*. Series DH1 No 29. London: HMSO, 1998
2 Isard P, Forbes J. The cost of stroke to the National Health Service in Scotland. *Cerebrovasc Dis* 1992; **2**: 47–50
3 Persson U, Silverberg R, Lindgren B *et al*. Direct costs of stroke for a Swedish population. *Int J Technol Assess Health Care* 1990; **6**: 125–37
4 Raftery J. Stroke services purchasing – present and future. In: Law S, Mant J. (eds) *Best Buy for Stroke*. Proceedings of a seminar for purchasers. London: London School of Hygiene and Tropical Medicine, 1995
5 Ebrahim S, Harwood R. *Stroke: Epidemiology, Evidence and Clinical Practice*. Oxford: Oxford University Press, 1999
6 Maynard A. The economics of hypertension control: some basic issues. *J Hum Hypertens* 1992; **6**: 417–20
7 Sekita Y. Cost-benefit evaluation of comprehensive medical care for cerebral strokes. *Med Inf (Lond)* 1985; **10**: 59–71
8 Gustafsson C, Asplund K, Britton M, Norrving B, Olsson B, Marke LA. Cost effectiveness of primary stroke prevention in atrial fibrillation: Swedish national perspective. *BMJ* 1992; **305**: 1457–60
9 Holloway RG, Benesch CG, Rahilly CR, Courtright CE. A systematic review of cost-effectiveness research of stroke evaluation and treatment. *Stroke* 1999; **30**: 1340–9
10 Lightowlers S, McGuire A. Cost-effectiveness of anticoagulation in non-rheumatic atrial fibrillation in the primary prevention of ischaemic stroke. *Stroke* 1998; **29**: 1827–32
11 Gage BF, Cardinalli AB, Albers GW, Owens DK. Cost-effectiveness of warfarin and aspirin for prophylaxis of stroke in patients with nonvalvular atrial fibrillation. *JAMA* 1995; **274**: 1839–45

12 Antiplatelet Trialists Collaboration. Collaborative overview of randomised trials of antiplatelet therapy – I: Prevention of death, myocardial infarction, and stroke by prolonged antiplatelet therapy in various categories of patients. *BMJ* 1994; **308**: 81–106

13 Diener HC, Cunha L, Forbes C, Sivenius J, Smets P, Lowenthal A. European Stroke Prevention Study. 2. Dipyridamole and acetylsalicylic acid in the secondary prevention of stroke. *J Neurol Sci* 1996; **143**: 1–13

14 CAPRIE Steering Committee. A randomised blinded trial of clopidogrel versus aspirin in patients at risk of ischaemic events (CAPRIE). *Lancet* 1996; **348**: 1329–39

15 Ebrahim S, Davey Smith G, McCabe C et al. Cholesterol and coronary heart disease: screening and treatment. *Qual Health Care* 1998; **7**: 232–9

16 European Carotid Surgery Trialists Collaborative Group. MRC European Carotid Surgery Trial: interim results for symptomatic patients with severe (70–99%) or with mild (0–29%) carotid stenosis. *Lancet* 1991; **337**: 1235–43

17 European Carotid Surgery Trialists. Randomised trial of endarterectomy for recently symptomatic carotid stenosis: final results of the MRC European Carotid Surgery Trial (ECST). *Lancet* 1998; **351**: 1379–87

18 North American Symptomatic Carotid Endarterectomy Trial Collaborators. Beneficial effect of carotid endarterectomy in symptomatic patients with high-grade carotid stenosis. *N Engl J Med* 1991; **325**: 445–53

19 Asymptomatic Carotid Atherosclerosis Study. Endarterectomy for asymptomatic carotid artery stenosis. *JAMA* 1995; **273**: 1421–8

20 Lee TT, Solomon NA, Heidenreich PA, Oehlert J, Garber AM. Cost-effectiveness of screening for carotid stenosis in asymptomatic persons. *Ann Intern Med* 1997; **126**: 337–46

21 Kuntz KM, Kent KC. Is carotid endarterectomy cost-effective? An analysis of symptomatic and asymptomatic patients. *Circulation* 1996; **94**: II194–8

22 Rothwell P, Warlow CP on behalf of the European Carotid Surgery Trialists' Collaborative Group. Prediction of benefit from carotid endarterectomy in individual patients. Lancet 1999; **353**: 2105–10

23 Jordan Jr WD, Roye GD, Fisher 3rd WS, Redden D, McDowell HA. A cost comparison of balloon angioplasty and stenting versus endarterectomy for the treatment of carotid artery stenosis. *J Vasc Surg* 1998; **27**: 16–22

24 Prospective Studies Collaboration. Cholesterol, diastolic blood pressure, and stroke: 13,000 strokes in 450,000 people in 45 prospective cohorts. *Lancet* 1995; **346**: 1647–53

25 Crouse JR, Byngton RP, Hoen HM, Furberg CT. Reductase inhibitor monotherapy and stroke prevention. *Arch Intern Med* 1997; **157**: 1305–10

26 Standing Medical Advisory Committee. *The Use of Statins*. London: Department of Health, 1997

27 Davey Smith G, Ebrahim S. Coronary risk assessment methods and cholesterol lowering. *Lancet* 1999; **353**: 1097

28 Rose G. *The Strategy of Preventive Medicine*. Oxford: Oxford University Press, 1992

29 Cook NR, Cohen J, Hebert PR, Taylor JO, Hennekens CH. Implications of small reductions in diastolic blood pressure for primary prevention. *Arch Intern Med* 1995; **155**: 701–9

30 Taubes G. The (political) science of salt. *Science* 1998; **281**: 898–907

31 Chalmers J for the WHO-ISH Hypertension Guidelines Committee. 1999 World Health Organization – International Society of Hypertension Guidelines for the Management of Hypertension. *J Hypertens* 1999; **17**: 151–85

32 MacMahon S, Peto R, Cutler J et al. Blood pressure, stroke, and coronary heart disease. Part 1, Prolonged differences in blood pressure: prospective observational studies corrected for the regression dilution bias . *Lancet* 1990; **335**: 765–74

33 Collins R, Peto R, MacMahon S et al. Blood pressure, stroke, and coronary heart disease. Part 2, Short-term reductions in blood pressure: overview of randomised drug trials in their epidemiological context . *Lancet* 1990; **335**: 827–38

34 Mulrow CD, Cornell JA, Herrera CR et al. Hypertension in the elderly: implications and generalisability of randomized trials. *JAMA* 1995; **272**: 1932–8

35 Ham C. Priority setting in the NHS. *Br J Health Care Manage* 1995; **1**: 27–9

36 Drummond M, Coyle D. Assessing the economic value of antihypertensive medication. *J Hum Hypertens* 1992; **2**: 495–501

37 Lightwood JM, Glantz SA. Short-term economic and health benefits of smoking cessation: myocardial infarction and stroke. *Circulation* 1997; **96**: 1089–96

38 Krumholz HM, Cohen BJ, Tsevat J, Pasternak RC, Weinstein MC. Cost-effectiveness of a smoking cessation program after myocardial infarction. *J Am Coll Cardiol* 1993; **22**: 1697–702

39 Smeeth L, Fowler G. Nicotine replacement therapy for a healthier nation. *BMJ* 1998; **317**: 1266–7

40 Silagy C, Mant D, Fowler G, Lancaster T. Nicotine replacement therapy for smoking cessation (Cochrane Review). Oxford: Cochrane Library, 1999

41 Wasley MA, McNagny SE, Phillips VL, Ahluwalia JS. The cost-effectiveness of the nicotine transdermal patch for smoking cessation *Prevent Med* 1997; **26**: 264–70

42 Ebrahim S, Davey Smith G. A systematic review and meta-analysis of randomized controlled trials of health promotion for prevention of coronary heart disease in adults. *BMJ* 1997; **314**: 1666-7

43 Dieppe P. Evidence-based medicine or medicines-based evidence? *Ann Rheum Dis* 1998; **57**: 385–6

Index

NEXT ISSUE   BRITISH MEDICAL BULLETIN   Volume 56 Number 3 2000

Human reproduction: pharmaceutical and technical advances

Scientific Editors: Robert P Millar and David T Baird